Dictionary of Communication Disorders

Fourth edition

Dictionary of Communication Disorders

Fourth edition

David W. H. Morris

M.A., B.Ling., Dip.C.C.S., MRCSLT (reg), MASLTIP

Independent Speech and Language Therapist, ChatAbility,
Cottesmore, Oakham, Rutland, UK, and
Chatting Independently Ltd, March, Cambridgeshire, UK.

W
WHURR PUBLISHERS
LONDON AND PHILADELPHIA

First published by Taylor and Francis in 1988
All right reserved by Whurr Publishers Ltd 1990
Reprinted 1990
Second edition published by Whurr Publishers Ltd 1993
Reprinted 1994
Third edition 1997
Fourth edition 2005 Published by Whurr Publishers Ltd
19b Compton Terrace, London N1 2UN, England and
325 Chestnut Street, Philadelphia PA19106, USA

British Library Cataloguing in Publication Data

A catalogue record for this book is available from the
British Library.

ISBN 1 86156 285 3

Printed and bound in the UK by Athenaeum Press Limited,
Gateshead, Tyne & Wear.

Contents

Dedication
To my parents

Preface

The *Dictionary of Communication Disorders*, formerly the *Dictionary of Speech Therapy*, was the first in the United Kingdom to be written with students of Speech and Language therapy in mind, since, having been such a student myself, I recognised a need for it. However, it was also written for Speech and Language Therapists working in the field as well as for those who, for whatever reason, were returning to it. It was written also to recognise the wide range of subjects about which a Speech and Language Therapist is required to know, such as Linguistics, Phonetics/Phonology, Psychology/Psychiatry, Hearing, Augmentative and Alternative Communication, Computing, Anatomy/Physiology, and Neurology, as well as Speech Pathology. The groupings for whom the Dictionary is required have not changed over the years nor has the need, in my opinion, for a book where Speech and Language Therapists and those in allied professions can find out about particular terms.

For many reasons, some personal and some professional, it has been eight years since the third edition of the Dictionary was published and so there was much which required to be updated as well as many additions to be made to it.

So, what is new in this 4th Edition of the *Dictionary of Communication Disorders*?

As with previous editions, all the main references have been updated, new references have been added to the bibliography, and the definitions of some terms have been rewritten while others have had information from the most recent research added to them. Some terms have been deleted such as those of older communication aids which are no longer used, and some basic computer terms have been omitted since using a computer is much more popular than it was sixteen years ago when the first edition was written. I owe a debt of gratitude to Professor Brian Moore, of the University of Cambridge, for his help in developing this fourth edition.

There are many new terms covering assessments and treatment programmes in Speech Pathology as well as information concerning new high-tech communication aids, computer software and symbol systems in the ever evolving field of Augmentative and Alternative Communication.

There have been changes to two of the appendices. Appendix I listing the assessments described in the text has been divided into assessments for children and adults and the assessments have been categorised by diagnostic category. In this way, I have tried to make it easier to find an appropriate assessment for a particular client just by looking in the Appendix. Appendix IV listing holders of trademarks and/or copyright for AAC devices, software and other hardware, gives the name of the manufacturer holding the trademark, the names of the trademarked products followed by the supplier and their website address.

The most significant change in society as a whole since the first edition of the Dictionary has been the increasing use of the internet and I wanted to reflect this in this latest edition of the Dictionary. So, you will find at the end of the list of references following the definitions particularly for medical conditions, the website address for Support Groups for those conditions in the UK or USA, as well as, in some instances, a website address to give more information concerning the conditions themselves. I have done this mainly for medical conditions so that you can have a quick reference to find a Support Group for the family of a client whom you may be treating with the condition. All website addresses have been checked and are active.

By making these changes to the fourth edition of the Dictionary of Communication Disorders, I hope I have maintained the aim, which I wrote in the preface to the first edition in 1986, of clarifying terminology which may mystify many entering or already working in the field of communication disorders.

David W. H. Morris
September 2004

AAC *see* AUGMENTATIVE AND ALTERNATIVE COMMUNICATION.

abdomen the lower part of the trunk that contains within its cavity the gut, liver, kidneys and urogenital system. The walls comprise muscles and bones. The roof of the abdomen is formed by the diaphragm that separates the thoracic and abdominal organs. This structure produces ABDOMINAL–DIAPHRAGMATIC RESPIRATION. *See* Tortora and Grabowski (2000).

abdominal–diaphragmatic respiration breathing produced by the movement of the diaphragm. In inspiration, the diaphragm decreases in size and pushes out the abdominal wall. In expiration, the opposite happens. This form of breathing is most common in men. It is opposed to THORACIC RESPIRATION (*see* CLAVICULAR). *See* Tortora and Grabowski (2000).

abducens nerve (cranial nerve VI) *see* CRANIAL NERVES.

abduction a description of movement away from the midline. It is opposed to ADDUCTION. *See* Tortora and Grabowski (2000).

aberrant a psychological description of behaviour that is found to be abnormal.

ability tests *see* INTELLIGENCE TESTS.

ABLB *see* ALTERNATE BINAURAL LOUDNESS BALANCE (ABLB) TEST.

abnormal behaviour behaviour that departs from the norm. Such behaviour can be found in those with conditions such as SCHIZOPHRENIA, AFFECTIVE DISORDERS, ANXIETY DISORDERS, personality disorders and drug-dependency. Treatment can include BEHAVIOUR THERAPY and PSYCHOANALYSIS although some disorders may be improved through drug therapy. *See* Smith et al (2003).

ABR *see* AUDITORY BRAINSTEM RESPONSE.

abreaction *see* PSYCHOANALYSIS.

abrupt release during the production of plosives, there is a sudden release of built-up pressure in the mouth. It is opposed to DELAYED RELEASE. *See* Cruttenden (1994).

AC an abbreviation for air conduction (*see* PURE-TONE AUDIOMETRY).

acalculia an arithmetic disorder that can present as a person's inability to cope with arithmetic processes or as difficulty in the spoken or written production of symbols used in calculation. It can be associated with APHASIA, especially if the client has a lesion in the right hemisphere producing problems of spatial orientation. *See* Eisenson (1984); Kolb and Whishaw (1996).

accent

1. The part of a word, phrase or sentence that is given increased loudness as well as a change to the intonation pattern. In English, the accent is regular in that the main accent is always on a specific syllable of each word. *See* Cruttenden (1994).

1

2. The regional variations of pronunciation of a language. These variations are caused by differences in the type of vowel and consonant used as well as in the phonological and prosodic patterns produced by the speaker. It is differentiated from a DIALECT. *See* Wells (1982).

acceptability an acceptable utterance made by one native speaker to another native speaker is one that follows the syntactic rules of that language. *See* Lyons (1968).

acceptable stammer the criterion of success used by speech therapists using the STAMMER MORE FLUENTLY approach.

access

1. The process by which the computer obtains data or other information from a disk in a disk drive or instructions from a memory so that they can be carried out (e.g. from a program in the computer's memory). *See* Brookshear (1991).
2. In AUGMENTATIVE AND ALTERNATIVE COMMUNICATION, access refers to the means by which a person uses a communication aid. This may be by direct manual selection, headpointing or by using switches. *See* Beukelman and Mirenda (1998).

accessory nerve (cranial nerve XI) *see* CRANIAL NERVES.

Acorn Computers Acorn produced the BBC series of microcomputers that were no longer produced in the mid 1980s but Acorn carried on building computers which use the RISC Operating System until it was taken over in 2000. However, the RISC Operating System still exists and uses windows and mouse selection in a similar way to Microsoft Windows and the Apple OS. *See* http://www.riscos.com; http://www.cjemicros.co.uk

acoupaedics *see* EDUCATION OF HEARING-IMPAIRED CHILDREN (1a).

acoustic method *see* EDUCATION OF HEARING-IMPAIRED CHILDREN.

acoustic neuroma *see* VESTIBULAR SCHWANNOMA.

acoustic phonetics the physical study of the ways in which sounds are heard. The three main acoustic features which describe the ways in which sounds are produced are frequency, intensity and time. Frequency is the complete number of repetitions of variations in air pressure that happen in a second. The unit used to measure frequency is the Hertz (Hz). A Hertz is the number of cycles per second used in producing a sound (i.e. the number of times the cords open and close). So, if a sound causes the cords to vibrate 550 times per second, then the frequency of the sound will be 550 Hz or 550 cps (cycles per second). The higher frequencies of the sound, which are whole multiples of the fundamental frequency, are known as harmonics. To work out the harmonic series of a sound, the fundamental frequency is multiplied by successive whole numbers. For example, if a sound has a fundamental frequency (i.e. 100 cycles per second) and a frequency of 300 cycles per second, this is the third harmonic of the sound. Frequency is the acoustic measurement of the pitch of a sound. The pitch is an auditory property that allows the listener to determine a sound on a scale going from low to high. Loudness depends on the size of the changes in air pressure that occur. Intensity is the measure of loudness and is proportional to the average size of the changes in air pressure. The unit used to measure intensity is the decibel (dB). Quality of a sound changes in relation to the change in frequencies between sounds. Thus, there is a difference in the quality of any two vowels that are held to be different. *See* Ladefoged (2001).

acquired agnosia *see* AGNOSIA.

acquired aphasia *see* APHASIA.

acquired apraxia a disorder caused by trauma to the brain after birth affecting the person's co-ordination. As a speech disorder, it is characterised by the person groping for the correct order of sounds which produces trial and error realisations of the required sounds. In the most severe forms of acquired apraxia, people may not even be able to start off a word with the correct sound. The programming of the movements required to make sounds in a particular order becomes disordered, particularly, though not exclusively, with polysyllabic words. There is also disruption to PROSODY, articulatory inconsistency and difficulties in initiating utterances. *See* Miller (1986).

acquired disorders any disorder not caused at birth (i.e. congenital disorders) in the PRENATAL or PERINATAL stages. Acquired disorders usually have an organic cause (e.g. CEREBROVASCULAR ACCIDENT, HEAD INJURY, etc.). The commonest acquired disorders of communication are APHASIA, DYSARTHRIA and DYSPRAXIA. They can occur at any time in the person's life. *See* Crystal (1981); Beukelman and Yorkston (1989) (AAC and acquired disorders); Fried-Oken (2001) (AAC and acquired disorders); Lasker and Bedrosian (2001) (AAC and acquired disorders).

acquired dyslexia occurs following damage to the brain caused by such conditions as CEREBROVASCULAR ACCIDENT, HEAD INJURY or brain tumour (*see* TUMOURS OF THE CENTRAL NERVOUS SYSTEM). There are four types:

1. Phonological dyslexia: the inability to read non-words (*see* NONSENSE WORD) aloud, e.g. 'dup', 'getuld' etc., while the ability to read everyday words aloud remains intact. Other symptoms such as 'visual errors' in reading aloud non-words e.g. [dek] for /desk/ can appear. Derivational errors are also present when reading words aloud, especially when they contain bound morphemes (*see* MORPHOLOGY).
2. Deep dyslexia: SEMANTIC errors are present when reading. Other symptoms can also be present e.g. visual impairment, function word substitu-

tion and derivational errors. Low-imageability words are harder to read aloud than high-imageability words; verbs are harder to read than adjectives, which are harder to read than nouns. However, deep dyslexia can only be diagnosed if a semantic error is present in reading aloud, even if there are none of the other symptoms.

3. Letter-by-letter reader (word-form dyslexia): what is being read aloud can only be understood by reading one letter at a time. This is the only acquired dyslexia that is produced by a focal lesion, the link between the ANGULAR GYRUS in the left cerebral hemisphere (*see* CEREBRAL HEMISPHERES) and the visual input system in both hemispheres being broken. Since the angular gyrus is unaffected per se, writing is relatively unimpaired. It is also known as Déjérine's syndrome after the neurologist who discovered the disconnection.
4. Surface dyslexia: a disturbance between the visual word recognition system and the semantic system. However, the word can still be spoken since the visual recognition system and phonemic system are still intact. *See* Patterson and Kay (1982); Ellis (1993); Nickels (1995).

acquired dysphasia *see* APHASIA.

acquired hearing loss a hearing loss produced by disease, tumours, natural ageing, excessive noise, toxic drugs and trauma at any time during a person's life after birth.

acquisition a learning process opposed to INNATENESS. The phrase language acquisition is used to describe the stages of language development in children between the ages of 9 months and 5 years. It can also be used to describe how children with specific learning difficulties, or adults with speech and language disorders, develop communication skills which they have hitherto lacked. *See* Clark and Clark (1977); Fromkin and Rodman (2003); Paul

(1997a, b); Calculator (1997); Light (1997); Romski et al (1997); Bedrosian (1997) (all articles concern language acquisition/development and AAC)

acrocephalosyndactyly *see* APERT SYNDROME.

Action Picture Test devised by Renfrew in 1966 (2nd edn, 1971; 3rd edn, 1989) it is a quick means of finding out if a child has a LANGUAGE DELAY or SPECIFIC DEVELOPMENTAL LANGUAGE DISORDER. Answers are sought to simple questions regarding what is being enacted in each of the 10 coloured pictures of everyday events. Responses are analysed for (1) amount of correct information given and (2) the grammatical forms used, which should include some irregular forms of verbs and nouns as well as complex and compound sentences. The test is standardised in the UK and can be applied to children from 3;6 to 8;6 years. *See* Renfrew (1989) in Appendix I.

active voice usually contrasted with PASSIVE voice, it refers to a grammatical construction in which the grammatical subject is typically the actor as in:

1. The dog bit the man.

    In earlier versions of transformational generative grammar (*see* TRANSFORMATIONAL GRAMMAR), active sentences and their passive equivalents were related by a transformational rule. *See* Clark and Clark (1977); Fromkin and Rodman (2003).

acuity the sounds which the ear can pick up. These can vary depending on how near to the sound source the person is. *See* Denes and Pinson (1993).

acute

1. A description of the sudden onset of an illness or disease. It is opposed to CHRONIC.
2. A distinctive feature used by Jakobson and Halle to distinguish sounds made towards the front of the mouth and produced using the high frequencies such as alveolar, dental and palatal consonants (*see* ARTICULATION) from

vowels made in a similar position. These are denoted as [+ACUTE]. *See* Hyman (1975).

acute laryngitis inflammation of laryngeal mucosa and of VOCAL FOLDS. The symptoms are hoarseness leading to DYSPHONIA, malaise, pain when speaking, redness and swelling of the LARYNX. Vocal rest is usually recommended and possibly a period of speech and language therapy. *See* Pracy et al (1974); Mathieson (2001).

adaptation *see* ASSIMILATION (1).

adduction a description of movement towards the midline. It is opposed to ABDUCTION. *See* Tortora and Grabowski (2000).

adenoidal facies *see* MOUTH BREATHING.

adenoids lymphatic tissue found in the posterior wall of the nasopharynx (*see* PHARYNX). At birth, the adenoids are small and as the child grows older, the adenoids grow until puberty when they atrophy. If they become large, they may block the eustachian tube (*see* EAR) causing hearing problems and/or nasal obstruction. Such obstruction results in mouth breathing and snoring. There is a particular facial appearance known as 'adenoidal facies' associated with the condition. The obstruction may become so significant that an adenoidectomy, in which the adenoids are removed, is necessary. *See* Pracy et al (1974).

adiadochokinesis an inability to produce rapid sequences of movement. In speech, this relates to rapid alternating movements of the articulators. It occurs as a feature of DYSPRAXIA and DYSARTHRIA. *See* Darley et al (1975); Robertson and Thomson (1986).

adjective adjectives appear in NOUN PHRASES and are also used as predicates. This is exemplified by the following sentences:

1. An interesting question.
2. The question is interesting.

    In noun phrases, the adjective comes between the determiner and the noun, as will be found in the discussion concerning CONSTITUENT ANALYSIS. However, when two or more adjectives are used in a noun phrase, they are placed in a particular order. Following analysis of sentences in which the noun is premodified by one or more adjectives, the following order can be found:

determiner – general – age – colour – participle – provenance – noun – denominal – head noun.

This order takes account of sentences such as those shown in the box below.

In all cases, the noun phrase will make sense by using any or none of these adjectives. *See* Strang (1968); Fromkin and Rodman (2003).

Adult Quick Learning Systems for ALS Patients (AQLS) a MINSPEAK software specifically designed for people with amyotrophic lateral sclerosis (ALS) or MOTOR NEURONE DISEASE. It allows people with ALS or MND to communicate spontaneously with a significant reduction in keystrokes. There are two formats: the iconic version which uses icon sequences and single hit words, and the alphabetic version which uses an enhanced QWERTY KEYBOARD plus quick-access words and phrases. The iconic version is based on the 128-location version of UNITY and has a vocabulary of 5000 words. There is a teaching programme of 15 lessons to teach those using the system. The alphabetic version is designed for people who are literate but need such a system to help them communicate. This system has quick access to 250 of the most common words and phrases, reducing the keystrokes required. The AQLS package includes both versions of the software

plus overlays, lesson plans and manuals. It can be used on the DELTA TALKER, PATHFINDER and LIBERATOR COMMUNICATION AID. Word prediction is available only on the Pathfinder and Liberator if it uses Liberator version 2 software. *See* Appendix IV (Semantic Compaction Systems).

adverb an adverb is usually an adjunct to the verb. The most common and most recognisable form of adverb is an adjective with '-ly' attached to it, e.g. quickly, slowly, etc. These adverbs are found in sentences such as:

1. He ran quickly.
2. The tortoise moves slowly.

However, adverbs can take other forms. They can mark time and place, e.g. here, now, there, perhaps, seldom, etc. These can only be used as adverbs. Other words such as yesterday, downstairs, first, etc. can be used as adverbs although they can function in other ways. Adverbs, like adjectives, can be used in the positive, comparative and superlative forms. They can be differentiated from adjectives by the use of 'than' which requires a comparative and 'of all' which requires a superlative. Consider, for example, the following sentences:

1. The World Cup is the greatest football competition of all [football competitions].
2. Stephen Hendry played better than Jimmy White.

See Strang (1968); Fromkin and Rodman (2003).

adVOCAte is a light-tech communication aid allowing for 16 minutes of DIGITISED

det.	gen.	age	colour	partic.	proven.	noun	head noun
The	large	old	grey	crumbling	English	country	house
A	small		blue				ball
The	great	young		battling	French	rugby	team.

(based on Quirk and Greenbaum, 1979)

SPEECH and up to 16 seconds recording time per location and an optional remote text display. It can be configured to use one to 16 locations and can be accessed by direct selection or switch scanning. It has five levels, four with single selections and one level with key linking. The device has also an infra red output to operate battery or mains powered devices. *See* Appendix IV (Toby Churchill).

affect the continuum of consciously experienced pleasure and displeasure. *See* Kolb and Whishaw (1996); Smith et al (2003).

affective disorders a group of disorders that produce abnormal moods in a person, e.g. DEPRESSION and MANIC-DEPRESSION. *See* Kolb and Whishaw (1996); Smith et al (2003).

afferent (motor) aphasia an APHASIA described by Aleksandr Luria in the 1960s. It is similar to ACQUIRED APRAXIA. The person is unable to predict where or how to position the articulators for sound production. A severe afferent aphasia results in a global problem; in a mild form, only similar sounds may be confused, e.g. bilabials /p,b,m/, alveolars /t,d,n/, etc. There may also be a disorder in the person's writing ability by confusing what Luria calls articulemes, i.e. sounds. The lesion causing such a disorder occurs in the secondary zones of the postcentral kinaesthetic cortex. *See* Eisenson (1984).

afferent system nerve cells that convey information from receptors in the periphery of the body to the CENTRAL NERVOUS SYSTEM. These nerve cells are called afferent or sensory neurones and are the first cells to pick up incoming information. *See* Taverner (1983); Tortora and Grabowski (2000).

affix a general term used in MORPHOLOGY to refer to the adding of morphemes (prefixes and suffixes) to the base form. *See* Allerton (1979); Fromkin and Rodman (2003).

affricate *see* ARTICULATION.

AFP an abbreviation for alpha-fetoprotein. *See* AMNIOCENTESIS.

age-equivalent scores scores that are obtained after working out the results of assessments by looking up tables in the manuals of the assessments concerned. Such tests have undergone standardisation and so these scores can be compared to the chronological age of the assessed person.

ageing the process of becoming older. During this process a person undergoes physical changes, e.g., anatomical, physiological and skeletal changes, increasing problems with vision and hearing; psychological changes, e.g., possible changes in intellectual levels; memory changes, e.g., memory loss in senile dementia, more generally, memory problems which occur with retaining material requiring full attention and ability to organise it. Neugarten (1968) (see Bromley 1988) showed that, as they grow older, people have different reactions to their old age. These reactions can be positive where a person substitutes other activities for lost activities, becoming less positive where a person gradually withdraws from the world, to one who is deeply pessimistic and no longer takes part in life. In a study of 87-year-old men, Reichard et al. (1962) (see Bromley 1988) found similar reactions to the ageing process. Davison and Neale summed up growing old as: '...the greatest challenge of old people is to cope with reality, the gradual loss of loved ones and friends, the deterioration of physical and psychological capacities, the low regard in which they are held by the culture at large' (Davison and Neale 2004). *See* Bromley (1988); Davison et al (2004); Balandin and Morgan (2001) (AAC and ageing).

aglossia *see* GLOSSECTOMY.

agnosia a disorder of understanding speech or knowing what objects are although speech can still be heard and objects touched. There are five main types which may be congenital or acquired:

1. Acoustic – difficulty in sound discrimination.

2. Pure word deafness – a specific difficulty in recognising speech sounds resulting in an inability to repeat what has been said but the patient, with difficulty, can use some spontaneous speech, read or write. At times, by watching the therapist's face intently, lip-reading may be possible for auditory comprehension.

3. Visual – inability to understand various situations by failing to recognise visual stimuli.

4. Tactile – inability to recognise objects by feel or touch.

5. Auditory verbal – the inability to understand spoken language.

See Eisenson (1984); Kolb and Whishaw (1996); Adams et al (1997).

agonist muscle a description of the contraction of one muscle against another that acts as an antagonist muscle. This muscle contraction is also known as a prime mover. *See* Tortora and Grabowski (2000).

agrammatism restricted use of grammar, often associated with aphasia. *See* APHASIA (1).

agraphia disorders of writing which may be neurological in origin. There are three types:

1. Phonological dysgraphia: impaired ability to write and spell non-words (*see* NONSENSE WORD) while the ability to write real words is preserved.

2. Surface dysgraphia: inability to write and spell real words.

3. Deep dysgraphia: semantic errors occur in writing.

See Rosenbek et al (1989); Kolb and Whishaw (1996).

AI *see* ARTIFICIAL INTELLIGENCE.

aided symbols those symbols` which require an external means of production such as objects or black and white line drawings, whereas unaided symbols require no such external means of production such as facial expressions, vocalisations, natural speech and so on. *See* Beukelman and Mirenda (1998).

air bone gap *see* PURE-TONE AUDIOMETRY.

air conduction *see* PURE-TONE AUDIOMETRY.

air-conduction hearing aid the main type of hearing aid given to those who have a hearing loss. There are also BONE-CONDUCTION HEARING AIDS. *See* Miller (1972); Graham and Martin (2001).

airstreams the source of power for the production of most sounds is made by air from the lungs. There are four types of airstream:

1. Pulmonic egressive airstream: the normal airstream used by all speakers using all varieties of English. The speaker uses ABDOMINAL–DIAPHRAGMATIC RESPIRATION or clavicular breathing (*see* CLAVICULAR) although the length of message which can be produced in the former will be more than that produced in the latter. Thus, if a deep breath is taken in and let out from the lungs producing a fricative (*see* ARTICULATION), e.g. /s/, a very long uninterrupted sound will be produced until the breath runs out. No other type of airstream allows the speaker such a long uninterrupted flow for producing speech.

2. Pulmonic ingressive airstream: this airstream works in the opposite way to the egressive airstream. The lungs are emptied of air followed by the speaker producing speech while drawing air into the lungs. If a similar fricative is produced as in (1), the sound will not be sustained for very long. Speech can become very distorted.

3. Glottalic airstream: an airstream produced by a movement of the larynx with glottal closure. An upward movement of the larynx produces a glottalic egressive airstream which produces an ejective, while a downward movement of the larynx produces a glottalic ingressive airstream which produces an implosive.

4. Velaric airstream: an airstream which produces velaric ingressive stops or clicks.

See Ladefoged (2001).

akinetic seizure a type of seizure that usually affects only children. It produces a loss of tone that may be generalised throughout the body or specific to the neck. In the former, the child collapses to the ground, while in the latter, the head falls forward onto the chest. It can be controlled by clonazepam or sodium valproate. Children may have other types of seizure. *See* Gilroy and Holliday (1982).

alexia *see* ACQUIRED DYSLEXIA and DEVELOPMENTAL DYSLEXIA.

alexia with agraphia a disorder of both reading and writing but EXPRESSIVE LANGUAGE and AUDITORY COMPREHENSION are intact. *See* Ellis (1993); Rosenbek et al (1989).

alexia without agraphia also known as pure alexia, it is a rare condition in which the person cannot read but can write. Oral expression, auditory comprehension and repetition are intact. Benson and Geschwind (1969) suggested the following specific symptoms: right homonymous hemianopia (a disorder of the right visual fields), inability to identify colours, an impairment in calculation, occasional problems with naming objects, severely impaired reading and relatively intact writing. *See* Rosenbek et al (1989).

allomorph *see* MORPHOLOGY.

allophone *see* PHONOLOGY.

AllWrite a word processing software for people with visual impairment that speaks as you type by letter, word or sentences as well as the actions of the cursor keys, menus and shift keys. It is compatible with mainstream word processors. *See* Appendix IV (Sensory Software International).

alpha-fetoprotein *see* AMNIOCENTESIS.

Alpha Talker a high-tech communication aid with digitised speech output. It uses MINSPEAK to organise vocabulary to store into the device. It has a memory of three minutes for standard speech and five minutes for extended speech. With an extra memory card this can be increased to 15 minutes standard and 25 minutes extended. It can be accessed using direct manual selection, optical headpointing, single, dual or two switch scanning. Overlays of 4, 8 and 32 locations can be used. Other features include icon prediction, which shows by illuminating a light on a symbol which symbols have messages stored under them and shows the others in the sequence; and predictive selection, which makes symbols with nothing stored under them inoperative when using with direct manual selection or optical headpointing, while with scanning, the scanning light jumps the unused symbols. The Alpha Talker also allows for auditory prompts to be stored. This allows for the person to hear the names of the symbols before they are activated. This feature can be used either with direct manual selection, optical headpointing or using a switch for scanning. The device's memory can be backed up on computer, and basic computer emulation is possible as well as attaching the DIRECTOR, an environmental control system. The Flash Eprom system means the device should never lose its memory. *See* Rumble and Larcher (1998); Appendix IV (Prentke Romich Company).

Alpha Talker II a high-tech communication aid with digitised speech output. It uses MINSPEAK to organise vocabulary to store into the device. It has a memory of six minutes for standard speech and 11 minutes for extended speech. With an extra memory card this can be increased to 37 minutes. It can be accessed using direct manual selection, optical headpointing, single, dual or two switch scanning. Overlays of 4, 8 and 32 locations can be used. Other features include icon prediction, which shows by illuminating a light on a symbol which symbols have messages stored under them and shows the others in the sequence; predictive selection, which makes symbols with nothing stored under them inoperative when using with direct manual selection or optical headpointing; while with scanning, the scanning light jumps the unused symbols. The Alpha Talker also allows for auditory prompts to be stored. This allows the person who uses the Alpha Talker to hear the names of the symbols before they are activated. This feature can be used either with direct manual selection, optical head-pointing or using a switch for scanning. The device's memory can be backed up on computer and basic computer emulation is possible as well as attaching the DIRECTOR, an environmental control system. The Flash Eprom system means the device should never lose its memory. *See* Rumble and Larcher (1998); Appendix IV (Prentke Romich Company).

alternate binaural loudness balance (ABLB) test a test for RECRUITMENT used with those who have a unilateral hearing loss. It matches the loudness level of two tones. It requires a two-channel audiometer to send a signal to each ear. The tester presents a tone of 20dB SL (*see* SENSATION LEVEL) to the better ear and the same tone to the poorer ear. The level of the tone is increased until it is heard at the same loudness in each ear.

alternate hypothesis the hypothesis must be proved by statistical analysis. This hypothesis states that a significant difference between scores does exist. The alternate hypothesis must be set out before the results of the experiment are known and be based on what is known about the subject under investigation from other experiments, surveys etc. It will be proved if the NULL HYPOTHESIS is rejected. Both hypotheses are used in inferential statistics. The alternate hypothesis is also known as the experimental hypothesis. *See* Miller (1984); Porkess (1988); Clarke and Cooke (1992).

alternative access *see* INPUT SYSTEMS; SCANNING DEVICES.

Alzheimer's disease a type of dementia. The cause is unknown but there is an increasing rate of loss of neurones in the brain. Atrophy occurs in both the white and grey matter of the BRAIN while the sulci widen and the gyri atrophy. A person with this disease will have a gradual loss of short-term memory which becomes worse while long-term memory (*see* MEMORY) is retained intact until the later stages of the disease. A change in personality occurs as well, e.g. a quiet person can become aggressive, and transient hemiplegias may also occur. Women are affected twice as frequently as men and death may occur 2–5 years after the original onset. The language impairment of someone with Alzheimer's disease reflects quite closely the disorders found in Wernicke's aphasia (*see* APHASIA (2)), especially in the later stages of the disease. However, in the early stages, there may be language problems such as the use of circumlocution in naming tasks and verbal PARAPHASIAS which may be self-corrected. In conversation, the patient in the early stages of the disease will digress quite frequently and will find difficulty returning to the subject and will often fail to answer a specific question but not a related one. This latter problem, as with others, gets worse as the disease progresses. The person will respond better to specific comprehension tests than in conversation and will succeed in repetition tasks when asked to repeat high probability phrases, e.g. near the table in the dining room, while they become confused and make paraphasic errors with low probability phrases, e.g. the Chinese fan had a rare emerald. As the disease progresses, all these problems become worse with an increase in verbal and literal PARAPHASIAS and circumlocution. Cueing strategies such as phonemic or semantic cueing have little effect. In conversation, the digression from the subject is much more marked. In the later stages, PRAGMATICS become a problem with the person becoming mute or using PALILALIA or ECHOLALIA. Jargon (*see* JARGON APHASIA) becomes more evident and discourse becomes empty. During a naming task, the correct label may be produced in the midst

ANS *see* AUTONOMIC NERVOUS SYSTEM.

antagonist a muscle contraction which is opposed to the contraction of the prime mover, i.e. agonist muscle. *See* Tortora and Grabowski (2000).

anterior a distinctive feature proposed by Chomsky and Halle. It is used to produce a distinction of sounds produced towards the front of the mouth. The sounds which are denoted as [+ANTERIOR] are dentals and labials (*see* ARTICULATION). *See* Hyman (1975).

anterograde often referring to a type of amnesia, it refers to the inability to acquire new information or remember what happens in the person's daily routine. *See* Smith et al (2003).

antidepressant drugs tricyclic drugs given to treat those who have endogenous DEPRESSION. The most commonly used antidepressant drugs are:

amitriptyline,	protriptyline,
imipramine,	dothiepin,
clomipramine,	trimipramine,
nortriptyline,	doxepin.

For the side effects of these drugs, *see* AMITRIPTYLINE. *See* Stafford-Clark and Bridges (1990); Kolb and Whishaw (1996); Smith et al (2003); Davison et al (2004).

anxiety a neurotic disorder. Abnormal anxiety is caused by acute fear which is often irrational and produces feelings of panic. Someone with such irrational anxieties may show some of the following features:

1. Anxiety may dominate their mental status.
2. Physical symptoms (e.g. tachycardia – abnormal heart rhythms).
3. Restlessness, sleeplessness and sweating, etc.
4. Choking, suffocation, collapse.
5. HYPOCHONDRIASIS.

Not everyone with anxiety has all of these symptoms. It will depend on severity of the anxiety condition. Treatment can be given by PSYCHOTHERAPY, ANXIETY DRUG THERAPY, BEHAVIOUR THERAPY and self-help groups. *See* Stafford-Clark and Bridges (1990); Smith et al (2003); Davison et al (2004).

anxiety disorders a group of disorders that produce abnormal behaviour. The main symptom is anxiety or anxiety-producing PHOBIAS or OBSESSIVE–COMPULSIVE DISORDER. *See* Smith et al (2003); Davison et al (2004).

anxiety drug therapy the main drugs used are benzodiazepines. They act partly on the brain and partly by decreasing the activity of the spinal reflex centres. The drugs, which take a long time to act, are diazepam, chlordiazepoxide, medazepam, clorazepate and oxazepam. The main side effect of these drugs is drowsiness. The drugs which take a shorter time to act are lorazepam, temazepam and triazolam. They can produce problems with the kidneys. The drug is taken at night so that the person can be fully aware of what is happening during the day. The only problem with such drugs is a growing dependence on them resulting in the person becoming unreceptive to other non-medication forms of therapy. Other drugs used in the treatment of anxiety are MONOAMINE OXIDASE INHIBITORS and tricyclic ANTIDEPRESSANT DRUGS. Beta-blocking drugs can also be given to reduce an abnormally fast heartbeat and for sedation during the night. *See* Stafford-Clark and Bridges (1990); Smith et al (2003); Davison et al (2004).

apathy a reaction (e.g. frustration) of certain people to various situations. They withdraw and become indifferent to certain situations whereas others react with aggression to similar situations. It is uncertain why this should happen but it may be learned behaviour, their in-born personality or due to their surrounding environment. *See* Smith et al (2003).

Apert syndrome a craniosynostosis syndrome involving an abnormal growth of the cranium and malformed fingers and toes. The face has a particular appearance with wide-set, bulging eyes, abnormally small maxillae, crowded teeth and a protruding mandible. The incidence is 1:100000 and it is caused by one of two mutations on chromosome 10. It is autosomal-dominant (*see* CHROMOSOMES). Usually, intelligence is within normal limits although there can be a degree of LEARNING DISABILITY. Shipster et al (2002) investigated the nature of the speech and language problems which those with Apert syndrome may have. It is also known as acrocephalosyndactyly. *See* Hosking (1982); Goodman and Gorlin (1983); Cohen et al (1993); Shipster et al (2002); http://www.faces-cranio.org/Disord/Apert.htm

apex in articulatory terms, the tip of the tongue which is used, for example, to produce dental and some alveolar sounds, known as apico-alveolar. *See* Catford (1989).

Apgar score devised by Virginia Apgar, it is a test given to newborn babies. If the numerical test scores remain low for a considerable time, the prognosis for the baby's life and possible neurological sequelae are poor. It gives a value of 0, 1 or 2 to the baby's heart rate, respiratory effort, reflex irritability, muscle tone and colour. It is repeated at 1 and 5 minutes of life. *See* Illingworth (1987).

aphasia also known as dysphasia. The commonest causes are CEREBROVASCULAR ACCIDENT (CVA), HEAD INJURY or brain tumour (*see* TUMOURS OF THE CENTRAL NERVOUS SYSTEM) which have affected part of the BRAIN, usually the left cerebral hemisphere (*see* CEREBRAL HEMISPHERES) which controls the use of language – both comprehension and expressive language. Both can be disordered to a lesser or greater degree. Both children and adults are affected. In most cases, it is more accurately termed acquired dysphasia as language has already been acquired. Those who are diagnosed as having acquired dysphasia can have word-finding difficulties, comprehension problems both auditory and reading, problems with reading out loud, repetition, serial speech and writing. Those who have word-finding difficulties are said to have a non-fluent aphasia while others who produce fluent speech which is syntactically correct but may be meaningless have a fluent aphasia. Different classifications have been used to describe different kinds of aphasia. They have been produced by among others the Boston School, Schuell and Alexsandr Luria. Probably the commonest classification in use presently is the Boston classification. The following types of aphasia are recognised by this school:

1. Broca's aphasia. Speech production is non-fluent. It is marked by phonetic disintegration and by reduced vocabulary, especially of function words, and by restricted grammar (agrammatism). Prosody and written language are affected. Auditory verbal comprehension is relatively intact. Luria's terms for this type of aphasia are 'afferent kinaesthetic aphasia' and 'efferent kinaesthetic aphasia'.

2. Wernicke's aphasia. Speech is fluent and grammatically and prosodically intact. It is interspersed with neologisms and paraphasias which may be semantic (inappropriate selection of words) or phonemic (deletion, addition, substitution, or mis-sequencing of sounds). Verbal comprehension is severely impaired. Both reading and writing are affected. Luria's term for this type of aphasia is 'acoustic amnesic'. Eisenson described it as being JARGON APHASIA.

3. Conduction aphasia. An inability to repeat words. Short bursts of speech can be fluent although there may be phonemic PARAPHASIAS. Auditory comprehension is good relative to the expressive deficit. Luria called this type of aphasia a 'dynamic aphasia'.

4. Anomic aphasia. Comprehension is good and speech is fluent and grammatical. There is however a marked word retrieval deficit. Recall of proper names and names of objects is most affected. Ideas are expressed through

circumlocution. Luria called this type of aphasia 'semantic aphasia'.

5. Transcortical aphasia:

   (a) Motor. A rare condition bearing certain similarities to Broca's aphasia except there is a disproportionate ability to repeat fluently. Spontaneous speech is dysfluent. Auditory verbal comprehension is good.

   (b) Sensory. Also rare. It shares certain features with Wernicke's aphasia. There is good ability to repeat. Propositional speech is empty and echoic. Auditory comprehension is impaired.

6. Global aphasia. A very severe disorder in which all language modalities are affected. Speech is fragmented and reiterative and may be unintelligible. Serial speech may be retained. *See* Mark et al (1992); Van Mourik et al (1992).

7. Pure aphasias. Rare conditions in which only one modality is affected leaving the remainder intact.

In a review of the literature concerning thalamic and striato-capsular aphasia, Kennedy and Murdoch suggest these can be seen as independent aphasic syndromes.

1. Acute thalamic aphasia (0–3 months post-onset): Lack of spontaneous speech (once speech is initiated syntax is intact); naming impairments with semantic and phonemic PARA-PHASIAS, neologisms (*see* JARGON APHASIA), circumlocutions and jargon (*see* JARGON APHASIA); PERSEVERATION; relatively intact repetitions; some degree of auditory and reading comprehension impairment; impaired writing abilities and fading or lowered voice volume.

2. Chronic thalamic aphasia (> 3 months post-onset): Relatively fluent language; naming deficit, mild auditory and reading comprehension impairment; disorder of writing.

In Kennedy and Murdoch's (1994) review of the literature concerning

striato-capsular aphasia, they found not all lesions in this area of the dominant hemisphere (*see* CEREBRAL HEMISPHERES) result in aphasia, and those people who do have an acute form of striato-capsular aphasia exhibit relatively intact abilities to severe impairment in language tasks such as spontaneous speech, naming, repetition, auditory and reading comprehension. There is no uniform type of language disorder: subgroups of aphasia based on lesion site have been proposed. However, distinct patterns of language deficit have been reported to occur.

3. Acute striato-capsular aphasia (0–3 months post-onset):
   Anterior lesion: Broca's type aphasia; transcortical motor aphasia; anomic aphasia
   Posterior lesion: Wernicke's type aphasia
   Anterior-posterior lesion: global type aphasia

4. Chronic striato-capsular aphasia (> 3 months post-onset):
   Anterior lesion: Broca's type aphasia; transcortical motor-type aphasia
   Posterior lesion: Wernicke's type aphasia; minimal/high-level aphasia
   Anterior-posterior lesion: global-type aphasia

The main assessments used to test for aphasia are the BOSTON DIAGNOSTIC APHASIA EXAMINATION (BDAE), the WESTERN APHASIA BATTERY (WAB), the MINNESOTA TEST FOR THE DIFFERENTIAL DIAGNOSIS OF APHASIA (MTDDA) and various screening tests such as those devised by Whurr, the APHASIA SCREENING TEST, or by Enderby and her colleagues, the FRENCHAY APHASIA SCREENING TEST or the SHEFFIELD SCREENING TEST FOR ACQUIRED LANGUAGE DISORDERS. With the advent of cognitive neuropsychology, Kay and her colleagues have devised the PSYCHOLINGUISTIC ASSESSMENTS OF LANGUAGE PROCESSING IN APHASIA (PALPA). See Satz and Bullard-Bates (1981); Eisenson (1984) (adult dysphasia);

Rosenbek et al (1989); Kay et al (1992) in Appendix I; Basso (1992) (prognostic factors); Martins and Ferro (1992) (recovery in acquired aphasia in children); *Aphasiology* 1993 7(5) (complete volume on acquired childhood aphasia); Kennedy and Murdoch (1994); Morris (1995a, 1995b) (AAC and aphasia); King and Hux (1995) (AAC and aphasia); Kolb and Whishaw (1996); Lasker et al (1997) (writing and severe aphasia); Beck and Fritz (1998) (aphasia and iconic codes); Beukelman and Mirenda (1998) (AAC); Garrett (1998) (adults with severe aphasia); Koul and Harding (1998) (AAC and aphasia); Cress and King (1999) (AAC and progressive aphasia); Reeves and Harris (2001) (AAC and aphasia).

Aphasia Screening Test devised by Whurr in 1974, it is a SCREENING TEST to assess the severity of APHASIA. It covers all modalities of communication in both comprehension (20 tests) and expressive language (30 tests). Each subtest is scored out of 5. The scores are plotted onto a profile chart to give an instant idea of the person's difficulties and where treatment can begin. In the revised test the new manual contains standardisation data and many examples of patient profiles. There is also included in the revised test a Short Form Aphasia Screening Test for a faster and less detailed assessment. *See* Whurr (1996) in Appendix I. In some cases, it may be necessary to use a more formal, standardised assessment such as the BOSTON DIAGNOSTIC APHASIA EXAMINATION (BDAE), the WESTERN APHASIA BATTERY (WAB), the MINNESOTA TEST FOR THE DIFFERENTIAL DIAGNOSIS OF APHASIA (MTDDA) or the PSYCHOLINGUISTIC ASSESSMENTS OF LANGUAGE PROCESSING IN APHASIA (PALPA). *See* Whurr (1996) in Appendix I; Beech et al (1993).

aphasiology the study of aphasia in all its forms.

aphemia the former (historical) term for APHASIA used by Broca to describe his patient, Leborgne. However, it seems to be thought of more as a term for describing APRAXIA rather than aphasia. *See* Eisenson (1984); Rosenbek et al (1989).

aphonia complete loss of voice. This may be organic in origin, e.g. vocal nodules, or psychogenic, e.g. conversion aphonia. *See* Greene and Mathieson (1989); Freeman and Fawcus (2001).

Apple Apple was founded in 1981 by Grant Martin and Simon Rowley. Apple can claim to have invented the PC in its business form in the early 1980s with the production of the Apple II. In response to the IBM PC, Apple produced the Macintosh. Apple popularised the concepts of windows, pull-down menus and mice devices although these had originated from Xerox. The original Macintosh, the Mac Classic, was slow and underpowered but as Apple recognised the strengths of the IBM PC, later versions have taken account of limited compatibility with the IBM PC. Since these early computers, Apple have become more commercially orientated and produced the Performa range followed by Power PC Macs. The newest Macs are iMacs and their laptop counterparts iBooks. http://www.apple.com/uk

applied linguistics putting theoretical linguistics into practice. This can happen in speech and language therapy when forming a treatment programme for those who have communication disorders. In such programmes, therapists have to use their knowledge of SYNTAX, SEMANTICS, PRAGMATICS, SOCIOLINGUISTICS and PSYCHOLINGUISTICS to assess the status of the person's linguistic systems. *See* http://www.humnet.ucla.edu/humnet/al/whatal.html; http://www.aila.ac

applied psychology *see* PSYCHOLOGY.

apposition a linguistic phenomenon which makes an implicit co-ordination of constituents without the use of a conjunction or pronoun:

1. Fred, the baker's son, went home.
2. Fred who is the baker's son went home.

(1) demonstrates apposition while (2) shows an explicit linkage with a pronoun. *See* Allerton (1979).

appropriateness the type of language people use differs from situation to situation. For example, informal language occurs at parties and among friends while much greater care is taken in the type of language used, say, in religious services. Variation occurs in both spoken and written forms of English. *See* Crystal and Davy (1969).

apraxia a severe form of dyspraxia. It may be developmental (*see* DEVELOPMENTAL APRAXIA OF SPEECH and DEVELOPMENTAL VERBAL DYSPRAXIA) or acquired (*see* ACQUIRED APRAXIA) and in the latter case is usually associated with CENTRAL NERVOUS SYSTEM impairment. There is a total inability to programme certain skilled purposeful movements in the absence of loss of motor power, sensation or co-ordination. It can appear in different forms including constructional, motor, ideomotor, ideational, verbal and dressing apraxia. Usually, two or more types appear together while it is very rare to find only one type in isolation. *See* Kolb and Whishaw (1996).

Apraxia Battery for Adults devised by Dabul in 1979, it is an assessment to diagnose the severity of ACQUIRED APRAXIA. There are six subtests:

1. DIADOCHOKINESIS.
2. Increasing word length (e.g. thick – thicken – thickening).
3. Limb and oral apraxia – 10 oral directions for the volitional manipulation of the oral structures and 10 oral commands requiring use of arms and hands.
4. Latency and utterance time for polysyllabic words – 10 polysyllabic words are represented in picture form and the person has to name them immediately after presentation; both latency and utterance times are measured.
5. Repeated trials test – the same pictures as used in subtest 4, each word is repeated three times.

6. Inventory of articulation characteristics of apraxia.

See Dabul (2000) in Appendix I.

Apraxia Profile devised by Hickman, allows the assessor to document children's oral-motor sequencing problems and establishes the level of oral movements and sequences which they can produce successfully. It is suitable for children in the age range of 2;00–12;00. *See* Hickman (1997) in Appendix I.

aprosody absence of appropriate nonsegmental parameters of speech, i.e. intonation, stress, rhythm, pause. *See* Crystal (1992).

aptitude tests tests that are designed to predict the client's future performance levels. Unlike achievement tests, that test what the person has already learnt, aptitude tests do not depend on past experience. Thus, intelligence tests can be called aptitude tests as they aim to predict the person's performance over a range of abilities and do not rely on memory recall or practised skills. *See* Smith et al (2003).

arcuate fasciculus a band of fibres that links Broca's area to Wernicke's area (*see* CEREBRAL HEMISPHERES). A disturbance in this area of the brain produces conduction aphasia (*see* APHASIA (3)). It is sometimes called the superior longitudinal fasciculus. *See* Barr (1988); Kolb and Whishaw (1996).

Armstrong Naming Test devised by Armstrong, this picture naming test was developed as part of a battery of single-word expressive and verbal memory tests that have been used to distinguish between healthy people who are elderly, people with mild fluent aphasia and people with language difficulties associated with ALZHEIMER'S DISEASE. It provides a naming score that can be used as a baseline measure of word finding; a measure of cueing responsiveness; error type analysis and it takes into account the effect of stimulus name length in syllables on naming success. *See* Armstrong (1996) in Appendix I.

Arnold-Chiari malformation *see* HYDRO-
CEPHALUS.

articulation the production of vowels and
consonants by the active and passive
articulators in the mouth. The active
articulators are the moving parts in the
mouth which modify the airflow as it
passes into and through the MOUTH to
produce sounds whilst the passive articulators are the non-moving parts of the
mouth against which, in the production
of many sounds but not all, the active
articulators come into contact. There
are three ways for describing articulations of sounds:

1. Place of articulation – the different
   places in the mouth where the constriction is greatest are:
   (a) bilabial – both lips are placed
   together, e.g. [p, b];
   (b) alveolar – the tongue comes either
   into direct contact with the alveolar
   ridge, e.g. [t, d] or close to it, e.g. [s, z];
   (c) interdental – the only time the
   tongue is placed between the teeth,
   e.g. [θ, ð];
   (d) dental – the tip of the tongue is
   placed against the top teeth, e.g. [t̪, d̪];
   (e) retroflex – the blade of the tongue
   is turned back to touch the hard
   palate, e.g. [t, ɖ, ʂ, ʐ, ɳ];
   (f) palatal – the flat of the tongue is
   placed against the hard palate, e.g. [c,
   ɟ, ɲ, ç, ʝ j, ʎ];
   (g) palato-alveolar – the sound is
   made in two places, both at the alveolar ridge and hard palate, e.g. [tʃ, dʒ];
   (h) labio-dental – the top teeth are
   placed over the bottom lip, e.g. [f, v,
   ɱ, ʋ];
   (i) labial-velar – the lips approximate
   to each other and move apart while at
   the same time there is a slight closure
   at the velum, e.g. [w];
   (j) velar – the back of the tongue
   comes into contact with the soft
   palate, e.g. [k, g, ŋ, x, ɣ];
   (k) uvular – the back of the tongue is
   placed close to the uvula, e.g. [g, G, N,
   R, χ, ʁ];
   (l) pharyngeal – the back of the
   tongue is pushed against the wall of
   the pharynx, e.g. [ħ, ʕ];
   (m) glottal – the vocal folds come
   together in the glottis producing a
   break in the production of a word,
   e.g. [ʔ, h, ɦ].

2. Manner of articulation – the different
   ways in which the articulators are
   moved in the mouth:
   (a) plosive – the articulators are
   brought firmly together, pressure is
   built up behind the closure followed
   by abrupt release, e.g. [p, b, t, d, t, ɖ, c,
   ɟ, k, g, q, G, ʔ];
   (b) fricatives – the articulators are
   brought close together without meeting and the airstream is allowed to
   pass though producing a hissing quality to the sound, e.g. [Φ, β, f, v, θ, ð, s,
   z, ʃ, ʒ, ʂ, ʐ, ç, ʝ, x, ɣ, χ, ʁ, ħ, ʕ, h, ɦ];
   (c) affricates – a combination of (a)
   and (b) which occurs in quick
   sequencing, e.g. [tʃ, dʒ];
   (d) lateral – the sides of the tongue
   are lowered while the tongue touches
   the alveolar ridge in the centre of the
   mouth, e.g. [l, ɫ, ɭ, ʎ, ʟ];
   (e) trill/tap – a trill is a series of taps
   whilst a tap is a very brief, loose contact
   with the alveolar ridge, e.g. [r, R, ɾ, ɽ];
   (f) nasal – the soft palate is lowered
   away from the back wall of the pharynx allowing the airstream to pass
   into the nasal cavities. There is also an
   obstruction in the mouth produced
   by the lips [m], the tongue against the
   alveolar ridge [n], and the back of the
   tongue against the soft palate [ŋ];
   (g) approximant – the articulators are
   brought close to each other and there
   is no abrupt release, e.g. [ʋ, ɹ, ɭ, j, ɥ].

3. Voicing sounds can be produced
   either with the vocal folds vibrating
   (i.e. voiced), e.g. [b, d, g, v,...] or with
   them at rest (i.e. voiceless), e.g. [p, t,
   k, f,...].

Consonants can be described as:
[p] – voiceless bilabial plosive;
[d] – voiced alveolar plosive;

[v] – voiced labiodental fricative.

The CARDINAL VOWEL SYSTEM is used to describe the production of vowels. *See* Ladefoged (2001).

Articulation Attainment Test devised by Catherine Renfrew, it is not meant to be used as a diagnostic test of a child's articulation problem but rather is intended to find out how many consonants a child can produce. The test uses 38 words made up of 100 consonants. The child has to name 38 objects spontaneously as well as produce some serial counting and phrases for repetition. *See* Renfrew (1971) in Appendix I.

articulation delay many children have an articulation difficulty, failing to produce sounds correctly because they cannot place their articulators in the correct position. An articulation delay occurs when a child's articulation development is below the child's chronological age (CA) and fails to acquire the adult articulatory patterns. However, the child will catch up with his CA with regular therapy and/or a home therapy programme. It is also called articulatory immaturity. *See* Grunwell (1987).

articulation disorder the deviant production of speech sounds. It may be structural, e.g. associated with orofacial abnormalities; neurological, e.g. cerebral palsy; or degenerative, e.g. ageing. A child who has this condition requires a very systematic programme to improve his articulation. In other words, unlike an articulation delay, it will not improve with ordinary therapy or in the fullness of time. *See* Grunwell (1987).

articulation tests assessments used by speech and language therapists to find out the severity of the articulation disorder or delay. Two of the most common tests used in the UK are the EDINBURGH ARTICULATION TEST (EAT) and the GOLD-MAN-FRISTOE ARTICULATION TEST. *See* Anthony et al (1971) in Appendix I.

articulatory dyspraxia *see* DEVELOPMENTAL APRAXIA OF SPEECH.

articulatory phonetics a study within phonetics of the way in which articulation of sounds takes place. For this study, introspection and observation of what is going on in people's mouths are carried out as well as the use of such techniques as electromyography (a technique to observe and record muscle contractions during speech), spirometry (a technique for measuring the maximum expiration and inspiration of the lungs) and palatography (a technique for observing articulation around the palate). These devices seek to find out how the vocal organs produce speech sounds such as those described under ARTICULATION. *See* Catford (1989); Fromkin and Rodman (2003).

artificial intelligence (AI) the attempt to make a computer or other machine make decisions using similar sensory techniques to human beings. The aim is to make the machine 'understand' the input and act upon it using some kind of reasoning processes. The 'intelligence' is written in the computer program and is not contained in the machine itself. *See* Brookshear (1991).

artificial larynx there are several artificial laryngae available to those who have undergone total LARYNGECTOMY. With the larynx removed, to produce voice the person requires artificial techniques such as the Bart's Vibrator, the Medici Speech Vibrator, the Siemen's Servox, the Rexton Laryngophone, the Weston Electronic No. 5A (male) and No. 5B (female). Each works by being placed next to the skin under the chin; a button on the side is pressed, which starts a diaphragm vibrating on top of the device; this produces a voiced sound as the person mouths the sounds. There are facilities to control volume, pitch and tone of voice produced. Most have rechargeable batteries. There are also two pneumatic devices – the Tokyo and Osaka. These consist of a tube that leads from the tracheostoma, passing through a cylindrical unit which contains a rubber membrane. The membrane is vibrated by air from the lungs as a sound source and directs the sound into the mouth by the mouth tube. *See* Edels (1984); Greene and Mathieson (1989).

arytenoids cartilages and muscle found in the LARYNX which control the vocal folds. *See* Tortora and Grabowski (2000).

ASCII abbreviation for American Standard Code for Information Interchange. The computer uses codes to represent alphabetic, numeric and punctuation characters that are stored in memory or put on the screen. The ASCII characters are those found on the tops of the keys on the keyboard. *See* Brookshear (1991).

asemantic jargon *see* JARGON APHASIA.

ASHA *see* AMERICAN SPEECH–LANGUAGE HEARING ASSOCIATION.

asomatognosias the loss of knowledge or sense of one's own body and bodily condition. There are a variety of conditions including: anosognosia – the unawareness or denial of illness; anosodiaphoria – indifference to illness; autotopagnosia – an inability to localise and name body parts; and asymbolia for pain – the absence of normal reactions to pain. These may be for one or both sides of the body but are most commonly for the left side as a result of damage to the right hemisphere. *See* Kolb and Whishaw (1996).

aspect grammatical aspect signals features of the 'temporal contour' of actual states or events. In English, progressive aspect, signalled by a form of the auxiliary 'be + -ing' inflection, conveys a durative timing for the verb to which it is attached as in:

1. The boy went to the factory.
2. The boy is going to the factory.
3. The boy was going to the factory.

See Huddleston (1976).

Asperger's syndrome a neurobiological disorder documented by Hans Asperger in 1944 when he found people who were developing language and intelligence normally but were exhibiting autistic-like (*see* AUTISM) behaviours such as a lack of social and communication skills. Those who have Asperger's syndrome show marked deficiencies in social skills, have difficulties with changes and prefer sameness. They often have obsessive routines and may be preoccupied with a particular subject of interest. They have a great deal of difficulty reading nonverbal cues (body language) and very often have difficulty determining proper body space. By definition their IQ is normal. *See* Wing (1996); http://www.udel.edu/bkirby/asperger/; http://www.nichcy.org/pubs/factshe/fs20txt.htm

aspiration the airflow which follows the release of a plosive sound before the onset of voicing for the following vowel. It is marked with the diacritic [H] placed above the sound with which it is made. *See* Ladefoged (2001).

assertive training a form of treatment given during social skills training. It exists for those who allow themselves to be dominated either, in the case of children, by younger children, or, in the case of older people, by those with less authority.

Such people are placed in situations in which they have to assert themselves either gradually, by giving step-by-step training, or very quickly by placing them in the situation and not allowing them to leave the situation until they show themselves to be sufficiently assertive. *See* Trower et al (1978); Smith et al (2003); Argyle (1994); Davison et al (2004).

Assessment and Therapy Programme for Dysfluent Children devised by Rustin in 1987, this programme allows for the assessment of dysfluent children, aged between 2.5 and 11 years of age, and provides a comprehensive therapy and monitoring programme. The initial assessment is carried out using a structured interview with both parents and their child. A two-week intensive therapy programme follows, incorporating parental involvement and follow-up sessions. Workbooks for both parents and children are provided which contain the exercises related to programme modules. Parents fill in a homework sheet regularly during the initial two-week course and each week after the end of the course. *See* Rustin (1987) in Appendix I; Rustin et al (1996) in Appendix I; Beech et al (1993).

Assessment of Comprehension and Expression 6–11(ACE 6–11) devised by clinicians and practitioners at the University of Manchester, ACE 6–11 provides a quick assessment of language development for children between the ages of 6;00 and 11;00. There are two versions of the test: the Main Test comprising 5 subtests and the Extended Test comprising the Main Test and 2 additional subtests. The seven subtests cover the following aspects of language development: sentence comprehension, inferential comprehension, naming, syntactic formulation, semantic decisions, non-literal comprehension and narrative. ACE 6–11 has been standardised on a sample of 790 children aged between 6;00 and 11;00 in the UK and the Republic of Ireland.

Assessment of Language-Related Functional Activities (ALFA) devised by Baines and her colleagues, ALFA assesses a different functional activity in each of the 10 subtests such as telling the time, counting money, addressing an envelope, solving daily maths problems, writing a cheque/balancing a cheque book, understanding medicine labels, using a calendar, reading instructions, using the telephone and writing a phone message. Those being assessed actually carry out each activity and their performance is recorded objectively and quantitatively. Its subtests require use of all language modalities – auditory comprehension, verbal expression, reading and writing as well as cognitive and motor skills. *See* Baines et al (1999) in Appendix I.

assessment of phonological processes tests that show the number of PHONOLOGICAL PROCESSES a child produces at a particular age.

assessments measures used by various professionals throughout the rehabilitation process. Speech and language therapists use them to find out what communication disorders a person may have and the severity of the disorder. There are assessments for almost all disorders but since some people may have a mixture of problems, e.g. dysphasia with dyspraxia, two or more tests may be required. Most assessments are made up of smaller tests called subtests. The two main types of assessments are formal and informal assessments. The former types have been published like those described in this book. They themselves have been tested to check their reliability and validity. Some assessments also undergo standardisation. These assessments have been administered to a large number of the population covering the age range for which the test is intended to be used. In this way, the author of the test can discover the most frequent and normal responses of the different age groups and, thus, be enabled to compare the scores obtained from those tested with those of the norm for that age range. The informal assessments are tests made up by the therapist to assess certain parts of a particular treatment programme or to assess a communication disorder in a more relaxed environment than that in which a formal assessment takes place. *See* Aiken (1988); Kersner (1992); Beech et al (1993); Beukelman and Mirenda (1998) (AAC assessments).

assimilation

1. The process whereby one sound is changed because of the influence of another sound next to it. For example, [n] becomes [ŋ] because of [ð] in the phrase 'in the' (based on Ladefoged 1993). There are three types of assimilation:
   (a) anticipatory (or regressive) where the sound is influenced by the next sound; this is the most common form of assimilation in English;
   (b) progressive where the sound is influenced by the preceding sound;

(c) coalescent where two or more sounds can come together to form one sound. For example, 'got you' becomes [gɔtʃa] where the 't' and 'y' sounds come together to form [tʃ].

See Fromkin and Rodman (2003); Cruttenden (1994).

2. A phenomenon proposed by Piaget to explain the development of the child's ability to 'understand'. He introduced the notion of schema or schemata which are 'well-defined sequences of actions...their chief characteristic, whatever their nature or complexity, is that they are organised wholes which are frequently repeated and which can be recognised easily among other diverse and varying behaviours' (Beard, 1969). Assimilation occurs when the child brings new experiences into schemata which already exist. Accommodation occurs when a child has to work out a response to a new experience which allows him to modify his schema continually. Eventually the child can organise all this information into a whole and so one schema can be subordinated to another. Piaget called assimilation, accommodation and organisation invariant functions. There are three types of assimilation:
   (a) reproductive – the child assimilates an experience to a schema but cannot fit it into an organisation, so keeps assimilating the experience, getting nowhere;
   (b) generalisation – the child begins to extend the range of objects or experiences to a schema;
   (c) recognitory – as the child generalises his range of objects into a schema, he realises he has to accommodate certain actions to the object, e.g. there is only one way to hold a cup.

See Beard (1969).

astereognosis an inability to recognise shapes by tactile means. Oral stereognosis is the recognition of differing shapes and textures intraorally. *See* Kolb and Whishaw (1996).

Aston Index devised by Newton and Thomson at Aston University in 1976, it is a screening test to assess the use of children's language between the ages of 5 and 14 years. It has two levels of which level 1 is suitable for the screening of 5–6 year olds while level 2 is for use with the older age range. It contains six tests to measure general ability; the results provide age-equivalent scores and 10 performance tests that measure the ability necessary for learning to read and write. All the results are plotted onto graphs provided on the score sheets. Thus, the therapist or teacher can discover any delay in development or the most significant difficulties a child may possess. *See* Newton and Thomson (1976) in Appendix I.

astrocytomas *see* TUMOURS OF THE CENTRAL NERVOUS SYSTEM.

ataxia *see* CEREBRAL PALSY.

ataxic dysarthria speech disorders resulting from this type of DYSARTHRIA are caused by a lesion in the CEREBELLUM. It is primarily a disorder of pitch, time and stress. Speech gives the impression of being scanning and monotonous because of disintegration of syllabic structure. Vowels are prolonged and there is lengthening of word segments so that the duration of words is greatly increased. Phonation and articulation are also affected. *See* Darley et al (1975).

athctosis *see* CEREBRAL PALSY.

atrophy the wasting away of structures in any part of the body. It is often used in referring to the wasting of part of the brain, which may produce such communication disorders as DYSARTHRIA or APHASIA. *See* Gilroy and Holliday (1982).

attachment the way in which children bond with their parents, usually their mother or the person who provides the initial care and security. Children tend to explore unknown environments when this person is with them. It has been suggested that a failure to develop such bonding may lead to failure in making close personal relationships in later life. Ainsworth (1979) set up a laboratory experiment called the 'Strange Situation' in which the child was faced with the mother and a strange female, and the researchers tried to find out the type of attachment the child made in different situations. They found three groups: those who were 'securely attached'; those who were 'insecurely attached: avoidant'; and those who were 'insecurely attached: resistant'. From these results, they could conclude all babies become attached to their mothers by 1 year of age but the quality of the attachment depends on the mother's responses to the child. While most babies are securely attached, some form insecure attachments often because the mother will only respond to the baby's cries when she wants to and fails to respond at other times. The avoidant behaviour is related to maternal hostility and rejection while resistant behaviour is related to the unresponsiveness of the mother. (*See* Smith et al, 2003.) Further studies have shown that those children who are securely attached by 2 years of age are better equipped to cope with new experiences and relationships. Erikson (1963) suggested eight stages of psychosexual development which people go through from birth to old age. He believed a person's psychological development depended on the kinds of social relationships made at various times in their lives but each relationship had problems that had to be faced. He produced them as opposites: trust vs mistrust (1 year old); autonomy vs doubt (2 years old); initiative vs guilt (3–5 years); industry vs inferiority (6 years–puberty); identity vs confusion (adolescence); intimacy vs isolation (early adulthood); generativity vs self-absorption (middle adulthood) and integrity vs despair (after 65 years). *See* Smith et al (2003).

attention the selection of relevant stimuli from the environment as part of the process of comprehension. The stimuli may be auditory, visual or tactile kinaesthetic. *See* Smith et al (2003).

Attention-deficit hyperactivity disorder (ADHD) a disorder in which the child cannot attend for any significant period of time to a particular activity especially when asked to sit still, for example at school or at mealtimes. The diagnosis is reserved for those children who behave in an extreme way, not for those who are just overactive and slightly distractible. There has been a move away from a variety of different symptoms to separating those children with attention-deficit disorder (ADD) only and those with both attention deficit and hyperactivity. The latter group, ADHD children, seem more likely to develop CONDUCT DISORDERS, whilst the former group, those with ADD, have more problems with focusing attention or speed of information processing, which can lead to academic problems in such subjects as maths, reading or spelling. Both drug therapy and BEHAVIOUR THERAPY have been used to treat the condition. *See* Davison et al (2004); http://www.pavilion.co.uk/add/english.html.

Attitudes and Strategies towards AAC a training package for AAC users and carers providing a ready-to-use resource for training people who are involved in AAC. It is workshop-based and focuses on attitudes to AAC and strategies used in AAC conversations. These priority areas have been highlighted by the many AAC users and their communicative partners whom the authors have known. There is a manual and a video. *See* Murphy and Scott (1995).

audiology a science concerned with the hearing mechanism used by humans. Audiologists study the development, anatomy, physiology, and pathology of the auditory system. This is done mostly by the use of tests, the results of which are analysed by audiologists. They are also concerned with the psychological aspects of hearing loss as well as with treatment strategies used in the rehabilitation of the client's hearing loss. *See* Katz (1985).

audiometric tests tests that are carried out by an audiologist to find out if a person has a hearing loss or degree of hearing loss. The most common test is PURE-TONE AUDIOMETRY. If people are found to have particular problems in the hearing mechanism other tests are used specifically for the problem.

When younger children are presented to have their hearing tested, the audiologist may use DISTRACTION TESTS or FREE FIELD AUDIOMETRY. *See* Katz (1985); Graham and Martin (2001).

audiometric zero the sound pressure level required to make any frequency barely audible to the average person with normal hearing. It is also the hearing threshold level setting on an audiometer marked at 0 dB. *See* Katz (1985); Graham and Martin (2001).

audiometry the process used by audiologists to test a person's hearing. The most common test is PURE-TONE AUDIOMETRY.

auditory aphasia *see* APHASIA (2).

auditory brainstem response (ABR) an audiometric test to diagnose the neurological causes of hearing loss and to find the site of lesion and to detect a hearing loss in children. Electrodes are placed on the earlobes or the mastoids and on the vertex. Testing begins at 60 dB SL or 90 dB sound pressure level. The audiologist compares the results from the testing with normal responses. Disorders of the cranial nerve VIII or brainstem will show up in the ABR. It is a non-invasive technique, does not affect the state of the client and is regarded as providing a good objective test of the client's hearing threshold level. Providing an electrical stimulus to produce an ABR has come about with the advent of COCHLEAR IMPLANTS. See Josey (1985); Ramsden and Axon (2001).

auditory comprehension the processing of incoming auditory stimuli leading to recognition. It involves sound discrimination, perception of sequence and retention. Auditory comprehension is a subtest of the main language tests for those with acquired and developmental language delay or disorder. If it is found that auditory comprehension is a particular problem, more specific tests can be used to assess this further. *See* Riedel (1981); Rosenbek et al (1989).

Auditory Discrimination and Attention Test devised by Morgan-Barry for children from 3 to 12 years of age with a speech deficit. It assesses the child's ability to discriminate between 17 minimal pairs, i.e. words that are minimally differentiated by a single phoneme (see PHONOLOGY). The minimal feature contrasts are voiced/ voiceless, place of articulation, manner of articulation (*see* ARTICULATION) and constituents of CONSONANT CLUSTERS. The child is presented with a page showing two pictures. The child places a counter below the correct picture named by the therapist. Each pair of pictures is presented six times to prevent a random response. Norm tables to convert error scores into percentages and standard scores are provided. The test was standardised on 650 children. The manual reports extensive research studies comparing the results of those with a language disorder, those with a hearing loss and children with a LEARNING DISABILITY, as well as children without language or cognitive problems. It was developed in the UK. *See* Morgan-Barry (1988) in Appendix I; Beech et al (1993).

Auditory Discrimination Screening Test devised by Catherine Renfrew, it assesses the phonological feature contrasts and semantic confusions often found in children with speech and language problems. It can be used with children of 5 years and upwards but if it is to be used with younger children, the therapist must cover up the bottom row of pictures. In scoring, errors in auditory discrimination must be distinguished from vocabulary errors. *See also* ACTION PICTURE TEST.

auditory method *see* EDUCATION OF HEARING-IMPAIRED CHILDREN (1a).

auditory phonetics the perception of sounds or how sounds are heard and interpreted. In the communication act there are two parties involved – the speaker and the listener. It is what happens in the latter that is described in auditory phonetics. There are two processes that happen at almost the same time. The first of these processes is the perception of sounds by the auditory apparatus or the EAR while the second is how the sound, after it goes through the ear, transforms the information into a format that can be understood by the BRAIN and how the message is decoded.

auditory speech perception a learnt skill for accepting auditory information. The various parts of this skill which have to be learnt by the child are:

1. Awareness of the presence of the sound.
2. Localisation of the sound, so that the child knows where it comes from and so can pick up on linguistic cues as well as seeing the person producing the sound.
3. Cutting out of background noise and focussing his attention solely on the sound he perceives.
4. Extraction of linguistic information from the acoustic phonetic characteristics of the phonemes produced.
5. Use of memory, particularly the short-term memory, to retain and process the utterances produced by the speaker.

However, if the person has a hearing loss during this period, these skills are more difficult to acquire:

1. Those with a conductive loss have a problem receiving information and so will require a hearing aid or will ask the speaker to speak louder to enable information to be received.
2. Those with a sensory hearing loss have a problem in receiving information and also in discrimination.
3. Those with a neural/central hearing loss have a problem in obtaining meaning from the information they receive.
4. hose with a mixed hearing loss will have elements of (1)–(3).

See Sanders (1977); Hazan (2001).

augmentative and alternative communication (AAC) the forms of communication offered to those who cannot speak or whose communication attempts are unintelligible, and to those who require help to overcome word-finding difficulties. Systems which are described as being high-tech are operated by mechanical, electronic or computerised means. Low-tech systems comprise sign languages, such as MAKATON, BRITISH SIGN LANGUAGE or PAGET-GORMAN SIGN SYSTEM, gesture systems and communication books or boards. The International Society of Alternative Augmentative Communication (ISAAC) promotes the use of AAC techniques throughout the world. *See* Enderby (1987); Zangari et al (1988); Lloyd et al (1990) (AAC model of communication); Jones (1995a) (training in the use of AAC systems); Schlosser and Lloyd (1991); Panton (1993) (comments on Lloyd et al. 1990); Lloyd et al (1993) response to Panton (1993); Zangari et al (1994) (historical perspective); Glennen and DeCoste (1997); Beukelman and Mirenda (1998); Mirenda (1998a, b); Rumble and Larcher (1998); http://www.isaac-online.org; http://www.communicationmatters.org.uk

augmentative communication aids *see* AUGMENTATIVE AND ALTERNATIVE COMMUNICATION; Rumble and Larcher (1998).

aural rehabilitation *see* EDUCATION OF HEARING-IMPAIRED CHILDREN.

autism a PERVASIVE DEVELOPMENTAL DISORDER. It is a syndrome the diagnosis of which is characterised by a triad of social, communication and imagination impairments and repetitive behaviour. These are crucial to any diagnosis of a person who is thought to have autistic spectrum disorders. Studies of the prevalence of autism have varied from around 2–3 in 10000 children up to 16 in 10000 children. In the 1970s a study carried out by Gould and Wing showed that 22 in every 10000 people had the triad of impairments. It is often diagnosed or suspected between 2;00–3;00 years of age.

1. Impairments of social interaction:

   (a) The aloof group – this is probably the most common group which is characterised by behaving towards other people as if they do not exist. Those in the aloof group will totally ignore any means used to attract their attention and will ignore the presence of others around them with expressionless faces. It is as if they are in their own little world.

   (b) The passive group – probably the least common type of social impairment. While they will not move away or totally ignore other people, they do not initiate social interaction and may have poor eye contact, although they will look at the person when reminded so to do.

   (c) The 'active but odd' group – those in this group will make active approaches to other people but the rest of the social interaction will be inappropriate, such as staring at the other person for too long or touching or hugging the other person.

   (d) The over-formal, stilted group – people in this group will be adolescents or adults. They will have a good level of language because they are extremely polite and formal in their behaviour. Since they stick very closely to the rules of social interaction as they understand them, they fail to adapt appropriately to the subtle changes in behaviour required in different situations and so they can make mistakes because of a lack of true understanding.

2. Impairments of communication – while language may or may not be impaired, it is the way in which people with autism use language that is the problem.

   (a) Using speech – while some children with autism, perhaps as few as 1:4 or 1:5 may never develop language, others will develop language although the starting point may be delayed. Aspects of their problems in developing language include the following: ECHOLALIA or delayed echolalia (*see* ECHOLALIA); 'I/you' reversal; robotic voice and flattening of affect; use of platitudes or idiosyncratic language; misuse of prepositions and conjunctions; confusion of the positive and the opposite and words which appear in pairs; content of speech is often repetitive and not conversational; some may speak a lot but have no colloquialisms which makes their speech sound pedantic and old-fashioned; monologues are used or the same questions are asked regardless of the answers given previously.

   (b) Understanding speech – most people with autism have some understanding. Understanding can be at a very literal level in the following ways: lack of flexibility in word meaning; words that sound the same but have different meanings; tendency to react to one or two words in the sentence and ignore the rest; misunderstanding of idiomatic use of language e.g., 'pull your socks up' which the person with autism will understand as a command rather than he/she needs to improve whatever; lack of understanding of jokes particularly with verbal ambiguity; they may try to make jokes without understanding why they are funny.

   (c) Intonation and voice control – intonation can be monotonous or inappropriate in inflection; volume can be too loud or less commonly too quiet; some may use a 'special' voice different from their own.

   (d) Using and understanding non-verbal communication – people with autism have significant difficulty in using augmentative, alternative communication systems to communicate such as signing, gesture and facial expression. Similarly, they also have a problem with understanding such forms of communication.

3. Impairment of imagination – children with autism have difficulty in developing pretend play. Some may just handle toys while others may use them appropriately as well as not joining in play situations with other children. For example; Some children may look as though they are playing imaginatively by 'being' an object or character from a book they have read or a TV programme they have seen but they seem to be living the character rather than imagining they are the character. This inability to use their imaginations in such situations affects them in later life and so they are not able to share in other's emotions nor are they able to share ideas with others about the past or present. People with autism find pleasure from their own special interests.

4. Ritualistic and stereotyped phenomena. By looking at this behaviour as the opposite to having poor imagination, the only way to compensate for not having flexible, creative thinking, not being able to share ideas with others, having no interest in other people is to rely on the reassurance of repeating those activities that do give some pleasure.

(a) Simple repetitive activities – these involve tasting, smelling, feeling, tapping and scratching different surfaces, listening to mechanical noises, staring at lights or shiny things, twisting and turning hands or objects near the eyes, staring at things from different angles, switching lights on and off, watching things spinning round or self-spinning. This behaviour may also include self-mutilation.

(b) Elaborate repetitive routines – these routines are often invented by people with autism themselves such as rituals before doing something, e.g., tapping the chair three times before sitting down; placing objects in the same order which must not be disturbed; routines that must be the same every time they are performed or else there will be temper tantrums; attachments to particular objects such as a teddy bear or doll; collections of various domestic objects and going to any length to continue the collection; resisting change; repetitive acting out of characters on TV or videos; repetitive playing of music. In more able children such as those with ASPERGER'S SYNDROME, these repetitive activities develop into fascination for special subjects such as railway timetables, dinosaurs, the weather and so on.

There are other behaviours that may or may not appear and are not crucial for a diagnosis of autism. These include stereotyped movements, abnormalities of gait and posture, imitating movements, responses to sounds and visual stimuli, responses to proximal sensations, and appetite and thirst as well as anxiety and special fears, attention and motivation, special skills and inappropriate behaviour.

There is uncertainty as to the cause of autism. It may arise from some difficulty in forming a relationship with the natural mother. Young children with autism are more sluggish at sucking, tend not to smile, may not respond to the human voice and are undemanding. While not completely rejecting environmental causes, investigations are being made into organic causes of autism. Researchers are looking for possible brain pathologies such as ENCEPHALITIS in early years, complications for rubella passed to the child by the mother during pregnancy, TUBEROUS SCLEROSIS, untreated PHENYLKETONURIA, infantile spasm (severe epileptic attacks during the first year) and complications in the perinatal stage. These causes have been found in one-third of children suffering from autism. Site of lesion in the brain is another possible cause, but no conclusive evidence has been provided although proposed sites are in the dominant hemisphere, RETICULAR SYSTEM or BASAL GANGLIA. The different psychological behaviours of the autistic and non-autistic child may lead to a possible cause. However, the most likely outcome of all this research will be to provide a group of interrelated causes and not just one cause for autism. Treatment is aimed at improving the child's socialisation and providing him with socially acceptable behaviour. Such treatment is aimed at removing the child's 'self-encapsulation in an isolated world' (Jaspers 1963 in Wolff 1981). See Wing and Gould (1979); Wolff (1981); Wing (1980, 1996); Ellis (1990); Fay (1993); Peterson et al (1995); Glennen and DeCoste (1997) (AAC and autism); Beukelman and Mirenda (1998) (AAC and autism); Reynolds (2001) (AAC and autism); http://www.nichcy.org/pubs/factshe/fs20txt.htm; http://www.nas.org. uk/

Autistic Continuum: An Assessment and Intervention Schedule devised by Aarons and Gittens in 1992, the schedule is designed to look at various developmental areas. There is no time limit or complex scoring. The authors' approach looks at autism as a continuum and not as a particular disorder existing within its own boundaries. It is a revision of an earlier publication *Is this Autism? See* Aarons and Gittens (1992) in Appendix I.

Autistic Spectrum Disorders the name given in the UK to PERVASIVE DEVELOPMENTAL DISORDERS.

autonomic nervous system (ANS) part of the nervous system which innervates smooth muscle. It is divided into two parts:

1. SYMPATHETIC NERVOUS SYSTEM
2. PARASYMPATHETIC NERVOUS SYSTEM.

The ANS supplies the HEART, sweat glands and digestive glands. *See* J.H. Green (1982); Tortora and Grabowski (2000).

autosomal dominant *see* CHROMOSOMES.
autosomal recessive *see* CHROMOSOMES.
autosomes 22 of the 23 pairs of CHROMOSOMES which are morphologically similar while the twenty-third pair are the sex chromosomes. *See* Hosking (1982); Tortora and Grabowski (2000).

auxiliary verb auxiliary verbs such as 'be', 'have', 'do', 'can', 'shall', etc., subordinate to lexical verbs in English (in declarative sentences), and help to convey distinctions in tense, aspect and modality. They also have an important syntactic role in negation and in forming interrogative structures. For example:

1. John **is** singing.
2. Mary **might** arrive soon.
3. Bill **didn't** finish the job.
4. **Can** Sophie come out to play?

See Strang (1968); Fromkin and Rodman (2003).

babbling an early stage of language acquisition (*see* ACQUISITION and Appendix II). The child will babble when he is comfortable and this is reflected in the type of sounds the child produces, e.g. velars, sounds made by the tongue against the top of the mouth, and open vowels. By nine months, babbling has become more adult-like. Strings of sounds follow, put together in a CVCVCV structure. The pitch pattern is similar to the one used in adult English, with cooing and vocal play where the child experiments considerably with voice quality, and airstreams are also produced. It is also an indication of the development of motor co-ordination, of audition and of cognition. Absence of babbling may be associated with subsequent speech disorder although this is not absolutely established. *See* Cruttenden (1970); Adams et al (1997); Fromkin and Rodman (2003).

Babinski reflex a reflex obtained as part of the plantar response during a neurological examination. The reflex takes the form of the great toe being extended with extension of other toes which separate in the shape of a fan. *See* Gilroy and Holliday (1982); Tortora and Grabowski (2000).

baby talk a phenomenon which occurs in language development (*see* ACQUISITION and Appendix II) which refers to the special use of a simplified language used by a mother to communicate with her child. At first, she may use simple words to refer to objects, animals or people, e.g. [brm, brm] = 'car'; [horsie] = 'horse'; [doggie] = 'dog'; [mama, dada] = 'mummy', 'daddy', etc. As children's language develops, they begin to use two-word phrases, e.g. [cake allgone] = 'there is no more cake'; [dada shoe] = 'there are daddy's shoes'. The mother seems to know intuitively at what level to pitch her language, so that she is always one step ahead, thus encouraging children to reach another stage in his language development. It is also described as parental speech, motherese or parent talk. *See* Cruttenden (1979).

back-up in computer terms, a copy of one program, document, graphic etc. from an original, in case the original is lost or corrupted. The original may be kept on a hard disk while the back-up copy is kept on a floppy disk, CD, Zip drive etc. *See* Bishop (1985).

Bangor Dyslexia Test devised by Miles as a screening test to find out if a child's difficulties in reading and/or writing are those typically found in dyslexia or not. There are 10 subtests: (1) Knowledge of left/right body parts; (2) repetition of polysyllabic words; (3) subtraction; (4) multiplication tables; (5) months forward; (6) months reversed; (7) digits forward; (8) digits reversed; (9) b/d confusion; (10) familial incidence. *See* Miles (1982) in Appendix I.

basal ganglia a mass of grey matter at the base of the BRAIN. The nuclei found in this structure include the corpus striatum (caudate, globus pallidus putamen) and the amygdaloid nucleus. If this structure becomes diseased, tremor and rigidity (*see* PARKINSON'S DISEASE) may occur. *See* Barr (1988); Kolb and Whishaw (1996).

base 10 devised by LaPointe, it is a therapeutic technique for showing the success of a treatment programme, usually in APHASIA therapy. It comprises a printed form on which the aims of the therapy are entered and baseline scores are recorded. Progress is shown graphically, thus giving positive feedback to the person and providing the therapist with a record of success. The activities can be modified if improvement occurs. It is very useful for intensive therapy. *See* LaPointe (1977) in Appendix I; Code and Müller (1989); Rosenbek et al (1989).

base form the part of a word that remains after all the affixes have been removed. For example, the base form of 'quickly' is 'quick' after the affix '-ly' has been removed. It is also described as the base word. It is used in the morphological study (see MORPHOLOGY) of word formation. *See* Matthews (1974).

BASIC an acronym for Beginner's All Purpose Symbolic Instruction Code. BASIC is one of several languages used for programming computers. *See* Bishop (1985); Brookshear (1991).

basilar membrane *see* EAR.

baud rate the rate per second at which data move from one processor to another, e.g. from computer to printer. *See* Bishop (1985); Brookshear (1991).

BBC microcomputers *see* ACORN COMPUTERS.

BC (bone conduction) *see* PURE-TONE AUDIOMETRY.

BDAE *see* BOSTON DIAGNOSTIC APHASIA EXAMINATION.

Beck's cognitive therapy an approach to producing acceptable behaviour by treating thought processes. Beck provided therapy that was aimed at making people aware of their thinking processes, teaching them to recognise maladaptive

thoughts in various situations, producing more normal thought patterns for such situations and, having accomplished this, the therapist gives praise and reinforcement to cognitive and behaviour changes during therapy. *See* Rachman and Wilson (1980); Smith et al (2003).

Beckwith–Wiedemann syndrome (BWS) discovered by Beckwith in the USA (1963) and by Wiedemann in Germany (1964), BWS is a congenital syndrome with an incidence estimated to be 1:13700–14300 births. Incidence is equal between males and females while in about 15% of patients with the syndrome there is an autosomal dominant (*see* CHROMOSOMES) inheritance. The three main diagnostic characteristics are exomphalos, MACROGLOSSIA and gigantism. Other common features are ear creases and pits, facial naevus flammeus, nephromegaly and hypoglycaemia. Rarer complications include hemihypertrophy, moderate to severe developmental delay, congenital heart defects, polydactyly and neoplasia. There may also be a CLEFT PALATE. MACROGLOSSIA can be very common at birth but it is not a universal feature and cases are known where it is absent. While there have not been many studies concerning the ARTICULATION of people with BWS, McManamny and Barnett (1985) found that consonant production in general was affected, but more particularly, the production of labiodental and linguodental sounds as well as alveolar fricatives were affected. *See* Beckwith (1963); Wiedemann (1964); McManamny and Barnett (1985); Van Borsel et al (1999); http://www.beckwith-wiedemann.org

Bedside Evaluation Screening Test – Second Edition (BEST-2) devised by West and her colleagues, BEST-2 is designed to assess the nature of language disorders resulting from APHASIA. It assesses language in three communicative modalities: auditory comprehension, speaking and reading. *See* West et al (1998) in Appendix I.

29

behaviour modification *see* BEHAVIOUR THERAPY.

behaviour therapy aims at the modification of abnormal patterns of behaviour which do not have a medical origin. It is sometimes called the two-factor model of learning as it consists of two learning procedures – CLASSICAL CONDITIONING and OPERANT CONDITIONING. In the former, several behaviour therapies have been evolved such as SYSTEMATIC DESENSITISATION, FLOODING, MODELLING, and ASSERTIVE TRAINING, while in the latter the behaviour therapies of individual conditioning paradigms (*see* OPERANT CONDITIONING) and TOKEN ECONOMIES have evolved. Behaviour therapy occurs also in the form of COGNITIVE BEHAVIOUR THERAPIES such as RATIONAL-EMOTIVE THERAPY (RET) (Ellis), SELF-INSTRUCTIONAL TRAINING (SIT) (Meichenbaum) and BECK'S COGNITIVE THERAPY. Sjödé et al described the most important aspect of behaviour therapy as 'being task-specific rather than based on personality. The therapist has respect for the client as a learning, striving and a coping person who is not sick but will benefit from guided experiences in dealing with particular specified situations' (Sjödé et al 1979). *See* Smith et al (2003).

Békésy audiometry a procedure used in PURE-TONE AUDIOMETRY. Earphones are placed over or in the listener's ears and the listener is given a button to control the intensity of the tones. The button must be pressed in order to make the tone audible and released when it is audible (causing the intensity to decrease again). The whole range of frequencies, from low to high, should be tested. The audiometer does the sweep automatically and different tracings indicate different pathologies. Two frequency sweeps are carried out – one with a continuous tone and another with a pulsed tone. The person's threshold is traced by a stylus linked to the audiometer. *See* Katz (1985); Ballantyne and Martin (2001).

Bell's palsy an acute facial paralysis of the peripheral type produced by a disorder of the facial nerve (*see* CRANIAL NERVES). Its cause is usually unknown but it can be a result of a viral infection which involves the geniculate ganglion. Bell's palsy occurs often in the middle-aged and elderly. There is a facial paralysis which progresses steadily to a severe weakness and even to total loss of power on one side of the face. The affected side may present with a sagging cheek and it may be impossible to close the eye; in fact, the eye can hardly close and, at times, it is impossible to close because of weakness in the orbicularis oculi (*see* MUSCLES OF FACIAL EXPRESSION). Involvement of the geniculate ganglion can produce loss of tears resulting in a dry eye. The eyes are kept moist with eye drops. *See* Gilroy and Holliday (1982); http://www.bellspalsy.net

Biber test an assessment for comprehension in APHASIA. In the single form of the test, a picture has to be selected showing single word comprehension. The stimuli can be presented auditorily or visually and the person has to indicate by whatever means whether the heard/seen word corresponds to the picture. A picture is presented with the stimulus word which may be the target word, a related word or an unrelated word and a 'yes/no' response is given if the word corresponds to the picture. In the 'threesomes' version, selection is made from three pictures, two semantically related and an unrelated distractor. The target word is presented auditorily or visually and the person points to the appropriate picture.

bifid uvula a condition in which two halves of the posterior part of the velum fail to unite. Also known as a uvular cleft, it may be submucous. Hypernasal resonance is often associated with structural malformation. *See also* CLEFT PALATE.

bifurcation a division into two parts or branches such as the point at the bottom of the TRACHEA where the two BRONCHI divide and lead into the LUNGS.

Big Red Switch a large single plate switch, 5 inches in diameter. It can be used also as a remote switch, i.e. without a cable attaching it to a particular device. When used with a battery-powered receiver or a small appliance receiver, it gives four modes of control – Direct Mode: activates the appliance only when the Big Red is activated; Timed Seconds Mode: by activating the Big Red, the appliance switches on for a predetermined length of time measured in seconds; Timed Minutes Mode: the same as the previous mode but the time is measured in minutes; Latch Mode: one activation of the Big Red turns the appliance on whilst a second activation turns it off. *See* Glennen and DeCoste (1997); Appendix IV (AbleNet)

BIGmack a small portable message system into which a message of up to 20 seconds can be recorded. It is accessed either by pressing the large plate on the top of the device or by a single switch. It can also activate any battery-operated device or toy and give an auditory reinforcement. It is 5 inches in diameter and 2.25 inches at its highest point and uses an ordinary battery. It is mountable on a wheelchair or desktop or can be carried by a shoulder strap. External speakers can also be attached to it. *See* Glennen and DeCoste (1997); Rumble and Larcher (1998); Appendix IV (AbleNet).

binaural a description of the functioning of the two ears.

Binet Alfred Binet (1857–1911) believed a child who was slow in learning was similar to a 'normal' child except for some retardation in his mental development. In 1881 the French government passed a law that all children, including those with learning difficulties, should go to school. Binet was approached to provide a test to ascertain which children required special education. Thus, the first edition of the STANFORD-BINET INTELLIGENCE SCALES was produced. *See* Smith et al (2003).

bit acronym for binary digit. This refers to one of the two numbers used in binary notation (i.e. 0, 1). A bit could just be a small part of the computer's memory. Each cell in a computer's memory can store one bit. *See* Bishop (1985); Brookshear (1991).

Blackhawk a small light-tech communication aid providing vocabulary on four levels each with 16 keys. Each message allows for 3.5 seconds of recorded speech giving a total of 37 minutes. The four levels are selected by four separate locations. It can only be accessed by direct manual selection although a separate device can be attached which allows for up to nine switches to be attached to it. *See* Rumble and Larcher (1998); Appendix IV (AdamLab).

blade in articulatory terms, the part of the TONGUE behind the apex or tip which is used to produce alveolar sounds (*see* ARTICULATION) such as /t,d,s,z/. *See* Ladefoged (2001).

blind experiment an experiment in which the tester and the subject are kept in ignorance of a particular variable.

Blissymbolics developed by Charles Bliss in 1965, it was based on the concept of semantography. Bliss, born in 1897, was brought up in Austria where 20 languages were spoken. He was concerned about the linguistic confusion produced by so many languages. In the 1960s, he started to devise 'logical writing for an illogical world' (Bliss 1965). Blissymbolics is a language conveying meaning through pictographic, ideographic and abstract symbols. It has become a popular means for those with communication problems to communicate their needs and wishes. The symbol system has nine shapes to form the basis of all symbols. When combined and drawn in various ways they make up a complete language. It fulfils Bliss's intention of forming a logical system. About 30 years later, it was discovered by Shirley McNaughton in Canada when working with children who were non-communicating and had physical disability. Her team took the commonest words required by children and set them out with the symbols on a chart, so that the children could indicate their needs by pointing. It consists of 100 basic symbols which can be used by themselves or in combination to produce whatever message is required. There are more than 2200 Blissymbols, more than 900 of which have been added since the original Blissymbol dictionary. Blissymbolics has been used with a multiplicity of disorders suffered by children and adults. As a system it can be used as an augmentative means of communication or to augment the child's unintelligible speech. It was introduced into the UK in 1973. The Blissymbolics Communication Resource Centre (UK) was founded in 1977. The system is very versatile as it can be used by people with various abilities in various different environments. Since the symbols are always presented with the words, even those unfamiliar with the system can understand it. Many studies have shown that Blissymbols are the least transparent, the most difficult to learn and the hardest to retain (Bloomberg et al 1990; Hurlbut, Iwata and Green 1982; Mirenda and Locke 1989; Mizuko 1987). However there are good reasons why it is so widely used which are noted by Vanderheiden and Lloyd (1986), including:

1. The principles and strategies for combining symbols enable expression of thoughts not on the communication board. The symbols are conceptually based and constructed using consistent, systematic rules.
2. The symbols can be introduced simply and later expanded.
3. The use of Blissymbolics is compatible with other techniques including reading and writing.
4. Initially intended for use with children with cerebral palsy, Blissymbolics has been used with varying degrees of success in remediation of virtually every known communication impairment (Musselwhite and St. Louis 1988;

Silverman 1995; Vanderheiden and Lloyd 1986). *See* Kiernan et al (1982); Bailey and Jenkinson (1982); Luftig and Beersani (1985); Yovetich and Young (1988); Shepherd and Haaf (1995); Soto and Toro-Zambrana (1995); Fuller (1997); Glennen and DeCoste (1997); Beukelman and Mirenda (1998); Carmeli and Shen (1998); Hetzroni and Lloyd (2000); Hetzroni and Belfiore (2000); Ferm et al (2001) (Blissymbols and Minspeak); http://www.home.istar.ca/~bci/

block modification a person who stammers is often described as exhibiting blocking behaviour. This is the actual act of stammering, i.e. the repetition of sounds. Van Riper proposed block modification as a therapeutic technique to reduce the amount of blocking behaviour. It is part of the STAMMER MORE FLUENTLY approach, so the criterion for success is not necessarily total fluent speech but an ACCEPTABLE STAMMER where the speaker is happy to speak despite DYSFLUENCY and where the listener is aware of some dysfluency but is not annoyed by it. The first stage of this technique is to identify the stammer, i.e. what it sounds like, then desensitise people's fear and panic when they anticipates a stammer. Block modification has three stages:

1. Cancellation: after the blocking behaviour has occurred, the speaker corrects what was said.
2. Pull-outs: during blocking behaviour, the speaker stops and repeats the word or phrase in which the blocking took place.
3. Preparatory blocks: blocking behaviour is anticipated and the speaker prepares to speak as fluently as possible.

See Dalton (1983).

Blom-Singer oesophageal prosthesis a device placed in the FISTULA following a LARYNGECTOMY. If successful, the voice can be regained and communication is almost normal. The voice is usually fluent and sounds more normal than OESOPHAGEAL VOICE. It is powered by pneumatic air pressure; the duration in speech is better; the voice is louder and greater change in pitch is possible than with a normal oesophageal voice, allowing greater scope and variability. If, however, the resulting voice is not liked, the prosthesis can be removed and the tracheo-oesophageal fistula will close completely. *See* Edels (1984).

blood–brain barrier an anatomical and physiological barrier to give protection to the brain cells from dangerous substances and pathogens. If there is any form of trauma to the BRAIN, this can lead to a breakdown of the barrier allowing such harmful substances to attack the brain cells. It could also affect the way in which therapeutic drugs enter the brain to help with tumours in the brain. *See* Tortora and Grabowski (2000).

Bobath method a method of treatment developed by Karl and Berta Bobath to help those with CEREBRAL PALSY. It is based on the inhibition of persisting infantile tonic reflexes and the replacement of these with learned patterns of normal neuromuscular activity. *See* http://www.bobath.org.uk/bobath.html

body language non-verbal form of communication such as gesture, facial expression, bodily movement, etc., which often accompanies speech. *See* Beukelman and Mirenda (1998).

Boehm-3 Preschool devised by Boehm, Boehm-3 Preschool is designed to identify rapidly children between the ages of 3;00–5;11 who lack an understanding of basic relational concepts. It can be adapted for use with children who have special needs. *See* Boehm (2001) in Appendix I.

Boehm Test of Basic Concepts (1971, revised 1986) devised by Boehm, it is a standardised assessment which is concerned with the comprehension of concepts. Fifty concepts are divided into four categories: space, time, quantity and miscellaneous concepts. The revised edition includes further subsections of antonyms, synonyms and one in which concepts are combined. The test can be given individually or on a group basis. Children are provided with a picture booklet and are given verbal instructions regarding each task to be carried out. There is also a preschool version which assesses for 26 basic language concepts. It is most appropriate for children between 3 and 5 years of age. By using the test in conjunction with the Boehm Resource Guide for Basic Concept Training, a complete therapeutic programme can be put together for individual children. *See* Boehm (1976, 1986a, b) in Appendix I.

Boehm Test of Basic Concepts 3rd Edition (Boehm-3) is a new edition of the BOEHM TEST OF BASIC CONCEPTS with new norms and full colour stimulus material of 50 basic concepts. *See* Boehm (2000) in Appendix I.

bone CONNECTIVE TISSUE in which collagen fibres are held together by ground substance impregnated with complex calcium salts for great strength. Bone has a matrix, i.e. its ground substance, formed in a concentric tubular pattern. The outer surface has a layer of fibrous tissue known as periosteum. The bones which appear denser are compact bones while those which are more open on the inside are cancellous bone. Classification of bone is according to shape of which there are five types: long, short, flat, irregular and sesamoid bones. *See* Tortora and Grabowski (2000).

bone conduction *see* PURE-TONE AUDIOMETRY.

bone-conduction hearing aid the sound comes through the air waves and is transmitted to a bone-conductor vibrator placed on the mastoid process behind the EAR. These vibrations produce a signal transmitted to the inner ear through the bones in the skull. It is used when an AIR-CONDUCTION HEARING AID cannot be worn or is ineffective. In the last 25 years bone conduction implants have been used, two of which are the bone-anchored hearing aid (BAHA) (1977) and the Audiant (1984). The BAHA has a direct contact between a screw-shaped implant placed in the bone of the mastoid process and the transducer through a skin-penetrating coupling. The Audiant comprises two parts, one of which is internal – a strong earth magnet in a titanium disc attached to the skull with an orthopaedic screw – while the external part is the sound processor which has another earth magnet and an induction coil.

The transmission of sound is transcutaneous. At present, the BAHA model is the only bone-conduction hearing aid available. Indications for using a bone-conduction hearing aid rather than an air-conduction aid include people who do not have any ear canals (*see* EAR) due to congenital malformations; people with chronic ear infection which drains intermittently or constantly and people in whom the material of the earmould causes irritation in the external ear canal. *See* Miller (1972); Tjellström (2001).

Boston Diagnostic Aphasia Examination (BDAE) devised by Goodglass and Kaplan in 1972 (revised 1983; 2000), it is an assessment for APHASIA. It is a formal, standardised assessment which incorporates what the authors describe as the 'three general aims of any aphasia test':

1. Diagnosis of presence and type of aphasic syndrome, leading to inferences concerning cerebral localisation.
2. Measurement of the level of performance over a wide range of both initial determination and detection of change over time.
3. Comprehensive assessment of the assets and liabilities of the patient in all language areas as a guide to therapy.

From a practical point of view, the test does not give hard and fast guidelines for therapy. It highlights all the possible areas where the person may find varying difficulties such as articulation, loss of verbal fluency, word-finding difficulty (*see* LEXICAL SYNTACTIC DEFICIT), repetition, serial speech, loss of SYNTAX, PARAPHASIA, AUDITORY COMPREHENSION, reading and writing. The authors do not accept that there is a disorder called dyspraxia and so they do not use this term. *See* Goodglass and Kaplan (2000); Eisenson (1984); Rosenbek et al (1989); Beech et al (1993); Glennen and DeCoste (1997).

Boston Naming Test devised by Kaplan, Goodglass and Weintraub in 1983, it is a 'wide-ranging naming vocabulary test'. Its aim is to assess the type of errors made by those with word-finding difficulties in spontaneous speech, and uses confrontation picture naming to this end. It can be used with children aged between 5;6 and 10;6 years of age, adults with APHASIA, and those with DEMENTIA and ANOMIA. There are 60 black-and-white line drawings, graded in difficulty. Stimulus CUES can be given. *See* Kaplan et al (1983) in Appendix I; Beech et al (1993).

Boston School a group of workers concerned with research into the diagnosis, nature and treatment of aphasic disorders. This research is based on a localisation model in which they believe aphasic patients can be categorised according to which part of the left CEREBRAL HEMISPHERES is damaged. The Boston School proposes seven major types of aphasia: (1) Broca's aphasia; (2) Wernicke's aphasia; (3) conduction aphasia; (4) anomia; (5) transcortical sensory aphasia; (6) transcortical motor aphasia; and (7) alexia with agraphia (*see* APHASIA (1–7)) and four PURE APHASIAS: (1) APHEMIA; (2) PURE WORD DEAFNESS; (3) PURE ALEXIA; and (4) PURE AGRAPHIA. *See* Goodglass and Kaplan (2000).

bottom-up (top-down) processes the use of context in perception. Bottom-up processes are driven only by the input (raw sensory data) while top-down processes are driven by a person's knowledge, experience, attention and expectations. *See* Smith et al (2003).

bound morpheme a morpheme (*see* MORPHOLOGY) which cannot exist on its own. For example, the affix 'de-' in a word like 'devise' is a bound morpheme as 'de-' cannot be used as a separate meaningful unit. It is opposed to free morpheme (see MORPHOLOGY). *See* Matthews (1974).

Bracken Basic Concept Scale - Revised (BBCS-R) devised by Bracken, the BBCS-R is designed to assess children's receptive knowledge of 301 basic concepts in 11 distinct conceptual categories including colours, direction/position, letters, self/social awareness, numbers/counting, texture/materials, size, quantity, comparisons, time/sequence and shapes. It is possible to plan lessons or therapy from the results of such an in-depth assessment. The BBCS-R is suitable for children between the ages of 2;06–8;00. *See* Bracken (1998) in Appendix I.

bracketing a mode of representation analysis for CONSTITUENT ANALYSIS. Each sentence which is either spoken or written can be analysed into several component parts with the hierarchical relations represented linearly by brackets (see boxed example below in which the abbreviations mean det = determiner, N = noun, NP = noun phrase, V = verb, VP = verb phrase and S = sentence). Another way of showing the constituent analysis of the sentence is by branching in a TREE DIAGRAM. *See* Lyons (1981).

bradykinesia *see* PARKINSON'S DISEASE.

bradylalia abnormally slow rate of speech.

brain comprises two CEREBRAL HEMISPHERES – the left and right – connected by the CORPUS CALLOSUM. The motor and sensory areas run in parallel regions on either side of the central fissure down to the lateral fissure. Below the cerebral cortex is the THALAMUS (acts as sensory relay station to the cerebral cortex), HYPO-THALAMUS (controls temperature, metabolism and endocrine balance), RETICULAR SYSTEM (arousal system which activates regions of cerebral cortex), CEREBELLUM (controls muscles, balance and co-ordination of voluntary movement) and the MEDULLA OBLONGATA (controls breathing, swallowing, digestion and heart beat). *See* Barr (1988); Kolb and Whishaw (1996); Tortora and Grabowski (2000).

brain abscess a collection of pus in the brain substance. It may be caused by bacteria from the ear, usually suppurative otitis media (*see* OTITIS MEDIA), resulting in an abscess occurring in the temporal lobe (*see* CEREBRAL HEMISPHERES). The bacteria can also come from the blood. It acts as a TUMOUR OF THE CENTRAL NERVOUS SYSTEM. It distorts the brain structures by compressing its various parts. The symptoms produced are those of raised INTRACRANIAL PRESSURE, fever, APHASIA, epileptic seizures (*see* EPILEPSY), coma and headaches. Diagnosis is by CT (COMPUTED TOMOGRAPHY) scan and a culture of bacteria from the areas given above. Treatment is by surgical drainage and appropriate antibiotic or other chemotherapy. *See* Gilroy and Holliday (1982); Kaye (1991).

brain death a diagnosis where there has to be no chance for the person to recover from BRAINSTEM damage and no evidence of brainstem function following tests which will show lack of pupil response to light, lack of corneal reflex to stimulation, lack of oculocephalic reflex, failure of vestibulo-ocular reflex, failure of gag or cough reflex on bronchial stimulation, no motor response in the face or muscles supplied by the CRANIAL NERVES in response to painful stimulus, and failure of response of respiratory move-

(	(	(THE)	(DOG)	)	((CHASED)	(	(THE)	(CAT)	)	)	)
		.	.	.	.		.	.	.	.	.
		.	.	.	.		.	.	.	.	.
		det	N	NP	V		det	N	NP	VP	S

ments when the patient is disconnected from a ventilator and the $PaCO_2$ is allowed to rise to 50mmHg. The tests should be carried out by two senior doctors. *See* Kaye (1991).

brain tumours *see* TUMOURS OF THE CENTRAL NERVOUS SYSTEM.

brainstem this structure within the brain comprises the MEDULLA OBLONGATA, the PONS and the MIDBRAIN. Each of these three parts has structures particular to each, as well as tracts and fibres which are common to all three. *See* Barr (1988); Kaye (1991); Kolb and Whishaw (1996).

brainstem evoked response audiometry *see* AUDITORY BRAINSTEM RESPONSE (ABR).

branch
1. A section of a computer program that is not part of the main routine. It is often called a subroutine. The branching part of the program appears between branch instructions that direct the program to carry out a particular branch and which then direct the program back to the main routine.
2. In linguistic discussion, a branch links constituents together into a TREE DIAGRAM. *See* Lyons (1981).

breath groups the length of utterance that a person can produce in one breath. Poor breathing may affect the syntactic, phonological and semantic content of what is said. In speech and language therapy, breath groups can be introduced into treatment programmes for those who have DYSARTHRIA or DYSPHONIA. The person is shown how to reduce the number of words used in one breath to a level at which communication is more intelligible. *See* Brosnahan and Malmberg (1976); Robertson and Thomson (1986).

Bringing Unity into Language and Learning Development (BUILLD) devised by Valot, BUILLD is a curriculum guide to the teaching of the MINSPEAK APPLICATION PROGRAM (MAP) – UNITY. It uses a variety of therapeutic techniques for teaching the program, with motivating, functional activities including cooking, art, reading books, writing, playing games and singing songs. Its main aim is to tackle the teaching of multiple associations which specifically address icon associations. The person using Unity will begin with single words and increase the number of words they can use into frequently used phrases and sentences across the different settings. The success of this program increases with the use of the team approach, i.e. those who work most frequently with the user, including parents, speech and language therapists, occupational and physiotherapists, teachers, etc. There are 11 units in the curriculum. *See* Valot (1995).

Bristol Language Development Scales devised by Gutfreund and her colleagues in 1989 for children between 15 months and 5 years with an expressive language difficulty, including those with a language and/or hearing impairment, as well as non-English speaking children. It gives a detailed analysis of the child's expressive language. The therapist has to elicit a language sample which is then transferred onto the transcription sheet. The sample is then analysed using three methods:

1. PRAGMATICS: how the child uses language.
2. SEMANTICS: the meaning of the child's language.
3. SYNTAX: the form of the child's language.

Items within each section are divided into 10 stages of development. The main scale enables the therapist to assess the developmental level of a particular child at a specific age, identify gaps in the overall expressive language profile and diagnose areas of deficiency in the child's expressive language development. There is a syntax-free scale for non-English speakers, hearing-impaired children and children with learning disabilities who use a mixture of words and signs to communicate. The therapy planning form is used to formulate individual treatment plans for each child. It is based on the Bristol Language Development Research

Programme led by Gordon Wells. The research 'Language at Home and at School' followed the language development of a group of children from infancy through primary school. Papers from the research project can be found in *Language, Learning and Education*. *See* Wells (1985); Gutfreund (1989) in Appendix I; Beech et al (1993).

British Ability Scales an extensive battery of tests for assessing general cognitive abilities. The battery produces IQ scores and a detailed profile of the child's cognitive abilities in 23 areas of cognitive development. These 23 areas are organised into six major process areas:

1. Speed of information processing.
2. Reasoning.
3. Spatial imagery.
4. Perceptual matching.
5. Short-term memory.
6. Retrieval and application of knowledge.

The test can be administered in separate parts to children in the age range of 2;6–17 years of age. *See* Elliott et al (1990) in Appendix I.

British Picture Vocabulary Scales devised by Dunn and colleagues, they comprise a formal, standardised assessment to test a person's auditory vocabulary. They are suitable for children with a LEARNING DISABILITY, children who cannot produce an oral or written response, or as a screening test for new school entrants. They should not be used with those with a hearing loss. The child is given a page of four pictures, only one of which corresponds correctly to the auditory stimulus – the child need only finger or eye point. A ceiling score and a basal score must be found. The assessment is quick to administer and can be given either as a detailed test using the 'long form' or as a quick screening test using the 'short form'. *See* Dunn et al (1982) in Appendix I; Beech et al (1993).

British Picture Vocabulary Scale; Second Edition (BPVS II) devised by Dunn and colleagues (originally in 1982), it is a formal, standardised assessment to test children's auditory vocabulary. It is suitable for children with LEARNING DISABILITY, children who cannot produce an oral or written response, or as a screening test for new school entrants and should not be used with those with a hearing loss. The child is given a page of four pictures, only one of which corresponds correctly to the auditory stimulus. The child need only finger or eye point. The test can be given to children in the age range of 3;00–15;08. A ceiling score and a basal score must be found. It is quick to administer and can be given either as a detailed test using the 'long form' or as a quick screening test using the 'short form'. *See* Dunn et al (1997) in Appendix I; Beech et al (1993).

British Sign Language (BSL) used by the hard of hearing in the UK. It is a natural language, which has been developed by deaf people, having a grammar of its own, unlike a sign system such as MAKATON, which is not grammatical in its structure. However, the grammar of BSL does not match that of spoken English. *See* Kiernan et al (1982).

broad transcription *see* TRANSCRIPTION SYSTEMS.

Broca's aphasia discovered by a French neurologist, Paul Broca, in the nineteenth century. A major APHASIA proposed by the BOSTON SCHOOL for a communication disorder caused by trauma to the brain. The area which Broca discovered, known as Broca's area, is in the left cerebral hemisphere in the third frontal convolution in the precentral gyrus. For a description of the communication difficulties found in Broca's aphasia, *see* APHASIA (1). *See* Goodglass and Kaplan (2000); Rosenbek et al (1989) (AAC and Broca's aphasia); Garrett et al (1989).

bromocriptine a dopamine receptor agonist for idiopathic parkinsonism. It is often given if sinemet is not having any effect or the on/off phenomenon continues while on sinemet. The side effects are the same as those of L-dopa (*see* LEVODOPA). It should not be given to those with severe dementia as it may increase confusion and agitation. It can be used with other anti-parkinsonian drugs. *See* Gilroy and Holliday (1982).

bronchi two divisions of the TRACHEA which lead to the left and right LUNGS respectively. There are three differences between the two bronchi:

1. The right bronchus is shorter than the left.
2. The right bronchus is vertical while the left is almost horizontal.
3. The right bronchus is wide while the left bronchus is narrower.

When the bronchi reach the lungs, they branch again into smaller bronchi or secondary lobar bronchi – one for each lobe of the lungs. These branch, in turn, into tertiary or segmental bronchi, which branch into bronchioles. These bronchioles divide, finally, into terminal bronchioles. The whole system from the initial division at the end of the trachea is known as the bronchial tree. *See* Joseph (1979); Tortora and Grabowski (2000).

Brown Attention-Deficit Disorder Scales devised by Brown in 1996, the Scales are designed to assess a broad range of cognitive and affective symptoms associated with attention deficit disorder in adolescents and adults (from 12 years through to adulthood). They identify a broad range of cognitive, affective and behavioural symptoms including activating and organising work, sustaining attention and concentration, sustaining energy and effort, managing affective interference and utilising working memory and assessing recall. *See* Brown (1996) in Appendix I.

BSER (brainstem evoked response audiometry) see AUDITORY BRAINSTEM RESPONSE.

buccal nerve *see* MOUTH.

buccinator *see* MUSCLES OF FACIAL EXPRESSION.

Buddy Button small single plate switches suitable for any device that needs to be activated by a switch from a communication aid to a computer. *See* Glennen and DeCoste (1997); Appendix IV (TASH).

buffer part of a peripheral unit where data are stored temporarily when transferred from the computer's memory. The buffer will hold information sent to it and act on it depending on the speed at which the information reaches the unit. *See* Bishop (1985).

bug any error or part of a computer program that does not work as it should. The process in which the bugs are removed from programs is known as debugging. *See* Bishop (1985).

BUILLD see BRINGING UNITY INTO LANGUAGE AND LEARNING DEVELOPMENT.

bulbar palsy a palsy caused by a disorder in the pathways of the nuclei which originate in the MEDULLA OBLONGATA. This disease produces weakness in the affected muscles which can deteriorate over a period of time. The disease affects four muscle groups: (1) MUSCLES OF MASTICATION; (2) MUSCLES FOR SWALLOWING; (3) muscles of the TONGUE; (4) muscles of the face. It is a progressive disease which begins with difficulty of tongue movement, progressing to immobility of the tongue. The orbicularis oris muscles (*see* MUSCLES OF FACIAL EXPRESSION) are affected in the early stages, making it difficult to close the lips and thus producing excessive drooling. The soft palate (*see* MOUTH) fails to close which allows food to be regurgitated down the nose. The final stage of the disease is a failure to swallow and close the jaw. The prognosis is poor and death occurs in 1–2 years due to aspiration pneumonia. If the muscles are affected by an upper motor neurone disease (*see* NEURONS) there is spastic rather than flaccid weakness. This is also known as pseudobulbar palsy. There is no cure. The major nursing problem is ensuring adequate nutrition due to the swallowing difficulty. *See* Ginsbergh (1999); http://www.mndassociation. org/

bunching a description of the production of sounds in which the tongue is placed towards the back of the mouth under the soft palate to produce back vowels (*see* CARDINAL VOWEL SYSTEM), velar and uvular fricatives [ɣ, x, X, ʁ] (*see* ARTICULATION). *See* Catford (1989).

Burns Brief Inventory of Communication and Cognition devised by Burns, the Inventory is designed to determine which skills are impaired and, therefore, which skills are to be treated. It is aimed at three types of skills: those controlled by the left hemisphere such as verbal expression, reading, writing and numerical reasoning; by the right hemisphere such as scanning and tracking, visuo-spatial skills, prosody and abstract language; those skills which can be affected by a complex neuropathology such as orientation and factual memory, auditory attention and memory, visual perception and visual attention and memory. The Inventory can be used with people in the age range of 18;00–80;00.

burst a phenomenon found in acoustic phonetics when there is a sudden peak showing a burst of energy when an abrupt release occurs in plosive sounds (see ARTICULATION). *See* Ladefoged (2001).

Bus Story devised by Renfrew in 1969 (2nd edition, 1991). The child is told a short story accompanied by 12 illustrations of a sequence of events in the form of a comic strip. The child retells the story, supported by a review of the pictures. This retelling is analysed in respect of the amount of correct information given, sentence length and complexity. The test is standardised in the UK and can be applied to children from 3;0 to 8;0 years. *See* Renfrew (1991) in Appendix I.

byte a group of eight BITS. *See* Bishop (1985); Brookshear (1991).

C

CA *see* CHRONOLOGICAL AGE.

CADL *see* COMMUNICATION ACTIVITIES OF DAILY LIVING (CADL) 2ND EDITION.

café-au-lait spots *see* TUMOURS OF THE CENTRAL NERVOUS SYSTEM.

Cameleon a range of high-tech communication aid systems which are both a Windows based PC and a communication aid when they have a communication package stored in them such as Words+ TALKING SCREEN FOR WINDOWS, Words+ EZ KEYS, WINSPEAK, HANDSOFF, WINDBAG, CHAILEY COMMUNICATION SYSTEM or INGFIELD DYNAMIC VOCABULARIES. The Cameleon 3 is designed in three bright colours and has internal batteries. The Cameleon II is similar to Cameleon 3 apart from the bright colours and it can only be used from the mains or linked to a battery pack on an electric wheelchair. Cameleon 4 is similar to its predecessors especially Cameleon 3. The Cameleon CV *express* is a hand-held system with internal batteries.

The various Cameleon models have the usual ports found on an ordinary PC, can be accessed using switches, touch screen, remote headpointer, mouse or keyboard and can learn infrared signals to operate various appliances in the home such as TVs, videos or opening/closing curtains, windows and doors. *See* Rumble and Larcher (1998); Appendix IV (Cambridge Adaptive Communication).

Cameleon CamPac2 a computer-based communication aid based on a standard notebook computer for those requiring a communication aid who can also use a keyboard. It has its own voice synthesiser and amplified speakers. It can be used with the same software as for the more advanced CAMELEON range of systems. *See* Rumble and Larcher (1998); Appendix IV (Cambridge Adaptive Communication).

canal any passage or tube-like structure within the body. For example, the ear canal situated in the outer ear (*see* EAR) is an air-filled tube closed at one end by the eardrum. *See* Joseph (1979).

cancellous bone *see* BONE.

cancer a layman's term used to describe the existence of a malignant tumour. There are various types of cancerous growths. They can occur in the brain, the larynx, and, commonly, in the female breast. *See* Kaye (1991); Tortora and Grabowski (2000).

Canon communicator a high-tech communication aid, it is a mini-electronic typewriter which can be used with those who have difficulty being understood because they have inadequate expressive language or none at all. The original keyboard had the 26 letters of the alphabet placed in frequency order, i.e. the most used letters placed around the outside of the keyboard with other less used letters placed towards the centre of the keyboard. The keys for the vowels and consonants are of different colours, i.e. consonant keys were on the light-grey keys while the vowels and 'y' were on dark-grey keys. In some models, there is an alphabetic keyboard with the same colour differentiation between the keys. Some models also have a memory capacity where messages are placed under the top row of keys on the keypad. Messages are printed out on thermal tape. In the latest device, messages can also be recalled using digitised speech output. There are up to a total of 240 seconds of recording time under the 26 alphabet keys (CC-7S model). The memory of the device can store up to 7000 characters under the 26 alphabet keys (CC-7S/CC-7P models). Phrases can be printed out and, with the CC-7S models, the memory message can be played back as well as printed out. There is also a calculator function. All the communicator's functions can be operated by a single key operation by designating a key at the intersection of a row and column. An optional large display can be connected to either of these models. It has two 26-character lines with a word wrap-around function. Alternative keyboard covers are available for those with a tremor who may press the wrong key. The communicator itself works off a battery pack which can be recharged. Straps for attaching it to the client's arm or wheelchair are also available. *See* Glennen and DeCoste (1997); Rumble and Larcher (1998); Appendix IV (Canon).

Capgras' syndrome a psychotic syndrome. The person has a delusion that a close relative has been replaced by his or her double. It is usually found in SCHIZOPHRENIA.

carbamazepine *see* EPILEPSY.

carcinoma a malignant growth that can appear in any part of the body. Treatment may require surgery, RADIO-THERAPY or chemotherapy. *See* Pracy et al (1974); Kaye (1991).

cardinal vowel system devised by Daniel Jones in about 1914, it provides a set of reference points on the periphery of the vowel area in the mouth to describe vowels in relation to each other. The system has eight primary vowels which act as reference points of tongue and lip position. The diagram for primary cardinal vowels is:

In the primary vowel system, the front vowels are unrounded, i.e. the lips are spread, while the back vowels are rounded, i.e. the lips are pouted. As the tongue moves from [i], it moves down and back for the production of the other vowels and is bunched at the back of the mouth for the back vowels. There are four classifications of vertical tongue positions used in this system:

1. Close – the highest position in the mouth [i, u], which allows the vowel to be produced without audible friction.
2. Half-close – the next level [e, o].
3. Half-open – the next level [ɛ, ɔ].
4. Open – the next level [a, ɒ] where the tongue is furthest from the roof of the mouth.

The secondary cardinal vowels are produced by reversing the lip positions which results in the front vowels becoming rounded and the back vowels becoming unrounded. The diagram for secondary vowels is:

front   back

y
  ø   ɣ
      æ   ʌ
                            ɑ

All vowels can be described within the framework of either primary or secondary cardinal vowels. *See* Ladefoged (2001).

Carhart's notch a special feature found on a pure-tone audiogram. It is represented on the audiogram by a dip in bone conduction threshold (*see* PURE-TONE AUDIOMETRY) at 2000 Hz and is associated with OTOSCLEROSIS.

carotid artery one of the main arteries in the neck. As it rises it branches into the external and internal carotid arteries. The external carotid artery serves superficial structures within the neck and head such as the LARYNX, TONGUE, external ear (*see* EAR) and MUSCLES OF MASTICATION. The internal carotid artery supplies the anterior two-thirds of the BRAIN and orbits. *See* Joseph (1979).

Carrow Elicited Language Inventory (CELI) devised by Carrow-Woolfolk in 1974, it is an imitation test which assesses the level of expressive language of children between 3 years and 7 years 11 months. It uses 52 phrase and sentence stimuli containing a range of syntactic constructions and grammatical morphemes presented to the child to imitate directly. It is standardised on a North American population. *See* Carrow-Woolfolk (1974) in Appendix I; Beech et al (1993).

carry-over using the therapeutic techniques in everyday situations, e.g. people who stammer and are given a technique to speak more fluently will need to have the confidence to use these techniques when communicating with friends, family and in the community.

cartilage a type of connective tissue. There are three types – hyaline, fibrous and elastic. Hyaline is found in the costal cartilages, fibrous is found in discs among the vertebrae while elastic is found in the pinna (*see* EAR) and the EPIGLOTTIS. See Tortora and Grabowski (2000).

case in case-marked languages such as Latin, inflections on nouns signalled grammatical relations such as subject, direct object and indirect object. Case survives in English pronouns, in the distinctions I/me, she/her, he/him, we/us, they/them. *See* Lyons (1968).

case grammar a generative model of grammar devised by Charles Fillmore in the 1960s. It involved a deep structure which was distinct from that in Chomsky's (*see* CHOMSKYAN LINGUISTICS) STANDARD THEORY in having as categories semantically labelled entities such as agent, benefactive and instrumental for the arguments of the verb. (These categories are the 'cases' of the title of the theory.) Deep-structure verb + case configurations then map onto conventional surface structures in well-defined ways. *See* Steinberg (1982).

case history a summary of the person's illness, disease or disorder from onset to the stage at which the person presents for treatment. In the case of communication disorders, the therapist records the progress of the disorder from its onset to the initial interview. This will include details of the relevant parts of the person's medical history, leisure activities and feelings about their present condition. The amount of information required for a case history is determined by the severity of the disorder which the person has. *See* Byers Brown (1981).

CASP *see* COMMUNICATION ASSESSMENT PROFILE FOR ADULTS WITH A MENTAL HANDICAP.

catarrh a mucinous discharge from a mucous membrane. A symptom of nasal irritation. The most common products in the atmosphere to cause nasal catarrh are dust, and smoke from tobacco. *See* Pracy et al (1974).

category

1. Most commonly used in relation to grammatical categories such as noun, verb, adjective, which are classificatory units crucial for the description of language. See Lyons (1968); Huddleston (1976).
2. In the field of AUGMENTATIVE AND ALTERNATIVE COMMUNICATION (AAC), category refers to the groupings of

vocabulary. For example, in a low-tech system such as a picture book, specific pages can be set up in different categories such as 'clothes' where the category picture is placed in the centre of the page and pictures of the specific clothing are placed around the category picture. In a high-tech system, a symbol can represent the type of vocabulary and the second hit or symbol represents the particular item of vocabulary. *See also* LANGUAGE, LEARNING AND LIVING (LLL). *See* Beukelman and Mirenda (1998).

catenative a lexical verb which in English pre-modifies another lexical verb is referred to as catenative in some grammatical descriptions, e.g. 'begin' in the following example: he began to despair.

CELF-R Scoring Assistant a software program which allows for scoring the CELF-R assessment on an IBM PC or compatible. It will provide a summary report. *See* Wiig (1988a) in Appendix I.

CELF-R Screening Test a short version of the CELF-R assessment to decide if a more in-depth assessment using the full CELF-R is necessary. As well as the parts which are similar to the CELF-R, there is an optional oral expression subtest for 5;0 to 7;0 years of age and an optional written expression subtest for ages 8;0–16;0. *See* Wiig (1988b) in Appendix I.

CELF-RUK *see* CLINICAL EVALUATION OF LANGUAGE FUNDAMENTALS (REVISED UK VERSION).

central hearing loss a hearing loss produced by a pathological condition occurring along the path of the auditory nerve from the BRAINSTEM to the cerebral CORTEX. It produces a problem in speech perception rather than just hearing.

central nervous system (CNS) the system within the body which produces reflexes when one part of the body is particularly stimulated. These responses come from the BRAIN via the SPINAL CORD. *See* Taverner (1983); Tortora and Grabowski (2000).

central processor a unit which is used to operate other units. For example, a computer can be described as a central processor for the information which appears on a monitor screen, or for information which goes to a printer. It can also be used to describe a unit which is used to operate environmental controls. *See* Bishop (1985).

central tendency a way of summarising the scores using a single figure in DESCRIPTIVE STATISTICS. There are three such measures:

1. Mean – the sum of scores of each person tested, divided by the number of people who took part in the experiment.
2. Mode – the most frequently occurring score.
3. Median – the middle score after all the scores have been put in order.

If all the measures are the same, i.e. mean = mode = median, it is called a symmetrical or normal distribution of scores and can be shown as such on a graph. If the scores diverge, the distribution is said to be skewed. *See* Miller (1984); Clarke and Cooke (1992).

centre in articulatory terms, the part of the tongue between the blade and its back. It is used to produce palatal sounds and is involved in the ARTICULATION of the palatoalveolar sounds as the centre of the tongue approaches the hard palate. A description of any vowel which appears in the middle of the CARDINAL VOWEL SYSTEM. The vowel which is right in the centre of the cardinal vowel space is the schwa vowel [ə]. To produce this vowel, the tongue takes up a central position in the mouth. *See* Ladefoged (2001).

centrencephalic epilepsy *see* CONGENITAL NEURONAL DYSFUNCTION.

cephalic usually a suffix to describe disorders in or of the head, for example, microcephalic (an abnormally small head, *see* MICROCEPHALY).

CERA *see* CORTICAL EVOKED RESPONSE AUDIOMETRY.

cerebellar a description of structures

found within the CEREBELLUM and of its disorders. These may produce dysarthric (*see* DYSARTHRIA) speech.

cerebellar dysarthria *see* ATAXIC DYSARTHRIA.

cerebellum comprises a cortex of grey matter, a central area of white matter and four pairs of central nuclei. The cerebellum is connected to the MEDULLA OBLONGATA, PONS and the MIDBRAIN by the inferior, middle and cerebellar peduncles respectively. The cerebellum organises the person's motor movements. The synchronous movements of muscles will be affected adversely if there is a lesion to this part of the brain affecting the person's speech, producing cerebellar DYSARTHRIA. *See* Barr (1988); Kolb and Whishaw (1996); Tortora and Grabowski (2000).

cerebral a description of structures or disorders that occur within the BRAIN.

cerebral abscess *see* BRAIN ABSCESS.

cerebral artery an artery which supplies the BRAIN. One of the most important is the middle cerebral artery which is situated in the lateral fissure between the frontal and temporal lobes (*see* CEREBRAL HEMISPHERES). Rupture of this artery or a branch produces a CEREBROVASCULAR ACCIDENT (CVA) as blood spreads over the brain and affects areas such as Broca's area (*see* CEREBRAL HEMISPHERES). This can cause APHASIA. *See* Barr (1988).

cerebral hemispheres the BRAIN has two hemispheres, right and left, connected by the CORPUS CALLOSUM. The folds and convolutions are known as gyri and the intervening grooves are known as sulci. Two of the sulci which appear in the fetus develop into the lateral and parieto-occipital fissures. These fissures with the central and calcarine sulci divide the hemisphere into four lobes – frontal, parietal, temporal and occipital. The frontal lobe extends forward from the central sulcus and upwards from the lateral fissure. The medial surface covers the anterior part of the corpus callosum. The parietal lobe, on the lateral surface, is bounded by the central sulcus and the lateral fissure. On the medial surface, the parietal lobe is bounded by the frontal lobe, corpus callosum, calcarine sulcus and parieto-occipital fissure. The temporal lobe, on the lateral surface, is bounded by the lateral fissure. The inferior surface of the lobe extends to the temporal pole. The occipital lobe starts where the temporal lobe ends and is separated from the parietal lobe by the parieto-occipital fissure. The left hemisphere in the majority of people is the dominant hemisphere (*see* DOMINANCE) and it controls the right side of the body. It contains the language centres of the brain. In particular, Broca's area can be found in the frontal lobe while Wernicke's area can be found in the parietal lobe. Both hemispheres have a motor and sensory region from which signals are sent to the nerves innervating the muscles of movement and touch. The occipital lobe is concerned with vision. The right hemisphere has centres controlling rhythm, artistry, arithmetic and the muscles used for speaking and eating. *See* Barr (1988); Kolb and Whishaw (1996).

cerebral infarction *see* CEREBROVASCULAR ACCIDENT.

cerebral palsy a group of disorders of movement and posture due to slow development and non-progressive disorders of the BRAIN. There are several possible causes of cerebral palsy which can occur at various times around the child's birth.

1. During the PRENATAL period, the possible causes are congenital infections, e.g. congenital malformations within the brain, radiation, nutritional deficiency or lack of oxygen.

2. During the PERINATAL period, the possible causes are periventricular haemorrhage, birth asphyxia, birth trauma, hyperbilirubinaemia or venous stasis/thrombosis.

3. During the POSTNATAL period, the possible causes are MENINGITIS, ENCEPHALITIS, trauma or metabolic disorders.

There are four types of cerebral palsy:

1. Spastic cerebral palsy: the most common type of cerebral palsy which accounts for about 70 per cent of children so affected. The damage to the brain, which produces both unilateral and bilateral hemiplegia, is centred on the corticospinal tracts (*see* PYRAMIDAL SYSTEM/TRACT). Bilateral hemiplegia produces a pseudobulbar palsy (*see* BULBAR PALSY) which produces dysarthric characteristics of speech (*see* DYSARTHRIA), impaired swallowing (*see* DYSPHAGIA) and a poor gag reflex.
2. Ataxic cerebral palsy: damage to the brain in the CEREBELLUM which produces HYPOTONIA, a broad base gait, TREMOR and DYSMETRIA. Speech becomes dysarthric (*see* DYSARTHRIA) while intelligence is usually within normal limits.
3. Dyskinetic cerebral palsy: damage to the BASAL GANGLIA, causing involuntary movements and reduced voluntary movements. There are three subtypes:
   (a) athetosis: slow, writhing movements and severely dysarthric speech caused by damage to the extrapyramidal system in the brain or asphyxia at birth or anoxia to the basal ganglia. There can also be a HEARING LOSS;
   (b) chorea: fast, jerky movements in the upper extremities caused by a disease to the basal ganglia;
   (c) dystonia: increase in muscle tone, no contractures and persistence of primitive reflexes. Distorted postures are maintained for long periods of time and produce rotation, adduction of limbs and extension of the spine. It affects the AGONIST and ANTAGONIST muscles.
4. Mixed cerebral palsy: a form of cerebral palsy which has features of (1)–(3). Those who may be involved with treatment will include the physiotherapist, speech and language therapist, occupational therapist, educational psychologist and, possibly, an ENT surgeon.

See Gilroy and Holliday (1982); Hosking (1982); Illingworth (1987); Kaye (1991); Kolb and Whishaw (1996); Glennen and DeCoste (1997) (AAC); Beukelman and Mirenda (1998) (AAC); http://www.scope.org.uk

cerebrospinal fluid (CSF) fluid that circulates round the BRAIN coming from the ventricles (*see* THIRD VENTRICLE and FOURTH VENTRICLE) in the brain and the central canal of the SPINAL CORD. Most of the CSF consists of water, protein and a few cells. It also contains sugar and sodium chloride. The CSF is used to diagnose diseases of the MENINGES and CENTRAL NERVOUS SYSTEM. *See* Barr (1988); Kaye (1991); Kolb and Whishaw (1996).

cerebrovascular accident (CVA) the medical term which encompasses all the different ways in which a stroke occurs. The functioning of the BRAIN is dependent on its blood supply and the oxygen carried in the blood. A quarter of the oxygen we breathe goes to the brain. If the brain is deprived of oxygen for greater than three minutes, cells are damaged. When a CVA occurs, there is interruption of the normal blood supply and irreversible cell damage takes place. There are two disorders which affect the blood supply to the brain – haemorrhage and thrombosis:

1a. Brain haemorrhage: a vessel ruptures either in the brain itself or in the subarachnoid space. About 10 per cent of all cerebrovascular accidents are due to haemorrhage. The resultant haematoma (blood clot) produces compression damage of the surrounding brain tissue and by raising the INTRACRANIAL PRESSURE may interfere with brain function at distant sites. In addition, subarachnoid bleeding can occur from a berry aneurysm. These form usually at junctions in the cerebral arteries (*see* CEREBRAL ARTERY). The vessel bonuleic acid (DNA) molecules) which provide the mental and physical characteristics which are inherited in a family. Genes exist in pairs like chromosomes with either gene being dominant or recessive. When both genes are dominant or when one is dominant and the other recessive, the dominant gene determines the inherited trait. Only if the gene from both parents is recessive will the recessive trait be inherited.

If there is an abnormality in the chromosomes, certain syndromes can result, e.g. DOWN SYNDROME. Some syndromes and diseases are described in terms of the autosomal or sex chromosome abnormality as follows:

1. Dominant autosomal disorder is inherited by several members of the family. There is a 50 per cent chance of children being affected as only one gene is abnormal.
2. Recessive autosomal disorder is inherited by fewer members of the family. There is a lesser chance of children being affected than in (1) as an abnormal gene from each parent is required. Both disorders can be produced by an abnormality of the X chromosome.
3. Sex-linked recessive disorder appears in males as they have only one X chromosome and so will have the abnormal gene while females who have an abnormal gene in one X chromosome have a second X chromosome which cancels out the first. For an X-linked disorder to be present in females both X chromosomes have to be affected. Disorders produced by this type of chromosomal abnormality include Duchenne muscular dystrophy (see DYSTROPHY).

See Hosking (1982); Smith et al (2003).

chronic a description of a disease or illness which has a slow progression or with symptoms that are slow to evolve. It is opposed to acute (see ACUTE (1)).

chronic non-specific laryngitis a condition caused by nasal discharge into the nasopharynx (see PHARYNX) and thence to the LARYNX, which becomes irritated. In many cases, the only symptom is persistent HOARSE VOICE. The primary problem, i.e. nasal disorder, should be treated before the secondary problem of the laryngitis. See Pracy et al (1974).

chronological age (CA) the natural age of a child or adult. It is used in assessments carried out by various rehabilitation professionals such as speech and language therapists, psychologists, etc. The child's CA can be compared to the AGE-EQUIVALENT SCORE obtained in certain assessments. Chronological age is also used by psychologists in the formula to work out an INTELLIGENCE QUOTIENT.

circle of Willis an anastomotic arrangement which joins together the blood supply brought to the brain by the internal carotid arteries (see CAROTID ARTERY) and the vertebral-basilar arteries. From this arterial circle come all the cerebral arteries (see CEREBRAL ARTERY) which supply the BRAIN. If obstruction occurs in one of the major input arteries, it is possible for blood to flow round the circle of Willis and supply the territory of the blocked artery. See Barr (1988); Tortora and Grabowski (2000).

circumvallate papillae see TASTE BUDS.

classical conditioning a learning procedure used in BEHAVIOUR THERAPY. It is based on the theory first proposed by Pavlov based on his experiments with dogs. He found that dogs could learn a conditioned response (CR – the learned or acquired response to a stimulus which did not provoke a response originally). He based his theory on the fact that people can learn certain reactions by giving an unconditioned response (UR – an innate or unlearned response produced by an unconditioned stimulus) to an unconditioned stimulus (US – a stimulus which automatically produces a response without prior conditioning). His experiments were aimed at finding out if a conditioned response could be learnt from a conditioned stimulus (CS – a stimulus which hitherto has been neutral produces a response when associated with the unconditioned stimulus). For example, Pavlov found dogs salivated (UR) when they smelled or tasted meat (US). Pavlov switched on a light when the dogs were given the meat (CS – dogs learn light is only on when given meat) and the dogs salivated (UR). However, he found if just the light was switched on, the dogs still salivated (CR – as they had been conditioned to salivate at the meat when the lights were on). There are three stages in learning a conditioned response to a conditioned stimulus starting from an unconditioned stimulus:

1. Simultaneous conditioning: both the light (CS) and the meat (US) are presented together, thus making the dogs salivate (UR).
2. Delayed conditioning: the light (CS) is switched on for a few seconds before the meat (US) is given to the dogs and is left switched on until the dogs salivate.
3. Trace conditioning: the light (US) is switched on, then switched off before the meat (US) is presented so that only a memory trace of the light remains for the conditioning process to take place. By repetition of placing the CS next to the the the US, the association of the two is reinforced. If reinforcement does not take place, extinction of the CR may take place.

See Smith et al (2003).

clause in some models of grammar, a clause is a grammatical unit which is smaller than, or co-terminous with, a sentence, but larger than a phrase. Its defining characteristic is that it contains a verb (although some grammatical descriptions would recognise reduced or verbless clauses). Clauses are normally identified as 'main' or 'subordinate' and the functions of subordinate clauses, e.g. adverbial, object, may also be identified. *See* Allerton (1979).

clavicular a description of the use of the chest. For example, some people who have dysarthria may not produce normal ABDOMINAL–DIAPHRAGMATIC RESPIRATION, but, instead, breathe from their chest. This is known as clavicular breathing.

clavicular respiration *see* CLAVICULAR.

CLEAR Phonology Screening Assessment devised by Keeling and his colleague, this screening assessment is designed to give a quick picture of a child's phonological development by testing one PHONEME in one position with one picture. The assessor uses a tick box form to give a visual analysis of the child's sound system. There are 24 consonant sounds individually tested in initial, medial and final word positions with 22 initial consonant clusters also tested. *See* Keeling and Keeling (2001) in Appendix I.

cleft palate a congenital condition in which there is failure of the palatal shelves to unite together with the nasal septum. In the normal development of the MOUTH the palatal shelves come together to form the hard palate or roof of the mouth as the TONGUE falls down into the cavity. A cleft palate is the embryological failure of the hard palate to fuse together while the child is in utero. A cleft lip is caused by failure of the tissue surrounding the lip to fuse together during the same period. A cleft lip and palate occurs when both the hard palate and lip have failed to form. Clefts can occur unilaterally or bilaterally. Most children who have this condition at birth can be helped by surgery. A cleft lip will be repaired around three months of age while a cleft in the palate will be closed at six months of age. Carrying out an operation at such an early age allows the surgeons to make use of the continual growth in the tissues of the affected areas. Thus, healing is more natural and few scars are left. A submucous cleft palate has a divided uvula or bifid uvula, a whitish line down the midline of the soft palate and a bony notch on the ridge between the soft and hard palates. The muscles of the soft palate do not function correctly and velopharyngeal incompetence (*see* VELOPHARYNGEAL) may result. Occult submucous cleft palate exists when the situation just outlined occurs but the white line is obscured by muscle, the bony notch is not evident and there is no bifid uvula. As surgical procedures have improved in closing a cleft lip and/or palate, the need for speech therapy to improve the child's articulation is not as great as in the past. However, the therapist's main purpose is to counsel the parents about the child's future speech, the efficacy of surgery and to give advice on the best types of feeding techniques available at the time. There may be problems of nasality as well as other articulation problems which will require speech therapy. While it is common for the speech of a child with a cleft palate to be described in terms of nasal resonance, nasal emission and compensatory articulations, a longitudinal study of children at different stages of surgical treatment showed a difference between passive and active cleft-type speech characteristics. The passive characteristics were thought to be caused by structural abnormality or dysfunction while the active characteristics were thought to be caused by specific articulatory gestures replacing intended consonants. The active cleft-type characteristics did not change as a direct result of surgery but the passive characteristics did disappear completely following surgery. *See* Watson et al (2001); Sell et al (1994) (screening assessment of cleft palate speech); Sell and Grunwell (1994) (speech and the unoperated cleft palate subject); Harding and Grunwell (1996, 1998); http://www.widesmiles.org/

Clicker 4 a powerful talking word processor with clicker grids, a curriculum graphic library of over 1000 pictures, which plays sound and video files and is available for both PC and Mac. Those using Clicker can write with speech feedback, have point and click access to an unlimited number of words and pictures, hear a word before they write it, build sentences using whole words, use talking wordbanks and writing frames and spellcheck their work with a talking spell checker with optional picture support. It is possible to create the child's own clicker grids in seconds to support any curriculum area. Grids can be linked together using customised pictures including digital photographs and recording customised sounds, and create integrated reading and writing activities and print out clicker grids of any size as well as printing documents. *See* Appendix IV (Crick Software).

client-centred therapy a type of PSYCHO-THERAPY proposed by Carl Rogers which assumes that each person has the motivation and ability to change and the person is the best qualified to decide how the change will occur. The therapist takes little part in the session and listens while individuals explore and analyse their own problems. *See* Smith et al (2003).

clinical audiology audiology used to evaluate the effects of a HEARING LOSS on the person's daily life and give him the means to cope with communication.

Clinical Evaluation of Language Fundamentals (revised UK version) devised originally by Wiig, CELF-R aims to assess school-age children to find out the nature and severity of the language difficulties. It comprises 11 subtests including: formulated sentences, word structure, listening to paragraphs, sentence structure, semantic relationships, sentence assembly, oral directions, word associations, word classes, recalling sentences and linguistic concepts. The UK version was put together by a team from the National Hospital's College of Speech Sciences and the Psychological Corporation and includes UK record forms, a manual supplement (written by the NHCSS panel) and amended stimulus manuals. *See* Wiig (1994) in Appendix I.

Clinical Evaluation of Language Fundamentals Preschool (UK Edition) devised by Wiig, CELF-Preschool[UK] measures a broad range of expressive and receptive language skills in young children in the age range of

3–6;11. It comprises six subtests including basic concepts assessing the ability to interpret oral directions containing references to attributes, size, direction, location, position and quantity; sentence structure examining the understanding of early developing sentence formation rules; word structure looking at the use of morphological rules and forms; formulating labels examining naming ability; and linguistic concepts letting the child follow directions that contain concepts requiring logical operations. CELF-Preschool[UK] has been standardised using UK norms. *See* Wiig et al (2000) in Appendix I.

Clinical Evaluation of Language Fundamentals – Third Edition (UK) (CELF-3[UK]) devised by Semel et al, (CELF-3[UK]) measures a broad range of receptive and expressive language skills in children and adolescents in the age range of 6;00-21;00. The subtests include: sentence structure; concepts and directions; word classes; sentence assembly; word associations; rapid automatic naming; word structure; formulated sentences; recalling sentences; semantic relationships and listing to paragraphs. It has been standardised on a UK population. *See* Semel et al (2000) in Appendix I.

clinical psychology a clinical psychologist assesses and treats EMOTIONAL DISORDERS and CONDUCT DISORDERS which occur among those with a LEARNING DISABILITY and/or physical disability, juvenile delinquents, drug addicts and in families where relationships have broken down. Such psychologists work in hospitals with inpatients and outpatients and in prisons. *See* MacKay (1975).

clonic *see* EPILEPSY.

close vowel *see* CARDINAL VOWEL SYSTEM.

cloze procedure a way of analysing reading processes. It takes the form of a passage of text with different types of words missing which have to be filled in by the client.

clumsy child syndrome a form of general DYSPRAXIA which manifests itself as impaired motor co-ordination. Difficulties arise in gross motor activities such as jumping, hopping and throwing, as well as in fine motor co-ordination. Written language may also be affected. It sometimes co-occurs with DEVELOPMENTAL VERBAL DYSPRAXIA. Dressing dyspraxia is also associated with this syndrome. The child has difficulty in orienting clothes when dressing so that shirts or jerseys may be put on upside down or back to front.

cluster reduction *see* PHONOLOGICAL PROCESSES.

cluttering a particular type of DYSFLUENCY in which the main feature is excessive speed of delivery. Resulting speech may at times be incoherent due to transposition and omission of sounds. PROSODY is also affected and there can be similar problems in the reading and writing of people who have this type of dysfluency. The individual is often unaware of the problem and unable to monitor his speech. Therapy for this disorder is aimed at relaxing the person and slowing down the speech RATE to a more acceptable level. *See* Dalton and Hardcastle (1989).

CNS *see* CENTRAL NERVOUS SYSTEM.

co-articulation an articulation which occurs almost simultaneously with another articulation. For example, in words such as 'eighth' and 'width', the [t] and [d] become dentalised as the speaker approaches [θ]. Thus, these two words would be pronounced [etθ] and [w+dθ]. Anticipatory co-articulation occurs where the articulators for both sounds move to the place of articulation (*see* ARTICULATION) of the second sound. For example, the word 'shoe' is pronounced with lip-rounding and even the [ʃ] is rounded, thus producing co-articulation. *See* Ladefoged (2001).

cochlea *see* EAR.

cochlear implants electronic devices implanted surgically in the cochlea (*see* EAR) of people who are profoundly or completely deaf to give them the sensation of hearing, while those who have bilateral acoustic neuromata such as neurofibromatosis type 2 which produces bilateral profound deafness have an auditory brainstem implant. The unit has a processor worn outside the ear which is linked to electrodes that are inserted into the cochlea where they transmit the signals to the nerve of hearing which are recognised as sounds by the brain. Cochlear implants are suitable for people who have profound SENSORINEURAL HEARING LOSS in both ears and who cannot benefit from conventional HEARING AIDS. Over 200 children a year receive implants in the UK usually between the ages of 1–5 years during the period when the child is developing language. A cochlear implant is not a cure for deafness and a child not wearing an implant will still be profoundly deaf when not wearing one. Even when wearing one the child may be considered hard of hearing or severely deaf just as a child with an ordinary hearing aid may be described as being hard of hearing. However, there are differences including the ability to hear high frequency speech sounds such as possessives, plurals, and ends of words and so children with cochlear implants can develop natural language, in a natural context with intelligible speech as well as having the ability to develop the processing of spoken language successfully through hearing, which is not possible for children with conventional hearing aids. It has been found that children implanted earlier in life usually do better than those implanted when they are older, and those with implants are more likely to go to mainstream schools than to schools for deaf children. In a longitudinal study of the first British congenitally deaf infant (without additional handicaps) to be fitted with multi-channel cochlear implants, it was found that the child's phonetic and phonological skills developed in the same way as a child with normal hearing or a child with a severe level of deafness using acoustic hearing aids would develop language. Children with implants also developed SUPRASEGMENTAL PHONOLOGY before including most of the back, central and front vowels (*see* CARDINAL VOWEL SYSTEM). Unlike many children with severe deafness and using acoustic hearing aids, this child was able to discriminate and moderate his own vocalisations to include high-frequency sounds within a year of implantation. He began to vary his vocalisations to use different voice patterns for different communicative purposes. After 2 years of using the cochlear implant, he had made the transition to spoken language through the auditory/vocal channel of communication and was at a comparable stage of development as his normally hearing cousin when matched for hearing age (HA). *See* Smith et al (2003); Tortora and Grabowski (2000); Allum-Mecklenberg (1996); Robinshaw (1996); Cooper (2001); RNID information sheet: http://www.rnid.org.uk/html/facsheets/med_cochlear_implants.htm implants. htm

cochlear nerve *see* EAR.

cochlear reflex *see* ELECTROCOCHLEOGRAPHY.

cochlear window *see* EAR.

cocktail party phenomenon the process of picking out what is said in a crowded room, setting aside all other linguistic information. This is known as selective listening. *See* Clark and Clark (1977); Smith et al (2003).

cocktail party syndrome described first by Williams in 1961, it was found in four unrelated children who had a learning disability, an unusual facial appearance and supravalvular aortic stenosis. It is also known as Williams' syndrome. Some of the most common abnormalities found by Williams and his colleagues were:

1. Mild prenatal growth deficiency and mild MICROCEPHALY.
2. Average IQ; friendly, loquacious personality, HOARSE VOICE and mild

neurological dysfunction. Perceptual and motor function is more reduced than verbal and memory performance.

3. Facial appearance is marked by prominent lips and open mouth.
4. Cardiovascular anomaly – supravalvular aortic stenosis.

During early infancy, these children tend to be fretful and have feeding problems. During childhood, they tend to be outgoing and loquacious, a personality referred to as 'cocktail party manner'. *See* Jones (1997).

Code–Müller Protocols (CMP) devised by Code and Müller, CMP is designed to gain information on the interpersonal perceptions of psychosocial adjustment between people who had APHASIA, significant others in their lives and the therapists working with them. It is a questionnaire of 10 items including ability to work, speak, be independent, to make relationships, to deal with frustration and embarrassment and so on. The result of the CMP is to evaluate the optimism concerning psychosocial adjustment by adding the scores together with higher scores giving higher optimism. However, as time has gone on, CMP has been used with other groups such as those who have had a LARYNGECTOMY and acquired deafness. *See* Code and Müller (1992); Code et al (1999).

coffee jar test a screening procedure developed by Gordon and McKinley (1980) to identify clumsy children. A number of common objects are included which the child is required to manipulate, e.g. threading beads is one of the tasks.

cognitive behaviour therapy a means of remedying behavioural and emotional disorders by trying to modify the person's thoughts. If cognitive methods are used to modify these thought processes, this is a cognitive therapy. Cognitive behaviour therapy or cognitive behaviour modification has been developed in the field of behaviour therapy. The basic premise is that emotional disorders are caused by maladaptive thought patterns and the main task of therapy is to remediate these processes. There are three main types of cognitive behaviour therapy:

1. Cognitive restructuring methods.
2. Coping skills procedures.
3. Problem-solving therapies.

It is the cognitive restructuring methods which make this type of behaviour therapy stand out from other psychological therapeutic techniques. There are three different cognitive restructuring methods commonly used:

1. Ellis's RATIONAL-EMOTIVE THERAPY.
2. Meichenbaum's SELF-INSTRUCTIONAL TRAINING.
3. BECK'S COGNITIVE THERAPY.

See Rachman and Wilson (1980); Smith et al (2003).

Cognitive Linguistic Quick Test CLQT devised by Helm-Estabrooks, the CLQT is designed to measure quickly strengths and weaknesses in five cognitive domains including attention, memory, executive functions, language and visuospatial skills. It can be used with adults, aged between 18 and 89, who have neurological problems as a result of a CVA, head injury or dementia. *See* Helm-Estabrooks (2001) in Appendix 1.

communicate a suite of vocabulary pages for the DYNAVOX. It has a large selection of core words, phrases and sentences with the following features: over 350 pop-up pages, phrases and single word vocabularies for 27 daily routines and 16 community-based situations as well as spelling and WORD PREDICTION. It comes in three formats – text-based, with DYNASYMS, or with PICTURE COMMUNICATION SYMBOLS for which PCS must be installed.

communication the ability to transfer information from one person either to another person or to a group of people. There has been much discussion as to the form the communication process takes. Thus, the speech chain came into being. When a link breaks in this chain, the result is a communication disorder and the therapist has to find ways to mend the links so the chain will function normally. *See* Denes and Pinson (1993).

Communication Activities of Daily Living (CADL) 2nd Edition devised by Holland and her colleagues, CADL is a test of functional communication which takes the form of a communication profile. There are 10 functional categories: (1) reading, writing and use of numbers; (2) SPEECH ACTS; (3) verbal and non-verbal contexts; (4) role playing; (5) divergencies; (6) relationship-dependent communicative behaviour; (7) non-verbal symbolic communication; (8) DEIXIS; (9) humour, absurdity; (10) use of metaphor. There is an attempt to relate CADL to type, cause and severity of APHASIA. The rating is on a three-point scale. Administration takes the form of a structured interview utilising props and situational contexts. It is designed for all age groups. CADL has two objectives: (1) to gain a valid reflection of communication skills; (2) to obtain a reliable assessment of these skills. It is a test of talking behaviour and communication, assessing more than just propositional and linguistic content. It does not discriminate against those who may use an augmentative and alternative communication system. *See* Holland (1980, 1999) in Appendix I; Eisenson (1984); Rosenbek et al (1989).

Communication Assessment Profile for Adults with a Mental Handicap (CASP) devised as a functional communication assessment for adults with a severe to mild LEARNING DISABILITY. However, it is unsuitable for those who have a profound learning disability or a severe visual impairment. The assessment is carried out by carer/key worker and speech and language therapist. There are three parts:

1. Carer's assessment: questionnaire concerning the client's communication abilities and requiring basic information about the client's daily life and environment.
2. Therapist's assessment: this concerns the client's communication abilities about event knowledge, hearing and auditory discrimination skills, vocabulary, comprehension of functional use of everyday objects, and comprehension and expression at sentence level.
3. Joint assessment: both the carer and therapist work together completing the summary of assessments, involving the client wherever possible.

The Communication Environment Rating Scale is completed, giving a broad outline of whether the client's different environments are enabling/encouraging him or her to use his or her communication skills. Priorities for change are also agreed. *See* Beech et al (1993).

communication board a low-tech form of augmentative and alternative communication. Thus, it can be used with those who have no or very limited verbal output which may be unintelligible or it may just be used as a temporary means of communication during therapy until the person's communication improves. The board can have pictures, symbols, words or phrases on it depending on what the person can understand best. *See* Fishman et al (1985); Glennen and Calculator (1985); Enderby (1987); Glennen and DeCoste (1997); Beukelman and Mirenda (1998); Robertson (2000).

communication disorder *see* COMMUNICATION.

communication profiles different types of assessment for testing the severity of APHASIA. The profiles examine in particular everyday situations in which those with aphasia may find themselves. Thus, people are tested in various situations such as 'greeting', 'understanding', 'social conventions' and so on. *See* Eisenson (1984).

Compact an all-in-one lightweight scanning environmental controller. It uses infra-red and radio control of appliances around the home and can have up to 31 definable functions as well as a unique sequencing mode which allows several functions to be accessed from a single selection. It has auditory tones to assist people who have visual problems. *See* Appendix IV (Possum).

compact a distinctive feature proposed by Jakobson and Halle for marking open vowels. They are denoted by [+COM-PACT] while other vowels are [−COMPACT]. The opposite is DIFFUSE. Chomsky and Halle described these vowels as LOW. *See* Hyman (1975).

compact bones *see* BONE.

Companion a sophisticated environmental controller allowing control of over 200 definable functions to control items in different rooms, home entertainment equipment, personal computer or communication aids. It can access a computer via its keyboard and mouse emulation. It has auditory prompts for people with visual problems and basic pre-recorded messages to assist with communication. *See* Appendix IV (Possum).

compatibility a phenomenon which, if it exists, would mean computer programs could be used on two different computers without having to be altered. Normally, it is impossible, for example, to write a program on a BBC computer using BBC BASIC and run it on an Apple microcomputer. However, wordprocessing documents can be copied from IBM PC computers to Apple Mac computers. Apple Macs with the Power PC chip can run any IBM PC computer software.

competence the knowledge individuals have of their own language. In Chomsky's view, competence, the normally implicit knowledge of the language, is opposed to PERFORMANCE, the implementation of this knowledge in speaking and understanding. *See* Lyons (1968); Nelson (1992) (competence and performance in AAC); Fromkin and Rodman (2003); Beukelman and Mirenda (1998).

complement the traditional sense is of an element of SENTENCE or CLAUSE structure which 'completes' the action of the verb. In this sense, it can refer to any obligatory post-verb element. In a more restricted sense, it refers to the 'completing' role of elements of structure following the verb 'to be' (or similar verbs), e.g. he is HAPPY, she was IN THE GARDEN, he is A TAXI DRIVER (the complement is shown in upper case). *See* Lyons (1968).

complementary distribution a type of phonological analysis. When two sounds belong to the same phonological unit or phoneme (*see* PHONOLOGY), they are in complementary distribution. In other words, there is no overlap between the distribution of the sounds, i.e. no overlap in the set of contexts in which the sound is found. *See* Hyman (1975); Fromkin and Rodman (2003).

compound racemose gland *see* SALIVARY GLANDS.

comprehension the process used by humans to understand forms of communication including speech, written language and gesture. Communication disorders such as APHASIA may have some elements of a comprehension disorder. In aphasia, there is often a distinction made between expressive and receptive disorders. The latter refers to comprehension problems as the way in which the person receives information either visually or auditorily. When children have an expressive language delay or disorder, their comprehension can still be better than their ability to produce utterances. Many people think that if the child can understand what is said to him, he will be able to produce a similar utterance which may not be the case. *See* Crystal and Varley (1998); Fromkin and Rodman (2003).

compulsion neurosis *see* OBSESSIVE-COMPULSIVE DISORDER.

compulsive rituals *see* AUTISM.

computed axial tomography *see* COMPUTED TOMOGRAPHY.

computed tomography (CT) a non-invasive X-ray technique used to locate space occupied by lesions. It differs from ordinary X-ray techniques in that it uses a narrow, moving beam which makes multiple scans of the brain. The results are processed by computer which distinguishes the different densities of brain tissue. Thus, lesions can be highlighted, some having a greater or lesser density than the surrounding brain tissue. A CT scan can pick out haemorrhages, tumours and cysts as well as atrophy, oedema, necrosis and changes due to MULTIPLE SCLEROSIS. *See* Barr (1988); Gilroy and Holliday (1982); Kaye (1991); Kolb and Whishaw (1996); Ginsbergh (1999).

concept keyboard an input device for operating software without having to use the computer's QWERTY KEYBOARD.

concord the grammatical phenomenon in which a form of one word in a sentence 'agrees' with a corresponding form in another word. For example, in English the subject of a sentence agrees with the verb in the present tense:

1. The dog runs away.
2. The dogs run away.

In (1), the singular form of the verb has the affix '-s' while in (2), the plural form has a zero morph (i.e. no affix) and is just 'run'. *See* Lyons (1968); Fromkin and Rodman (2003).

concrete operations the third stage of PIAGET's theory of the child's cognitive development during the 7–11-year-old period, having overcome the difficulties found during the pre-operational stage. The child's thought processes are now becoming more logical but he can still only understand relationships directly perceived by him (i.e., the child cannot yet think abstractly). During this stage the child can work out hierarchies of classes and sub-classes and can also place shapes in order by size without measuring them. *See* Beard (1969).

conditioned response *see* CLASSICAL CONDITIONING.

conditioned stimulus *see* CLASSICAL CONDITIONING.

conditioning tests tests used to assess the hearing of some young children (from about 2;6 years) who are too young to be tested by PURE-TONE AUDIOMETRY. It is based on OPERANT CONDITIONING. The children are told to do a specific action, e.g. put brick in box, put peg in peg board, when they hear a specific sound. The sounds are either pure tones (*see* PURE-TONE AUDIOMETRY) or warbles (*see* WARBLE TONE). When the child responds accurately and consistently then the intensity is reduced until the child's hearing threshold is reduced. The child should receive a reinforcement after a correct response.

conduct disorder persistent socially disapproved behaviour associated with social impairment. The prevalence is 3–9 per cent of school-age children. Conduct disorders are most common in boys (4:1); most children affected come from social classes IV and V. The causes arise from the child's experience of life:

1. Family factors – persistent conflict, divorce, etc.
2. Social factors – poor housing, etc.
3. Educational factors – one-third of these children have learning difficulties, especially with reading, etc.
4. Temperamental factors – unpredictable reactions, irritability, etc.

The most common symptoms include: fighting and bullying, aggression and temper tantrums, defiance and disobedience, destructiveness, lying, stealing, truancy, fire setting and arson. The major types of conduct disorder include:

1. Socialised conduct disorder: children who have failed to acquire socially approved standards of behaviour. However, within the family they can often make warm relationships and are often described as 'likeable rogues'.
2. Unsocialised conduct disorder: a more severe disorder in which children form poor peer relationships.

They are frequently self-destructive, aggressive and seem keen to be punished. Family life is always discordant, discipline harsh and little affection is shown to the child, who thus experiences rejection.

3. Mixed conduct and emotional disorder: children are indifferent to stress, resulting in abnormal behaviour.

Many children with a conduct disorder are restless and overactive for a short period of time but a small number are extremely and persistently overactive. Such children have problems from an early age. All psychotherapies (*see* PSYCHOTHERAPY) can be used to treat this condition. *See* Rutter (1975); Davison et al (2004).

conduction the transmission of sounds from one point to another.

conduction aphasia a major type of APHASIA described by the BOSTON SCHOOL. It is caused by damage to the ARCUATE FASCICULUS in the left hemisphere (*see* CEREBRAL HEMISPHERES). For a discussion of the communication problems in conduction aphasia, *see* APHASIA (3). *See* Goodglass and Kaplan (2000) in Appendix I; Rosenbek et al (1989).

conductive hearing loss a HEARING LOSS caused by a pathology affecting the conduction of sound through the outer ear and/or middle ear into the inner ear (*see* EAR).

confabulation a symptom of amnesia. The person who tries not to accept he has memory problems fills in the gaps in his memory with made-up information. *See* Davison et al (2004).

congenital disorder a disorder which appears at birth, perhaps as a result of a problem during the PRENATAL, PERINATAL or POSTNATAL periods or an inherited trait. It is opposed to a DEVELOPMENTAL DISORDER which occurs during childhood.

congenital hearing loss a hearing loss which occurs before the period of language development (*see* ACQUISITION). It can be caused by various diseases during the PRENATAL and PERINATAL periods.

congenital muscular dystrophy a congenital myopathy. A range of disorders of muscles which present as progressive weakness of muscles. The severe physical breakdown of the muscle is similar to other forms of DYSTROPHY. Treatment is given through PHYSIOTHERAPY. *See* Gilroy and Holliday (1982); Hosking (1982).

congenital neuronal dysfunction a condition which produces sudden, abnormal discharges of neurons in the brain, producing epileptic convulsions. This occurs in the RETICULAR SYSTEM in the centrencephalon. Thus, the type of EPILEPSY produced is known as centrencephalic epilepsy. *See* Ginsbergh (1999).

connected speech a particular type of speech. It describes the way in which conversation and different kinds of utterances are put together. It is opposed to speaking with single words and phrases which can function differently in general conversation. Prosodic features (*see* PROSODY) used in flowing speech are especially important. *See* Cruttenden (1994).

connective tissue (CT) tissue made up in a ground substance comprising fibres. There are two types determined by the type and quantity of fibres in the ground substance – packing connective tissue and supporting tissue. In the former there are two subgroups – reticular tissue and loose/dense CT, while the latter comprises BONE and CARTILAGE. *See* Tortora and Grabowski (2000).

consonant a speech sound which is not a vowel (*see* CARDINAL VOWEL SYSTEM). Such sounds have specific descriptions for the way they are articulated. They are described in terms of their voicing, place of articulation and manner of articulation (*see* ARTICULATION). *See* Ladefoged (2001).

consonant cluster a grouping of two or more abutting consonants in different parts of a word:

1. Word-initially – 'step', 'grape', 'blame', etc.
2. Word-medially – 'birthday', 'temper', 'ember', etc.
3. Word-finally – 'lamps', 'damp', 'jingle', etc.

Grunwell (1987) suggests rules for producing consonant clusters based on Cruttenden (1994). For example, for two-place initial clusters: C1, C2: '(1) where C1 is /s/, C2 must be one of /ptkmnwlj(f)/ (e.g. sphinx); (2) where C2 is one of /wrlj/, C1 may be one of a large number of consonants predominantly obstruents, including /ptkbdgfθ/ etc.' Other rules can be found for three-place clusters. *See* Grunwell (1987).

consonantal any sound or movement in the VOCAL TRACT which involves obstruction or some degree of constriction to the airflow. A DISTINCTIVE FEATURE used to differentiate sounds into two groups. [+CONSONANTAL] sounds are produced with an obstruction in the airstream when it reaches the mouth and are produced with low acoustic energy; [–CONSONANTAL] sounds are produced with little or no obstruction and high acoustic energy. *See* Hyman (1975).

constituent analysis the analysis of the hierarchical structure of sentences. The rules that follow exemplify a (highly simplified) account of the constituent structure of English sentences using phrase structure rules:

S $\longrightarrow$ NP + VP
NP $\longrightarrow$ (det) + (adj) + N
VP $\longrightarrow$ V + (NP)
PrepP $\longrightarrow$ Prep + NP

The rules define the hierarchical structure of English sentences. The symbols and abbreviations represent the constituents:

S = sentence
NP = noun phrase
VP = verb phrase
PrepP = prepositional phrase
det = determiner
adj = adjective

N = noun
V = verb
Aux = auxiliary
$\longrightarrow$ = 'consists of'

The first rule means a 'sentence consists of a noun phrase plus a verb phrase'. The brackets in the following rules mean the constituents in the brackets are optional. These rules are often called rewrite rules as the left-hand side of the formula can be rewritten in the form on the right-hand side. There may be only one symbol on the left while any number of symbols can appear on the right. The '+' symbol is the ordering symbol, so in the first rule a verb phrase must follow a noun phrase. This type of analysis can be shown graphically by use of branches in a TREE DIAGRAM or by BRACKETING. *See* Brown and Miller (1991).

constriction narrowing in the VOCAL TRACT. It is used when making a CONSONANT sound. *See* Catford (1977).

constructional apraxia impairment in producing two- or three-dimensional designs by copying, drawing or in construction either to command or spontaneously. There is difficulty with spatial orientation and body orientation. Difficulty with dressing, exemplified by putting clothes on back to front or inside out is related to an orientation problem rather than a motor disorder. Those who have right-sided lesions will neglect dressing the left side of the body or put both legs in the same trouser leg. *See* Kolb and Whishaw (1996).

constructs *see* PERSONAL CONSTRUCT THEORY.

contact ulcers growths that appear on the vocal folds producing a hoarse voice. The symptoms of contact ulcers are:

1. Extreme localised and generalised tension of the folds.
2. Explosive speech patterns.
3. Sudden glottal stops.
4. Restricted pitch.
5. Habitual throat clearing.

They are produced by the hard cartilaginous surfaces of the vocal processes hitting the opposite fold. Therapy takes the form of reducing the effort in phonation, reducing the pitch level of the voice, slowing down speech RATE with a relaxed mouth and jaw and at a lower volume, as well as stopping the use of hard glottal attack. *See* Greene and Mathieson (1989); Freeman and Fawcus (2001).

continuant a distinctive feature proposed by Chomsky and Halle to distinguish sounds produced from friction [+CONT] from those produced without [–CONT]. This phonological description is equivalent to the articulatory description of a fricative (*see* ARTICULATION). *See* Hyman (1975).

contour *see* SUPRASEGMENTAL PHONOLOGY.

contrastive analysis a phonological analysis of a person's sound system (*see* PHONOLOGY) which involves the comparison of one sound system with another. The sound system of a young child can be compared with that of an adult so as to find out what sound(s) the child is lacking. In the same way, it can be used with children whose sound system is disordered. By comparing the children's disordered sound system to a normal sound system, it is possible to find out what sounds they have and which are lacking in their system. However, Cruttenden (1972) believes this analysis is inappropriate, if not impossible, to use because the child's acquisition of sounds is so erratic. He states: 'Child language is so unfixed, so constantly changing that it is doubtful whether the term is appropriate'. If this type of analysis is used by the clinician, the variation in the child's acquisition of sounds should be taken into account. By using this form of analysis, it is possible to find out if there is a regular error pattern since the therapist can work out in which part of the word(s) the sound substitution, omission, distortion or addition takes place. *See* Grunwell (1987).

contrecoup effect *see* HEAD INJURY.

control group one of two groups which take part in an experiment, the other group being the experimental group. The control group is regarded as the group of subjects against which the performance of the experimental group will be compared. Control groups and experimental groups are used in INDEPENDENT GROUP DESIGN. It is also called the control condition. *See* Miller (1984); Porkess (1988).

conversion reaction the sudden impairment of muscular and sensory functions associated with psychological factors. The arms and legs can become weak, blindness can occur and those affected may no longer feel pain although they are physiologically normal. People may also become dysphonic (*see* DYSPHONIA). The effects of a stress-provoking situation produce these symptoms or a nervous reaction following a long period of excitement which suddenly ends. *See* Freeman and Fawcus (2001) (for conversion reaction and dysphonia); Davison et al (2004).

convulsion the sudden onset of seizure-like, involuntary movements, e.g. grand-mal epilepsy (*see* EPILEPSY), FEBRILE CONVULSIONS. *See* Gilroy and Holliday (1982).

coprolalia the significant increase of abusive and obscene language.

copula a grammatical description of a verb linking two parts of a sentence, usually the subject and the complement. In a majority of cases the copulative verb in English is 'to be':

1. The men are tall.

but there can be other verbs used in the same way:

2. He felt very well
3. You look great!

See Lyons (1968); Fromkin and Rodman (2003).

cordectomy the surgical removal of a VOCAL FOLD for tumours on the fold. When one fold is removed, the one which remains will usually compensate completely. If this does not happen, a TEFLON INJECTION might be required to enable this compensation to occur.

core vocabulary when choosing vocabulary for either a low or high-tech AAC system, there are two types of vocabulary – core and fringe vocabulary. The former comprises words or phrases which are used very frequently and very commonly by most people. Those working with people using AAC have relied on three sources of core vocabulary: word lists based on vocabulary-use patterns of other people who use AAC systems successfully; word lists based on the use patterns of the specific individual and word lists based on the performance of natural speakers or writers in similar contexts. Some AAC high-tech devices allow the person's low-tech systems to be stored into it and so they will have the same core vocabulary in both systems. See Beukelman and Mirenda (1998).

coronal a DISTINCTIVE FEATURE proposed by Chomsky and Halle to distinguish sounds produced with the tip of the tongue [+COR] from those which are not [–COR]. This phonological description is similar to the articulatory description of alveolar, dental and palatoalveolar consonants (*see* ARTICULATION). *See* Hyman (1975).

coronoid process *see* MANDIBLE.

corpus callosum the part of the BRAIN which links the two CEREBRAL HEMISPHERES and covers the lateral ventricle (*see* THIRD VENTRICLE). Its main body is about 8 cm long and it carries information from one hemisphere to the other. *See* Barr (1988); Kolb and Whishaw (1996).

correlation the statistical relationship of two variables. It is represented by the symbol 'r'. The range of the correlation is from -1 to $+1$. As one variable changes and the second variable changes in a similar way, they are said to be correlated. When the correlation coefficient is $+1$, the variables are said to have positive correlation while a -1 coefficient means the variables have a negative correlation and a 0 coefficient means there is no correlation. *See* Miller (1984); Porkess (1988).

cortex a layer of grey matter which covers the two CEREBRAL HEMISPHERES. It is shaped into folds. Its total weight accounts for about 40 per cent of the weight of the brain. It is full of neurons and fibres, and is 1–4 mm thick. *See* Barr (1988); Kolb and Whishaw (1996); Tortora and Grabowski (2000).

cortical a term for describing structures or disorders found in or near the cortex.

cortical evoked response audiometry (CERA) an audiometric test to check the late responses of the CORTEX. The results are displayed as stage III on the graph of auditory evoked responses. The electrodes have a similar placement to that for the AUDITORY BRAINSTEM RESPONSE (ABR). The person is given a series of tone bursts with slow rise and fall on each frequency. It is non-invasive, frequency specific and gives an objective measure of the person's response. Although it is a very slow test to administer, it comes very close to the hearing threshold. *See* Jacobson and Hyde (1985).

corticosteroids used for treating inflammatory diseases by reducing the inflammatory reaction and preventing the adverse effects of prolonged pressure. *See* Tortora and Grabowski (2000).

counselling a method of helping people to overcome their problems and help them to help themselves. The aim is to allow the person to come to terms with their own problems and work out what they can do rather than for the therapist to work out the solution to their problems. Often, the relationship between the person and the counsellor is particularly important rather than the type of counselling adhered to by the therapist. Carl Rogers proposed three important attributes for the counsellor:

1. Congruence, i.e. the counsellor has to demonstrate 'genuineness or authenticity'.
2. Unconditional positive regard, i.e. 'prizing, warmth, non-possessive warmth, or, most commonly, respect'.

3. Empathic understanding, i.e. 'a very special way of being with another person'. (Nelson-Jones 1982)

Communication is the all-important factor in helping people to come to terms with their problems. Other approaches have been considered but the therapist's personality is the most important factor. *See* Nelson-Jones (1982); Dalton (1994).

count nouns nouns which the language treats as separable entities, as evidenced by their use with numerals, e.g. one boy, two boys; one book, two books, etc. They are opposed to MASS NOUNS. *See* Palmer (1976).

counterbalancing a procedure used to try to overcome the order effect confounding the results of an experiment. When an experiment is carried out with two groups or more of subjects carrying out task A followed by task B, the results can be confounded by effects of fatigue, subtle changes in their instructions or familiarity with the situation. The way to overcome these difficulties is to counterbalance the groups where half of the subjects work under condition A first and half work under condition B. *See* Miller (1984).

CR conditioned response (*see* CLASSICAL CONDITIONING).

cranial nerves nerves that leave the BRAIN to innervate different muscles throughout the body. There are 12 nerves with the following functions:

I	Olfactory – sense of smell
II	Optic – vision
III	Oculomotor – supplies extraocular muscles
IV	Trochlear – supplies superior oblique muscles
V	Trigeminal – comprises three parts: i ophthalmic ii maxillary (upper jaw) iii mandibular (lower jaw)
VI	Abducens – supplies lateral rectus
VII	Facial – supplies muscles of facial expression (motor component)
VIII	Vestibulocochlear – supplies balance and hearing
IX	Glossopharyngeal – supplies general sensation and taste; supplies sensory component and pharyngeal plexus
X	Vagus – supplies parasympathetic component of cardiac oesophageal and pulmonary plexi; sensory component supplies the superior laryngeal nerves and recurrent laryngeal nerves
XI	Accessory – supplies the spinal and cervical areas of the spine
XII	Hypoglossal – supplies all intrinsic and extrinsic muscles of the tongue except the palatoglossus (*see* MOUTH).

Motor nerve fibres originating in the BRAIN cross over in the brain to supply muscles on the opposite side of the body. Thus, if a CEREBROVASCULAR ACCIDENT occurs in the left CEREBRAL HEMISPHERE, there will be a HEMIPLEGIA down the right side, as the nerves from the left hemisphere will be affected. *See* Gilroy and Holliday (1982); Tortora and Grabowski (2000).

creaky voice a description of a person's voice produced at a very low pitch. This occurs usually in males. The arytenoid cartilages (*see* ARYTENOIDS) hold one end of the folds tightly closed, which produces irregular vibrations at a low pitch. The sound produced may be called laryngealised. *See* Ladefoged (2001).

cretinism a congenital condition caused by an abnormality in the thyroid gland (*see* TRACHEA) and the amount of hormone it secretes. The clinical features may include: LEARNING DISABILITY, general sluggishness, anaemia, small stature, coarse skin, large tongue, low temperature, slow pulse and chronic constipation. Treatment consists of the provision of thyroid extract at an early stage which produces a good prognosis for physical development, but is probably of little value for improving the learning disability. *See* Clarke and Clarke (1974); Tortora and Grabowski (2000).

Creutzfeldt-Jakob disease a spongiform encephalopathy affecting the CENTRAL NERVOUS SYSTEM (CNS). It progresses slowly throughout the CNS and produces dementia. It affects people between the ages of 35 and 63 years of age and is found worldwide. It lasts for about 6 months to 3 years after diagnosis. The symptoms include a loss of short-term memory (*see* MEMORY), APHASIA and hallucinations. The person may also have cortical blindness, ataxia (*see* CEREBRAL PALSY) and myoclonus. There is a fast decline to DEMENTIA. However, in the 1990s in the UK there were reports of a new variant CJD which seemed to have its own clinical signs (see http://www.cjd.ed.ac.uk/lancet.htm). There is no effective treatment. *See* Gilroy and Holliday (1982); Kolb and Whishaw (1996); http://www.cjd.ed.ac.uk/lancet.htm; http://www.healthlinkusa.com/84A.asp

cri-du-chat syndrome a syndrome described first by Lejeune and his colleagues in 1963. The following disorders are found:

1. Low birth weight, slow growth and high-pitched cat-like cry (produced by abnormal laryngeal development which disappears gradually as the child becomes older).
2. LEARNING DISABILITY and hypotonia.
3. MICROCEPHALY, round face, epicanthal folds, strabismus (often divergent), low set and/or poorly formed, facial asymmetry.
4. Congenital heart disease.
5. Abnormal hands with simian crease, distal axial triradius and slightly short metacarpals.

See Hosking (1982); Jones (1997).

cricoarytenoid *see* LARYNX.

cricoid cartilage *see* LARYNX.

cross-hearing a phenomenon in which sounds heard in one ear could have come from the outer ear via bone conduction or the air around the head. This can cause confusion when testing a person's hearing.

Crowe's Protocols: A Comprehensive Guide to Stuttering Assessment devised by Crowe and his colleagues, Crowe's Protocols allow for establishing a prognosis and defining treatment goals for people of all ages who have fluency disorders. The following areas are evaluated by the assessor and those who have a fluency disorder themselves: cultural variabilities, physical measures of dysfluency, language-based assessment, personality measures, avoidance behaviours, attitudes, concomitant behaviours, anxiety, intelligence, knowledge of stuttering, aetiology, stimulability, counselling and prognosis. See Crowe et al (2000) in Appendix I (stammering).

CS (conditioned stimulus) *see* CLASSICAL CONDITIONING.

CSF *see* CEREBROSPINAL FLUID.

CT *see* CONNECTIVE TISSUE.

CT scan *see* COMPUTED TOMOGRAPHY.

cued speech devised by Cornett in 1966 as an augmentative and alternative communication system. It is not a sign language as such, but rather an oral approach supported by hand signs. The instructor can show the person the sound orally while the shape made by the hand clearly 'shows' which sound has been made. *See* Kiernan et al (1982); Beukelman and Mirenda (1998).

cues techniques used by the therapist to help the person succeed in therapy. These cues may be:

1. Signing, i.e. giving a clue to the correct response by gesture.
2. Semantic, i.e. giving the meaning of the word.
3. Phonemic, i.e. giving the first sound of the correct response.
4. Repetition, i.e. the therapist gives the response which is repeated.
5. Visual, i.e. the therapist produces a picture of the correct response, perhaps with some distractors, so that

there is certainty about the correct response.

See Rosenbek et al (1989); Glennen and DeCoste (1997) (AAC).

cuneiform cartilages found in the LARYNX. There are two cartilages. They look like small mounds and appear in the aryepiglottic fold. *See* Tortora and Grabowski (2000).

cursor the symbol (often a small flashing rectangle or horizontal or vertical line) which indicates the position on the screen where characters or graphics symbols will next appear. The cursor can move to any point on the screen. *See* Bishop (1985); Brookshear (1991).

Cushing's disease *See* DEPRESSION.

CV *See* PHONOTACTICS.

CVA *See* CEREBROVASCULAR ACCIDENT.

CVC *See* PHONOTACTICS.

CWLWM devised by Rees and Trythal, CWLWM is a phonetic screening assessment to indicate areas of difficulty in Welsh children's speech production.

There is a picture book to elicit 49 target words. It is suitable for children from 3;00 upwards.

cyanosis a condition due to the presence of more than 5g of reduced haemoglobin in the circulation. It imparts a blue colour to lips, tongue, nose and finger nails. It may be due to conditions such as chronic bronchitis, emphysema, pneumonia or heart disease. *See* Tortora and Grabowski (2000).

cytomegalovirus a highly infectious viral condition that affects nervous tissue. It is one of the diseases which can produce disorders in children, if the mother has it during the PRENATAL stage of the child's development. It can result in LEARNING DISABILITY, CEREBRAL PALSY and other disabilities. It is part of the TORCH classification of conditions which can affect the fetus during the prenatal period. *See* Hosking (1982); http://www.cdc.gov/ncidod/diseases/cmv.htm

dactylology *see* FINGERSPELLING.

DAF *see* DELAYED AUDITORY FEEDBACK.

daisywheel printer a type of printer that produces printouts or hard copy by means of a wheel or thimble placed on the print unit with spokes emanating from the centre with characters at their ends which are hit by a hammer against a ribbon. The print wheel looks like a daisy, hence the name daisywheel printer. *See* Bishop (1985).

damping a reduction of the amplitude of vibrations in a vibrating object. For example, a tuning fork begins to vibrate when it is struck against an object and resonates at a particular frequency. If the tuning fork is touched when it is vibrating, the amplitude of the vibrations is reduced and dies away. *See* Denes and Pinson (1993).

Dandy-Walker malformation also known as Dandy-Walker cyst, this is due to obstruction from birth of the foramina of Majendie and Lushka with resultant enlargement of the ventricles. This results in an abnormally large head and is associated with HYDROCEPHALUS while the brain tissue around it fails to grow adequately. *See* Hosking (1982); Kaye (1991); http://www.bcm.tmc.edu/pednsurg/disorder/wpdandy.htm

DDK rates *see* DIADOCHOKINESIS.

deaf a description of people who cannot use their hearing as a primary channel of communication even with amplification. *See* Martin (2001).

death instinct *see* PSYCHOANALYSIS.

debugging the process of finding and correcting errors in a computer program that may prevent it from being run. Errors can be of two types – those which are produced because of lack of logic in the writing of the program and those which are produced by a mistake in the codes used during the program. The latter are known as syntax errors. These can be caused by failing to use the correct command word or fail to use the correct punctuation in a line of the program. *See* Bishop (1985).

declarative sentence a sentence which makes a statement. It contrasts with interrogative and imperative in the classification of sentence types, e.g. 'the man went into town'. *See* Lyons (1968).

DECtalk SPEECH SYNTHESIS used with some high-tech communication aids including TOUCHTALKERS, DELTA TALKERS, the LIBERATOR COMMUNICATION AID, CAMELEON, ORAC and DYNAVOX. It produces 10 voices – four male, four female, a child's voice and one which can be either male or female. Each voice can be modified within specific parameters to allow inflection and other speech characteristics. *See* Keller (1994); Glennen and DeCoste (1997); Beukelman and Mirenda 1998);

Rumble and Larcher (1998); Appendix IV (Digital Equipment Company).

deep dyslexia *see* ACQUIRED DYSLEXIA.

deep structure *see* CASE GRAMMAR; TRANSFORMATIONAL GRAMMAR.

defence mechanisms processes, proposed by Freud among others, to allow people to protect themselves against anxiety-provoking situations. These mechanisms involve some degree of self-deception. Defence mechanisms are regarded as the 'normal' way of coping with stress (*see* HYSTERIA), as long as the person does face the stressful situation. They become an abnormal response when they become the dominant way of coping with problems. The defence mechanisms often cited are:

1. Repression: painful memories and various impulses are hidden by the person.
2. Rationalisation: where logical motives are worked out by the person so that they seem to have acted rationally.
3. Reaction formation: where a person tries to hide a motive by going to the opposite extreme.
4. Projection: where people, in trying to ignore their own undesirable qualities, project them to an extreme degree onto someone else.
5. Intellectualisation: where a person deals with undesirable topics, e.g. death, in an abstract and intellectual way to become detached from the situation.
6. Denial: where the person denies that the anxiety-provoking situation exists.
7. Displacement: where if a motive cannot be gratified in one form, the person tries to overcome it using another channel.

See Smith et al (2003).

degeneration the progressive wasting of part of the body or structures within the body caused by disease. Nerves in the peripheral nervous and CENTRAL NERVOUS SYSTEM can degenerate by Wallerian degeneration. Its opposite is regeneration. *See* Barr (1988); Kolb and Whishaw (1996).

deglutition *see* SWALLOWING.

degrees of freedom *see* *t*-TEST.

deixis a linguistic term for those features of sentence/clause structure which relate that sentence to specific temporal or locational features of the situation of the utterance. Deictic words include: here/there, now/then, I/you, etc. *See* Lyons (1968); Fromkin and Rodman (2003).

Déjérine's syndrome *see* ACQUIRED DYSLEXIA (3).

delayed auditory feedback (DAF) a means of interrupting the way we hear ourselves speak. In the treatment of people who STAMMER, an electronic device is used to interrupt the person listening to his/her own speech. While it can have the effect of making the dysfluent person more fluent, it has an opposite effect on the fluent person. Under normal conditions, when people speak they can hear it through their auditory feedback system as the sound travels to the ear through the bones in the skull. This chain of events is broken when using a DAF machine as there is a delay inserted between the person speaking and hearing what is said. This delay will slow down the RATE of speech so that the speaker can check what has been said before continuing. As DYSFLUENCY can be produced by a very fast rate of speech, if the person slows down, he can often speak more fluently. It can also be used with other communication disorders where the rate of speech may be very fast, such as some forms of DYSARTHRIA or DYSPHONIA.

delayed conditioning *see* CLASSICAL CONDITIONING (2).

delayed echolalia *see* ECHOLALIA.

delayed release a distinctive feature proposed by Chomsky and Halle. It describes sounds produced by gradual release as in the case of the fricative part of affricates (*see* ARTICULATION) which are all described as [+delayed release]. It is also used in ARTICULATORY PHONETICS. *See* Hyman (1975).

Delta Talker a high-tech communication aid with digitised speech output and synthetic voice. It uses MINSPEAK to organise vocabulary to store into the device. It has a memory of two and a half minutes for digitised speech and 256K of memory for synthetic voice. It has similar features to the ALPHA TALKER and the LIBERATOR COMMUNICATION AID in that it uses icon prediction to show where messages are stored and predictive selection where locations without messages are dead. This allows the device to have a predictive scan facility. There are also auditory prompts for those who have visual impairment. It has a visual display unit of two lines where accessed vocabulary will appear whether stored using digitised or synthetic outputs. The overlays can be reduced to 8 and 32 locations. The device allows for direct selection either manually or by optical headpointing, single, dual or two-switch scanning as well as using a multi-switch such as a joystick. *See* Glennen and DeCoste (1997); Rumble and Larcher (1998); Appendix IV (Prentke Romich Company).

delusion false, unreasonable belief which the person holds and will not waver from under any amount of reasoned argument. Such delusions have a strong element of meaning to them. These are often called primary delusions. If people have secondary delusions, they follow a similar pattern but they try to find a reasonable explanation for other abnormal experiences such as HALLUCINATIONS, illusions, etc. *See* Stafford-Clark and Bridges (1990); Smith et al (2003); Davison et al (2004).

dementia the progressive loss of function of brain cells producing changes in a person's character especially in old age. The damage may be caused by trauma, infections to the CENTRAL NERVOUS SYSTEM, tumours (*see* TUMOURS OF THE CENTRAL NERVOUS SYSTEM), metabolic disorders, infarctions or haemorrhages (*see* CEREBROVASCULAR ACCIDENT). The principle dementias are ALZHEIMER'S DISEASE or senile dementia, MULTI-INFARCT DEMENTIA, PICK'S DISEASE, NORMAL PRESSURE HYDROCEPHALUS, CREUTZFELDT-JAKOB DISEASE and HUNTINGTON'S DISEASE. There is global loss of functioning affecting intelligence, learning, memory, motor skills and social skills. Its progress is slow but inexorable. The prevalence of dementia is 5 per cent of people by 65 years of age and 15–20 per cent of people by the age of 80 years. It can occur in children although rarely. *See* Stafford-Clark and Bridges (1990); Gilroy and Holliday (1982); Davison et al (2004); Kolb and Whishaw (1996); Bourgeois et al (2001) (AAC and dementia).

demonstrative pronouns deictic words which refer the person reading or hearing them to a specific object or person near to or removed from the speaker. Such pronouns include 'this/that'. *See* Lyons (1968).

dendrite part of a neuron which is short, chubby and has many branches emanating at one end while at the other there is a long axon. Dendrites conduct nerve impulses toward the cell body. *See* Kolb and Whishaw (1996); Tortora and Grabowski (2000).

dental *see* ARTICULATION.

dependent clause *see* CLAUSE.

depression an affective disorder. Its precise cause is unknown but it is thought it could be due to a combination of factors including genetic, sex, life stress, biochemical as well as cognitive problems, with one or two being more prominent than the others. It affects three areas: mood, response to stimulation and functioning of the AUTONOMIC NERVOUS SYSTEM. These problems have all been summed up succinctly by Stafford-Clark: 'Unable to sleep, to eat, to work efficiently, to hope or to enjoy any of the simple pleasures of life, he may all too often despair of his plight, to die may then seem to him to be all that is left' (Stafford-Clark and Bridges, 1990). There are three types of depression:

1. Simple/minor depression: a general slowing down in activity with people

feeling sad, miserable, and worried, resulting in a loss of interest in everyday activities. It does not appear as a medical problem.

2. Endogenous/major depression: the person has a permanently depressed mood, feelings of hopelessness, helplessness, worthlessness, poor sleep and appetite regimes, due to anxiety.

3. Psychotic depression: a major characteristic is delusions plus a severely depressed mood, severe weight loss and a high risk of suicide. Psychotic depression has as a contributory factor Cushing's disease which is a disorder of the adrenal glands producing an abnormal amount of cortisol.

Depression in itself is a unipolar disorder while manic-depression is a bipolar disorder. It can be treated by tricyclic ANTIDEPRESSANT DRUGS, MONOAMINE OXIDASE INHIBITORS, ELECTROCONVULSIVE THERAPY, PSYCHOSURGERY, LITHIUM and various forms of PSYCHOTHERAPY. *See* Stafford-Clark and Bridges (1990); Kolb and Whishaw (1996); Smith et al (2003); Davison et al (2004); http://www.depressionalliance.org/Contents/index.htm

depressor anguli labii inferioris *see* MUSCLES OF FACIAL EXPRESSION.

Derbyshire Language Scheme (DLS) devised by Masidlover and Knowles in 1977 (revised 1987) for use with children who have a language delay/disorder. It has non-standardised assessment procedures to test the severity of the delay and teaching procedures based on the preceding assessment. It is based on the natural communication of the child by playing with toys and looking at pictures. Language is taught and assessed through play. The criterion for success is the child using what he has learnt during the therapy sessions at home and in the community. The assessment is divided into two parts: the Rapid Screening Test and the Detailed Test of Comprehension. The results of these assessments can be placed onto an assessment summary. There is a progress record to show graphically the child's performance, and to reveal areas of language development which still require therapy. *See* Masidlover and Knowles (1987) in Appendix I; Beech et al (1993).

descriptive grammar a person's basic linguistic knowledge of a language. It does not prescribe how one should speak but how it is possible to speak and understand as well as about the sounds, words, phrases and sentences of a particular language. *See* Fromkin and Rodman (2003).

descriptive statistics a part of statistics which analyses the scores obtained from experiments using bar charts, HISTOGRAMS, measures of CENTRAL TENDENCY, STANDARD DEVIATION, PERCENTILE SCORES and Z SCORES. *See* Miller (1984); Porkess (1988).

Detailed Test of Comprehension (DTC) an assessment procedure used in the DERBYSHIRE LANGUAGE SCHEME. It is used after the RAPID SCREENING TEST has been administered so that the therapist can assess more accurately the problems which the child has in comprehension and expressive language. These two aspects of communication are tested in natural contexts using everyday toys and pictures. The authors introduce the concept of information-carrying words, i.e. how many words the child requires to understand a command. In the example below, the sentences are from different levels of the DTC. In other words, the child has to show his comprehension at different levels by ignoring similar distractors. When testing the child's expressive language, the therapist writes down everything the child says during the test even if it is unconnected with the toys or pictures used in the test – see boxed example over leaf. *See* Masidlover and Knowles (1987) in Appendix I.

determiner a constituent which precedes a noun to show differences in meaning between nouns, e.g. quantity and number. Usually a determiner is one of the

Instruction	No. of item	Comp. level
Wash the teddy	TEDDY	0
WASH the TEDDY	CLOTH, BRUSH, TEDDY, DOLL	2
WASH the TEDDY'S FOOT	SAME AS ABOVE	3
WASH the LITTLE TEDDY'S FOOT	LITTLE TEDDY, BIG TEDDY	4
	LITTLE DOLL, CLOTH, BRUSH	

articles, either definite or indefinite ('a', 'an', 'the'), but it can also be a personal, possessive or demonstrative pronoun or a word signifying quantity. The determiner marks a NOUN PHRASE and usually appears at the beginning of a noun phrase. *See* Strang (1968).

Developing Language devised by Rinaldi in 2000, Developing Language is a metacognitive approach to teaching grammar and meaning. It is a comprehensive teaching/therapy programme for professionals working with individuals or groups of children who have language difficulties. Two manuals cover the developmental period of 10 months to 7;00+. Manual 1 covers the early stages of language development (10 months to 2;06) in comprehension and use from single words to four word combinations while manual 2 covers aspects of grammar and meaning acquired in the relatively later stages of communication development. *See* Rinaldi (2000) in Appendix I.

developmental aphasia *see* APHASIA.

developmental apraxia of speech (DAS) a disorder found in children with symptoms similar to those found in ACQUIRED APRAXIA. Research into developmental apraxia of speech has shown a consensus on its symptoms including deviant consonant and vowel productions, sequencing difficulties with phonemes and syllables, groping and trial-and-error behaviours and inconsistency in articulation. In 1997, Thoonen et al set out to create a standardised procedure to assess quantitatively this speech disorder. The authors had three aims in their study: to examine a standardised procedure of speech elicitation (i.e. single word-imitation) to assess symptoms that are relevant for the diagnosis of DAS; select a set of speech parameters that form a quantitative score for the severity of DAS and characterise the patterns of consonant errors that are specific to DAS. The results showed that the children assessed with their procedure produced similar types of consonant errors as had been reported previously, there was a large quantitative difference between children with DAS and children who did not have DAS, in that those with DAS produced an overall higher rate of singleton consonant errors (substitutions, omissions, distortions) and cluster errors (cluster reductions (*see* PHONOLOGICAL PROCESSES (5)); and the substitution-rate in the same group of children, particularly in real words as opposed to nonsense words, was significantly correlated with severity as rated by two speech and language pathologists which could suggest substitution-rate is an adequate measure of DAS. Finally, a qualitative difference between both groups emerged in that children with DAS did not benefit from the lexical status of the utterance (real versus nonsense words) to the same extent as those children without DAS. *See* Miller (1986); Adams et al (1997); Culp (1989) (AAC and developmental apraxia); Stackhouse (1992); Stackhouse and Snowling (1992); Glennen and DeCoste (1997) (AAC); Thoonen et al (1997); Beukelman and Mirenda (1998) (AAC); Cumley and Swanson (1999) (AAC).

developmental disorder any disorder which occurs after birth and progresses during childhood. *See* Davison et al (2004); Romski et al (1997) and Sigafoos (1999) (AAC and developmental disorders).

developmental dyslexia a reading and writing disorder which occurs in children who have average or above average intelligence. In general, the child has difficulty in learning to spell. The term dyslexia is used to describe only a child whose reading and spelling are unexpectedly poor. Assessments to find out the severity of dyslexia include the BANGOR DYSLEXIA TEST, the DYSLEXIA SCREENING TEST, and the DYSLEXIA EARLY SCREENING TEST. *See* Hornsby (1995); Ellis (1993).

developmental psychology the study of human development and behaviour from birth through childhood, adolescence and into adulthood and old age, perhaps concentrating on a particular part of the developmental process, e.g. language development. *See* Smith et al (2003).

developmental verbal apraxia *see* DEVELOPMENTAL APRAXIA OF SPEECH.

developmental verbal dyspraxia a term used to describe articulatory dyspraxia in childhood more precisely. It looks at this problem in a holistic way and the child as a complete person. It is seen as a syndrome which has some of the following symptoms:

1. Soft neurological signs (e.g. clumsiness).
2. Delayed lateralisation of cerebral function.
3. Predominance in males.
4. Some feeding problems.
5. Oral apraxia – poor lip posture, tongue control, slow diadochokinetic rates (*see* DIADOCHOKINESIS), and problems with oral sensorimotor feedback.
6. Speech – delayed speech development, resistant to therapy and unintelligible.
7. Articulation – inconsistent vs rigid pattern, phonetic experimentation, non-English articulation, errors in polysyllabic words, breakdown in continuous speech, perseveration, intrusive schwa, sound omissions, voice, place and manner errors (*see* ARTICULATION), vowel distortion and some dysarthric features.
8. PROSODY – inappropriate stress and intonation, variable speech, use of monotone.
9. Resonance – fluctuating nasality.
10. Incoordination of the VOCAL TRACT – DYSPHONIA, dysprosody, disorder of resonance.
11. Language – history of delayed language development, verbal comprehension often ahead of expressive language skills, phonological disability, restricted use of syntax and disordered language development.
12. Learning difficulty – often significant discrepancy between verbal and performance tasks, problems with reading, spelling, writing and drawing, poor auditory memory, sequencing difficulties, cross-modality difficulties and selective attention problems.

See Gordon and McKinley (1980).

deviant language language which does not fit into a normal developmental sequence. Abnormalities may relate to phonation, SUPRASEGMENTAL PHONOLOGY and/or segmental features (*see* PHONOLOGY), SYNTAX or SEMANTICS or a combination of all these.

deviation *see* CONDUCT DISORDER; STANDARD DEVIATION.

devoiced sounds which are devoiced are those which are usually voiced but because of their environment lose some of their voicing. This often occurs with the voiced plosives /b,d,g/ (*see* ARTICULATION) when used WORD-FINALLY, e.g. big, bad, etc. In narrow transcription (*see* TRANSCRIPTION SYSTEMS (2)), this process is represented by the DIACRITIC placed under the affected sound. *See* Cruttenden (1994).

diachronic linguistics one of the types of

69

descriptive linguistics proposed by de SAUSSURE in 1913. It studies the historical changes in language over time. Thus, a linguist studying language using this procedure would look at the progression of English from Old English to Middle English to Modern English. This is also known as historical linguistics. It is opposed to synchronic linguistics (*see* SAUSSURE). *See* Lyons (1968); Culler (1986).

diacritic in narrow transcription (*see* TRANSCRIPTION SYSTEMS (2)), markings have to be placed above or below the sound to show any particular features which are used in its production. For example, [ʰ] is the diacritic placed above and in the gap between the sounds to show aspiration, e.g. [pʰin]. These diacritics also show intonation contours and mark stress in a word or sentence in SUPRASEGMENTAL PHONOLOGY. In transcribing the speech of either children with phonological delay/disorder or those with DYSARTHRIA, the speech therapist will have to know the diacritics used to mark the characteristics of such speech. *See* Abercrombie (1967); Fromkin and Rodman (2003); Ladefoged (2001).

diadochokinesis (DDK) the average rates used by people to move their articulators in producing certain sequences of sounds and facial movements. The sequences are produced in all positions in the mouth, e.g. /p,p,p,/, /t,t,t/, /k,k,k/, /p,t,k,p,t,k/, oo..ee..oo..ee, etc. This test can be used with both adults and children. Its opposite is ADIADOCHOKINESIS. *See* Canning and Rose (1974) (children); Robertson and Thomson (1986) (adults).

diagnosis the identification of the person's presenting condition by the therapist after thorough examination, investigation and assessment. It is important to make sure that the decision is correct and no other diagnosis is likely. If it is uncertain which communication disorder the person has, a differential diagnosis takes place. For example, if the person has had a stroke (*see* CEREBROVASCULAR ACCIDENT),

he/she could have, among others, either APHASIA, DYSARTHRIA or dyspraxia (*see* ACQUIRED APRAXIA). To make sure the correct treatment is given each of these conditions would have to be assessed and the results analysed. *See* Byers Brown (1981).

diagnosogenic theory of stuttering a theory proposed by Wendell Johnson that stuttering behaviour is the result of the attitude of the listener to the normal dysfluencies of the child.

diagnostic audiometry the testing of a person's hearing to find out the severity and type of HEARING LOSS, e.g. CONDUCTIVE HEARING LOSS, SENSORINEURAL HEARING LOSS, etc. *See* Katz (1985); Miller (2001).

Diagnostic and Statistical Manual (DSM) the classification of mental disorders used in the USA. The latest edition is DSM-IV. In its expanded form this stands for *Diagnostic and Statistical Manual of Mental Disorders*, 4th edition. It is published by the American Psychiatric Association and is the official diagnostic system used extensively by mental health professionals. The first diagnostic system was published in 1952 (DSM-I) with successive versions in 1968 (DSM-II), 1980 (DSM-III), 1987 (DSM-IIIR); 1991 (the DSM-IV options book) and a draft version of the complete DSM-IV in 1993. The main change in DSM-IV is the introduction of a multi-axial classification system with five axes concerning clinical syndromes, personality disorders, general medical conditions, psychosocial and environmental problems and axis 5 which is a global assessment of functioning scale (GAF Scale) where consideration has to be given to psychological, social and occupational functioning on a hypothetical continuum of mental health/illness. There are places on the scale of 0/1 (inadequate information), 10 persistent danger of severely hurting self or others (e.g. recurrent violence) OR persistent inability to maintain minimal personal hygiene OR serious suicidal act with clear expectation of death) up to 100 (superior functioning in a wide range of activities, life's problems never seem to get out of hand, is sought out by others because of the many positive qualities. No symptoms.). *See* Davison et al (2004); http://www.psych.org/clin_res/dsm/ dsmintro81301.cfm

dialect language variations in grammar and vocabulary used in particular areas of a country or by particular social groups within an area. It may include regular usage but it will also contain elements which are peculiar to that region of the country. For example, in Aberdeenshire (Scotland), all wh- words begin with /f/. Thus, 'what' becomes /fit/. Common everyday phrases change, e.g. 'how are you' becomes 'fit like'. Other dialectal variations include 'loon' for 'boy' and 'quine' for 'girl'. *See* Trudgill (1995); Fromkin and Rodman (2003).

diaphragm *see* ABDOMINAL–DIAPHRAGMATIC RESPIRATION.

diastematomyelia a rare condition in which a bony projection produces a cleft of the spinal cord. There is a weakness in the muscles of the legs and deformity of the feet. Sensory impairment may also exist. Surgery can provide relief from some of the symptoms in some cases. *See* Gilroy and Holliday (1982); Kaye (1991).

diazepam a drug used for therapy with people who have spasticity or spinal cord lesions. Its side-effects include sleepiness, lightheadedness and increased muscle weakness. In the long term side effects can be lack of sleep, anxiety, HALLUCINATIONS, hostility, increased spasticity and addiction. *See* Gilroy and Holliday (1982).

dichotic listening stimulation of two ears with different stimuli. Dichotic listening was studied extensively by Doreen Kimura in the early 1960s while working at the Montreal Neurological Institute. She presented spoken digits simultaneously, one of which was heard in each ear through headphones connected to a stereo tape recorder. Each person was given three pairs of digits and asked to recall as many of the six digits as possible in any order. Kimura was interested in the auditory processing of those with temporal lobe lesions. She found that all subjects, regardless of the site of lesion, recalled more of the digits which had been presented to the right ear than those presented to the left ear. The same was found in normal control subjects. Thus, Kimura concluded that, when different stimuli are presented simultaneously to each ear, the pathway from the right ear to the speaking hemisphere has preferred access, and the ipsilateral pathway from the left ear is relatively suppressed. *See* Fromkin and Rodman (2003); Kolb and Whishaw (1996).

diencephalon a structure in the brain also known as the forebrain, which appears immediately above the MIDBRAIN. It has two segments which become the CEREBRAL HEMISPHERES. As they grow forwards, they form the frontal lobes (*see* CEREBRAL HEMISPHERES), growing backwards to form the occipital lobes (*see* CEREBRAL HEMISPHERES) and to the sides to form the temporal lobes (*see* CEREBRAL HEMISPHERES). The structures of the THALAMUS, HYPOTHALAMUS and THIRD VENTRICLE are also found in this area. *See* Barr (1988); Kolb and Whishaw (1996); Tortora and Grabowski (2000).

difference limen for intensity (DLI) the smallest change in the intensity of a sound which can just be heard. Those who have normal hearing usually have difficulty in detecting small changes in intensity when the intensity level is near threshold. As intensity increases, the DLI decreases. *See* Katz (1985).

differential diagnosis *see* DIAGNOSIS.

diffuse a distinctive feature proposed by Jakobson and Halle for marking close vowels [+DIFFUSE] (*see* CARDINAL VOWEL SYSTEM). It is opposed to COMPACT. Chomsky and Halle changed it to HIGH. *See* Hyman (1975).

digastric muscles *see* MUSCLES FOR SWALLOWING.

Digimax a high-tech communication aid which uses DIGITISED SPEECH allowing for 16, 34, 70, 106 or 142 minutes of messages to be stored into it using a touch membrane with 2, 3, 8, 12, 32 or 48 locations. Vocabulary can be divided into six different groups with eight levels for each group giving the potential for a total of 48 levels. When sequences are stored into the device, after pressing the first location only those which are valid selections are shown by LEDs. It can be accessed by direct manual selection, one or two switches, a joystick or multi-switch. The memory will not be lost if the batteries are removed or they lose charge. *See* Rumble and Larcher (1998); Appendix IV (Active).

digital subtraction angiography a modern technique in which a radio-opaque contrast medium can be injected into an arm vein. By computer enhancement the background can be subtracted leaving good quality pictures of the arteries alone. This avoids having to inject into arteries directly – a technique which can be dangerous to the person. *See* Kaye (1991); Tortora and Grabowski (2000).

digitised speech an electronic form of speech used by light-tech and high-tech AAC systems. It differs from synthetic speech (see SPEECH SYNTHESIS) in that it is a human voice which is stored onto a computer chip inside the device. However, it does take a lot of memory in the device although it does replicate closely the human voice which is used for the storing. Devices which use solely digitised speech include the ALPHA TALKER and MACAW. Other devices such as the DELTA TALKER and the ORAC have a combination of digitised speech and synthetic speech (see SPEECH SYNTHESIS). *See* Beukelman and Mirenda (1998); Rumble and Larcher (1998).

Digivox 2 a high-tech communication aid which uses DIGITISED SPEECH allowing for 16, 34, 70, 106 or 142 minutes of messages to be stored into it using a touch membrane with 2, 3, 8, 12, 32 or 48 locations. Vocabulary can be divided

into six different groups with eight levels for each group giving the potential for a total of 48 levels. When sequences are stored into the device, after pressing the first location only those which are valid selections are shown by LEDs. It can be accessed by direct manual selection, one or two switches, a joystick or multi-switch. The memory will not be lost if the batteries are removed or they lose charge. *See* Glennen and DeCoste (1997); Rumble and Larcher (1998); Appendix IV (Active).

diglossia a label proposed for the linguistic situation in some countries, e.g. Greece. It refers to a situation in which two varieties of a language co-occur. However, the two varieties have different uses. Usually one is used for formal occasions while the other is used colloquially. *See* Trudgill (1995).

digraph the actual visual shape of a vowel sound [œ]. *See* Cruttenden (1994).

diphthong a type of vowel in which the tongue and/or lips and jaw move during the duration of the vowel segments within the same syllable. In received pronunciation (RP) there are many diphthongs, e.g. /meɪk/, /tʃeə/, whereas in Scottish-English such diphthongs are produced as pure vowels. However, they do have diphthongs in common with RP such as /naɪn/, /haʊs/, /naɪf/ etc. The production of diphthongs can be explained using the CARDINAL VOWEL SYSTEM. The phonetician can start at one sound, e.g. [a] and show the glide to another, e.g. [ɪ] to produce [aɪ]. *See* Catford (1989).

direct object in CONSTITUENT ANALYSIS, a term applied to the syntactic relation that obtains between the main verb and, usually, the noun phrase that follows it within the VP and that is dominated by a VP node in a TREE DIAGRAM. In (1), the 'cup' is the direct object of 'broke':

1. The child broke the cup.

See Lyons (1968); Fromkin and Rodman (2003).

Director an environmental control system which can be operated by communication aids. It can be operated by the ALPHA TALKER, DELTA TALKER, TOUCH-TALKER, LIGHTTALKER and LIBERATOR COMMUNICATION AID. The Director learns any infra-red signal from an infra-red hand control. In this way, the communication aid user can have total control of their environment from accessing a few symbol sequences. For example, it can learn all the functions to operate a television, i.e. switch on/off, turn volume up/down, change channel, use teletext etc. In conjunction with the X-10 system, it is possible to turn on and off lamps, radiators or any devices which work off mains electricity. The Director can also open and close curtains or doors, etc. *See* Appendix IV (Prentke Romich Company).

discontinuous a distinctive feature proposed by Jakobson and Halle to distinguish sounds which are made with a complete closure in the vocal tract [+DISCONTINUOUS], i.e. plosives (*see* ARTICULATION), from those which are not [–DISCONTINUOUS], i.e. fricatives (*see* ARTICULATION) or vowels (*see* CARDINAL VOWEL SYSTEM). *See* Hyman (1975).

discourse analysis the analysis of linguistic units larger than a sentence. A discourse is a continuous utterance in which more than one sentence is represented, e.g. a story told by a child or adult. The data are analysed in an attempt to identify linguistic regularities about the discourse. *See* Fromkin and Rodman (2003).

disintegrative psychoses *see* CHILDHOOD PSYCHOSES.

dissimilation a process in which a neighbouring sound influences another sound but, unlike assimilation, the influence changes the sound. This occurs in DIACHRONIC LINGUISTICS to show phonetic changes in language. *See* Brosnahan and Malmberg (1976); Fromkin and Rodman (2003).

dissociative disorders those who have these types of disorders find it difficult to recall important personal events or may temporarily forget their identity or even assume a new identity. They are also liable to wander far away from their customary environment. There are four main dissociative disorders: dissociative amnesia where the person is suddenly unable to recall important personal information especially after a traumatic event – this forgetfulness is quite different from normal forgetfulness; dissociative fugue where the person not only forgets totally what is happening but suddenly moves from home and work and takes on a different identity; multiple personality disorder where a person can have at least two separate ego states, which can act in different ways or have different feelings either independently of each other, or together at different times; depersonalisation disorder where the way the person perceives the self is disconcertingly and disruptively altered. *See* Davison et al (2004).

distinctive feature phonological descriptions of the way in which sounds are produced. The terms placed in square brackets are in binary notation which shows two polar ends, e.g. [+CONTINUANT], [–CONTINUANT]. Jakobson and Halle (1956) and Chomsky and Halle (1968) proposed many such features. Jakobson and Halle's distinctive features were acoustic in nature:

acute	grave
compact	plain
diffuse	sharp
flat	checked
lax	unchecked
mellow	tense
discontinuous	strident

Chomsky and Halle's distinctive features follow articulatory positions for producing sounds:

coronal	high
continuant	low
anterior	back
strident	nasal
voice	lateral
sonorant	round
delayed release	distributed

See Hyman (1975); Fromkin and Rodman (2003).

distocclusion a type of malocclusion (*see* ORTHODONTICS) found in a person's teeth.

distraction tests tests used with very young children (6–18 months of age) who are unable to cope with PURE-TONE AUDIOMETRY. Children sit on their mother's knee. A person sits in front of the child and produces toys to attract his/her attention while the audiologist stands behind him and produces tones by a warble device, rattle, etc. The tester has to observe the child's reaction to the tones. This reaction usually involves the child turning his head to the side on which the tone is presented. One problem is that the child could respond to other stimuli in his immediate environment. *See* Hodgson (1985).

distributed a distinctive feature proposed by Chomsky and Halle to distinguish sounds produced with a stricture such as bilabial and palatoalveolar fricatives (*see* ARTICULATION) [+DISTRIBUTED] from those which are not made at this place of articulation [–DISTRIBUTED]. *See* Hyman (1975).

disyllable two syllables which make up a phonetic unit. It is contrasted to monosyllable. *See* Catford (1977).

divergent thinking a thinking process which allows the person to move off in different directions encompassing several aspects of a particular subject. This can often lead to novel or original ways of thinking. *See* Taylor et al (1982); Kolb and Whishaw (1996).

dizygotic twins twins who are not identical since they come from different egg cells and are not genetically similar, whereas identical twins come from a single egg cell and have the same genetic makeup. The latter are also known as monozygotic twins. *See* Smith et al (2003); Tortora and Grabowski (2000); Davison et al (2004); http://search.bellaonline.com/articles/art2778.asp

DLS *see* DERBYSHIRE LANGUAGE SCHEME.

dominance the two CEREBRAL HEMISPHERES are important because they contain Dparticular centres to allow humans to communicate, become artistic or read and write and so on. However, one of these hemispheres is more dominant than the other – this is the hemisphere which contains the language centres. In 98 per cent of right-handed people, language skills are in the left hemisphere, and in 60 per cent of left-handed people language skills are controlled by the left hemisphere. So, four out of five people with damage to the left hemisphere are likely to have their language affected. Sperry (Nobel Prize winner, 1981) carried out experiments where the two hemispheres were split so that he could find out accurately the specialisation of each hemisphere. In one of his experiments, he flashed the word 'nut' onto the left side of a screen for one-tenth of a second. The subject's gaze was fixed on the centre of the screen. The visual image goes to the right side of the brain which controls the left side of the body. He was able to pick up the nut with his left hand but he could not say what the word was because the left hemisphere did not receive any information. The subject could not report what his left hand had picked up because of the same lack of information to the left hemisphere and his hands were hidden from him by the screen. By carrying out similar experiments, Sperry was able to highlight the specialisation of the two hemispheres of the brain. *See* Smith et al (2003).

dorsum the back of the tongue which produces sounds such as velars and palatals (*see* ARTICULATION) by coming close to the hard and soft palates (*see* MOUTH). *See* Catford (1977).

dot matrix printers printers which form letters or graphics with a system of dots on the paper made up by a matrix of wires or styluses. Thermal paper as well as ordinary paper can be used with these printers with an ink ribbon. *See* Bishop (1985).

double blind procedure a procedure used when carrying out experiments.

Neither the subject of the experiment nor the person administering the test procedures knows what the experiment is about or when the experimental condition is taking place. This procedure is often used in research into the effectiveness of drugs when a placebo or a drug is given. In such cases, neither the subject nor the person conducting the test procedures knows if the subject is being given the placebo or the drug. *See* Smith et al (2003); Davison et al (2004).

Down Syndrome in the mid-1860s, Langdon Down identified the characteristics of this syndrome to which he gave his name. It is produced by Trisomy 21. In other words, an extra part of a chromosome is present on the long arm of chromosome 21. Thus, a person who has Down syndrome has 47 chromosomes instead of 46. People who have this condition comprise 22 per cent of the whole population of those with learning disabilities in Great Britain. There is an equal distribution throughout the world. 1 in 666 live births results in Down syndrome. The physical features which characterise Down syndrome are:

1. Epicanthic folds, i.e., slanting eyes.
2. HYPOTONIA, i.e., floppy limbs.
3. Square-shaped face.
4. Small noses and ears.
5. Tongues which come forward more than in those who do not have Down syndrome.
6. Teeth appear later.
7. Little fingers curve inwards.
8. A wide gap between big and second toes.

Intelligence is low, there are heart malformations and they are prone to upper respiratory tract infection. The same developmental sequences in babbling are similar between those who do not have Down syndrome and those who have. As far as phonological development is concerned, the rate of acquisition is slower in Down syndrome although the sound system follows a similar sequence of development. It has been found that development of one-word utterances is delayed by about one year in Down syndrome. Down syndrome children usually produce their first words around 2 years of age. At this age the proportion of meaningful utterances in the Down syndrome child is less than 5%, which increases slightly at around 4 years of age. When Down syndrome children reach the 2–3 word utterances, these children express similar semantic relations as other children. This stage is reached at about 4–5 years of age. When producing more complex utterances, the Down although it does seem to increase using MEAN LENGTH OF UTTERANCE as the child grows older. It has been found also that children who have Down syndrome and speech can 'fast map' (i.e. learn new words after as little as one exposure) at a level commensurate with age-matched and language-matched children. (Chapman et al 1990). When considering PRAGMATICS, the main types of illocutionary sentences used are declaratives, imperatives and questions. Clibbens et al (2002) carried out research into the use of signing between parents and four children with Down syndrome. *See* Cunningham (1982); Chapman et al (1990); Bishop and Mogford (1993); Davison et al (2004); Glennen and DeCoste (1997) (AAC); Beukelman and Mirenda (1998); Chan and Iacono (2001) (gesture and word production in Down syndrome); Clibbens et al (2002); http://www.dsa-uk.com

drive often described as an internal motivational force. *See* Smith et al (2003).

DTC *see* DETAILED TEST OF COMPREHENSION.

duration the length of time, in milliseconds, used to produce sounds. *See* Catford (1977).

dynamic display a general term for communication aids that use displays which change following each hit. The symbols are electronically generated on the touch screen. For example, if the user hits the symbol for 'clothes', the screen will change to a page of symbols for 'clothes'. There are various devices which use this system, such as the CAMELEON and the DYNAVOX. A second type of dynamic display is where the symbols remain static but the indicators for choosing the symbols change. For example, if the user chooses the 'drinks' symbol, the only symbols which will light up are those associated with the 'drinks' category. This system operates on the ALPHA TALKER, DELTA TALKER and the LIBERATOR COMMUNICATION AID. *See* Glennen and DeCoste (1997); Beukelman and Mirenda (1998); Rumble and Larcher (1998).

Dynamo a high-tech communication aid with almost 25 minutes of digitised speech and a black and white dynamic touchscreen. The Dynamo uses pages in which vocabulary is organised with the number of symbols per page required by the person using the system. The Dynamo has 3300 DynaSyms. It can be accessed by single switch or direct manual selection. It can learn infra-red signals to control appliances in the home such as TVs, videos or opening/closing curtains, doors or windows. See Appendix IV (DynaVox Systems Inc.).

DynaMyte a high-tech communication aid with synthetic speech (DECtalk) and digitised speech recorded using the in-built microphone, a dynamic display and the DYNAVOX SYSTEM SOFTWARE. In most respects it is the same as the DYNAVOX apart from being smaller and more portable for people who use AAC and are ambulant. *See* Rumble and Larcher (1998); Appendix IV (DynaVox Systems Inc.).

DynaSyms based on PICSYMS and developed by the author of PicSyms for the DYNAVOX, there are over 2000 symbols. They are both black and white and in colour with the label for the symbol appearing above the symbol. *See* Beukelman and Mirenda (1998); Glennen and DeCoste (1997); Appendix IV (DynaVox Systems Inc.).

DynaVox a high-tech communication aid with synthetic speech (DECtalk) using a dynamic display and the DYNAVOX SYSTEM SOFTWARE. Graphic symbols designed exclusively for the device, DynaSyms, are used with the device. These symbols change each time they are touched. The symbol appears on the top area of the touch screen. When the complete phrase or sentence is accessed, the top line is pressed and the device speaks out the whole message. DynaWrite is a software package which allows the user to spell in longer messages using word prediction. It follows grammatical rules, personal preference and a built-in 40000 word dictionary. A combined software package using DynaSyms and DynaWrite is also available. DynaCard is a credit card sized memory card providing up to 4 million characters of memory. The DynaVox 3100 has a 30.5cm (12") diagonal active matrix colour LCD display. It can be accessed by direct manual selection using the touch screen, one or two-switch scanning, multiswitch and joystick scanning as well as autozoom selection mode which magnifies the display area around the person's first selection. DynaVox 2 has a coloured display as well as a monochrome version, 8 MB and 20 MB memory cards, built-in infra-red environmental control unit with word prediction and word processing and is lighter in weight. *See* Glennen and DeCoste (1997); Rumble and Larcher (1998); Appendix IV (DynaVox Systems Inc.).

DynaVox System Software the proprietary software which operates all DynaVox products including the DYNAVOX and DYNAMYTE. It allows people to use dynamic displays and fast page changes with hundreds of ready to use communication pages for both children and adults. There is word prediction to speed up spelling and a list of 128000 word forms with about 4000 DYNASYMS and a built-in infra-red system which learn infra-red signals. There is a song manager to create songs on the DynaVox and DynaMyte and an alarm system. *See* Appendix IV (DynaVox Systems Inc.).

DynaWrite a high-tech communication aid using both synthetic and digitised speech and QWERTY, ABC or scanning keyboards allowing the person using the system to spell messages on a full-size computer keyboard. The DynaWrite has word prediction and has a built-in environmental control unit allowing the person using it to operate appliances around the home. It is lightweight at about 1 kg (2.16 lbs) and is portable or can be mounted on a wheelchair. Its synthetic speech system is VeriVoice which features two voices for male and female. The DynaWrite allows the person to talk on a mobile phone. *See* Appendix IV (DynaVox Systems Inc.).

dysarthria a group of disorders which stem from defined neurological conditions and which manifest abnormalities of RESPIRATION, PHONATION, RESONANCE and ARTICULATION. There are four main types although clear differentiation is not always possible:

1. Dyskinetic dysarthria.
   (a) Hyperkinetic type: this occurs in myoclonic and choreiform disorders. PROSODY is severely affected particularly in relation to rate and rhythm. There is deletion of sounds and word segments due to incoordination of the articulators. Reduced velar movement gives rise to hypernasal resonance.
   (b) Hypokinetic type: this occurs most frequently in PARKINSON'S DISEASE. Articulation is poor but this is due more to the difficulty in controlling rate and range of movement in ongoing speech rather than to specific articulatory weakness. On a word to word basis, speech may be clear but there is rapid deterioration in connected speech.
2. Spastic dysarthria: originates in the upper motor neurons. All parameters of speech are affected; respiration is poor, spasticity of the vocal folds results in hoarseness, intonation patterns are restricted and stress

is equal and excessive. The congenital form is associated with CEREBRAL PALSY when it is also known as congenital supra bulbar paresis.

3. Peripheral dysarthria: also known as flaccid dysarthria and lower motor neuron dysarthria. The principal speech characteristics are: hypernasality; nasal emission of air; continuous breathiness during phonation and audible inspiration. The consonants are also distorted and the person speaks in short phrases because of breathing problems.
4. Mixed dysarthria: occurs in those who have an impairment in more than one motor system. Possible causes of this condition are tumours, trauma and degenerative conditions such as MOTOR NEURONE DISEASE and MULTIPLE SCLEROSIS etc.

The speech disorders in those who have these forms of dysarthria will be characteristic of the motor speech disturbances characterised in the individual motor system disturbances outlined in 1–3 above. *See* Darley, Aranson and Brown (1975); Ferrier (1991) (AAC); Murdoch and Hudson-Tennent (1994) (acquired dysarthria in childhood); Beliveau et al (1995) (linguistic cues and severely dysarthric speech); Glennen and DeCoste (1997) (AAC); Hustad (2001); http://www.rcslt.org/leaflet-dysarthria.shtml

Dysarthria Examination Battery devised by Drummond, the Dysarthria Examination Battery is a quick assessment of motor speech disorders. It provides information on five speech processes: respiration, resonation, prosody, phonation and articulation. It is suitable for children and adults. *See* Drummond (1993) in Appendix I.

dysequilibrium syndrome a neurological condition resulting from renal dialysis. It is thought to occur when dialysis rapidly alters the blood comportment and there is production of a gradient of electrolytes from brain to blood. This results in fluid shift into the brain. It happens towards the end of the dialysis process and is characterised by signs and symptoms of increased intracranial pressure followed by spontaneous recovery. *See* Gilroy and Holliday (1982).

dysfluency the general term used to describe stammering/stuttering behaviour as well as cluttering. It can describe either the speech of someone who stammers or has other types of disorder, e.g. parkinsonian speech. It can also describe other forms of speech which include a lot of repetitions, hesitations and so on. It is also called non-fluency. When a speaker hesitates during a conversation for effect or while thinking of something else to say, this is described as normal dysfluency or normal non-fluency. *See* Dalton (1983, 1994).

dysgraphia as an ACQUIRED DISORDER caused by a trauma to the brain such as stroke or head injury, it affects writing and is associated with APHASIA. Such disorders in writing may mirror other disorders caused by aphasia, e.g. anomia, agrammatism. However, the condition may involve only minor spelling mistakes or difficulty in copying and writing to dictation. Writing disorders are not always associated with aphasia. As a developmental disorder, it is usually associated with DYSLEXIA. *See* Eisenson (1984); Hornsby (1995); Ellis (1993).

dyskinetic cerebral palsy *see* CEREBRAL PALSY.

dyslalia a historical term for articulation disorder which is no longer in use.

dyslexia a widely used description for someone who has difficulty with reading, writing and spelling. For a child, it is the unexpected failure to learn to read and write as he reaches the appropriate age (*see* DEVELOPMENTAL DYSLEXIA) while for an adult, it refers, usually, to the difficulty found in reading after a stroke or head injury or other trauma to the brain (*see* ACQUIRED DYSLEXIA). *See* Eisenson (1984); Ellis (1993); Hornsby (1995); Kolb and Whishaw (1996).

Dyslexia Adult Screening Test (DAST) devised by Fawcett and Nicolson, DAST is designed as an easy-to-use, quick way of finding out if further testing is required. It comprises 11 subtests which put an emphasis on fluency as well as accuracy such as rapid naming, phonetic segmentation, nonsense passage reading, verbal fluency, one minute reading, two minute reading, non-verbal reasoning, semantic fluency, postural stability, backwards digit span and one minute writing. It is suitable for people from 16;05 upwards. *See* Fawcett and Nicolson (1998) in Appendix I.

Dyslexia Early Screening Test (DEST) devised by Nicolson and Fawcett, it assesses children in the age range of 4;06–6;05 for dyslexia with the following subtests: rapid naming, phonological discrimination, rhyme detection/first letter sound, digit naming, bead threading, postural stability, forwards digit span and sound order and shape copying. *See* Nicolson and Fawcett (1996) in Appendix I.

Dyslexia Screening Test (DST) devised by Fawcett and Nicolson, it assesses children and adolescents in the age range of 6;06–16;05 for dyslexia with the following subtests: rapid naming, phonemic segmentation, nonsense passage reading, bead threading, two minute spelling test, one minute writing, one minute reading test, backwards digit span, verbal fluency, semantic fluency and postural stability. *See* Fawcett and Nicolson (1996) in Appendix I.

dysmetria the loss of the ability to work out the distance between the person and the object. It is caused by damage to the CEREBELLUM. *See* Gilroy and Holliday (1982).

dysphagia a disorder in swallowing caused by a trauma to the brain such as a stroke or head injury or brain tumour, etc. It can also be caused by degenerative diseases or lesions to the upper motor or lower motor neurons. These causes produce difficulty in swallowing liquid. Dysphagia can also be caused by organic and anatomical disorders such as structural abnormalities, e.g. cleft palate, disease, radiography, surgery (e.g. partial/total glossectomy), neck or facial trauma and burns. When these occur the person can have difficulty swallowing solids. Therapy depends on what the client cannot swallow and which part of the swallowing system does not function. *See* Silverman and Elfant (1979).

Dysphagia Evaluation Protocol devised by Avery-Smith and her colleagues, the Protocol is designed to evaluate quickly the factors which may be causing swallowing difficulties. It provides guidelines for conducting a feeding assessment at bedside and when to start, continue or stop assessing the person's swallow. The Protocol can also suggest if someone should have a VIDEO-FLUOROSCOPY, define what has to be investigated further by videofluoroscopy, identify the possible causes of the swallowing problem and classify and standardise treatment for specific types of DYSPHAGIA. *See* Avery-Smith et al (1997) in Appendix I.

dysphasia *see* APHASIA.

dysphonia disorders of respiration, pitch intensity and/or resonance which impair communication. Aetiology may be organic, behavioural or psychogenic. Organic-based disorders include structural anomalies, neurological and endocrinological disease. Behaviourally based disorders include excessive muscular tension misuse and abuse. Psychogenic disorders include conversion dysphonia, delayed pubertal voice and transsexual conflict. *See* Greene and Mathieson (1989); Dalton (1994); Freeman and Fawcus (2001).

dyspraxia *see* APRAXIA; ACQUIRED APRAXIA; DEVELOPMENTAL APRAXIA OF SPEECH; DEVELOPMENTAL VERBAL DYSPRAXIA.

dysprosody inappropriate production of suprasegmental features of speech, i.e. intonation, pause, stress and rate.

dystonia the abnormal movement or posture caused by a disorder affecting the agonist and antagonist muscles. Dystonia musculorum deformans is a movement disorder in the axial and limb muscles. It can be inherited as an autosomal dominant or recessive trait (*see* CHROMOSOMES). The condition progresses from a mild movement disorder to involvement of the lower limbs and in its final form to inability to walk. There is no specific drug therapy. However, there is often spontaneous remission. Acute dystonic reaction is caused by the sudden onset of dystonic movements in the facial muscles and a movement disorder in the eyes. Meige's disease affects movements of face, mouth and jaw. This is also known as Breugel's disease. *See* Gilroy and Holliday (1982); Kaye (1991); http://www.dystonia.org.uk/dystonia-societyh.html

dystrophy usually describes the weakness and degeneration of muscle fibres caused by genetically controlled myopathies. There are several dystrophies all of which have different characteristics:

1. Duchenne muscular dystrophy: a sex-linked recessive disease (*see* CHROMOSOMES) which is progressive. It occurs in 20 per 100000 male births. Children are normal at birth and reach their early milestones at a normal rate although there may be some delay in standing and walking. The child develops a clumsy, waddling gait and has difficulty in climbing stairs. GOWER'S SIGN appears at this stage. By about 10 years of age, the child may be confined to a wheelchair. Prognosis is not good; death can occur in the person's teens or early 20s.
2. Facioscapulohumeral dystrophy: an autosomal dominant disease (*see* CHROMOSOMES). It begins between 10 and 20 years of age. The person has minimal disability. There is progressive weakness affecting the lower face followed by trapezius (hand/

wrist area), the sternal head, shoulder girdle, spinal muscles and pelvic girdle. It is slowly progressive but many cases show minimal disability.

3. Scapuloperoneal dystrophy: an autosomal dominant or sex-linked recessive disease (*see* CHROMOSOMES). It occurs in early childhood. There is weakness around the shoulder girdle, the proximal upper limb and distal lower limb. No treatment is required as there is a full life expectancy.

4. Limb girdle dystrophy: an autosomal recessive disease (*see* CHROMOSOMES). It occurs between 10 and 20 years of age. There is weakness of the muscles of the shoulder girdle or pelvis and later both. The person may be confined to a wheelchair after 40 years of age.

5. Distal dystrophy: an autosomal dominant disease (*see* CHROMOSOMES). Weakness is in the distal muscles of upper/lower limbs. It occurs in adults. There is full life expectancy.

6. Oculopharyngeal dystrophy: an autosomal dominant disease (*see* CHROMOSOMES). There occurs bilateral ptosis followed by facial weakness, later onset weakness of masseters, pharynx, hands and feet. It occurs in the middle years and is slowly progressive.

See Gilroy and Holliday (1982); Kaye (1991); http://www.muscular-dystrophy.org/

E-tran frame *see* EYE TRANSFER COMMUNICA-
TION SYSTEMS.

ear the ear comprises three parts:

1. Outer ear: it comprises three parts:
   (a) Auricle or pinna: while the most visible part of the ear, it is the least important for hearing in humans. It is formed by elastic CONNECTIVE TISSUE which is covered by skin. It gathers sound waves from the environment and is most efficient at gathering high-frequency sounds.
   (b) The external auditory canal extends inwards from the auricle to the tympanic membrane. In adults, it goes inwards and at a slightly upward angle while in children it goes downwards at an acute angle. This canal is lined with skin while the outer third has glands that secrete wax which protects its lining and reduces the possibility of infection. The inner two-thirds is encased in bone and is also lined with skin. Its function is to act as a resonator for frequencies between 2000 and 5500 Hz and it helps to transport sound to the tympanic membrane.
   (c) Tympanic membrane: the external auditory canal ends in a concave disc made up of three layers. The first layer comprises skin continuous with the auditory canal; the second layer is rough fibrous connective tissue and contributes most to the vibrating of the tympanic membrane when sounds hit it; the third layer consists of mucous membrane continuous with the middle ear. The normal tympanic membrane is a pearly grey, semi-transparent ring of tissue held together by the annulus. Its function is primarily a mobile link in the auditory chain. The surface of the tympanic membrane is greater than that of the round window (see below).

2. Middle ear: this part of the ear transmits sound waves from the medium of the air from the outer ear to the fluid of the inner ear. It comprises six walls. The inner wall contains the basal turn. It opens into the Eustachian tube (anterior side). It is connected to the nasopharynx (*see* PHARYNX). It is covered by a mucous membrane while the Eustachian tube is lined with hair follicles. The tube is usually closed in adults and opens only when the person sneezes or swallows etc. In children, it is shorter and more horizontal and open. As it is open, infection can get into it quite easily. There are two windows linking the middle and inner ears: the oval window is above the promontory while the round window is below the promontory. The stapes rests in the oval window while there is a tough elastic membrane in the round

window. The canals in the inner ear all extend from the oval window. The three ossicles in the middle ear are the malleus (hammer), the incus (anvil) and the stapes (stirrup). These are the smallest bones in the body and are formed at birth. The action of the ossicles provides amplification for the middle ear. They bring the vibrations from a large area (the tympanic membrane) and focus them on a small area (the oval window). The size of the tympanic membrane is 27 times that of the oval window. There are two main muscles in the middle ear:

(a) The stapedius muscle attaches to the neck of the stapes. When it contracts it pulls it out of the oval window and to the side, tenses the oval window and causes less vibration at low frequencies. The nerve supply comes from the facial nerve (CRANIAL NERVE VII).

(b) Tensor tympani: it is attached to the malleus. When it contracts it tenses the tympanic membrane causing less sound to be transmitted. It is supplied by the trigeminal nerve (*see* CRANIAL NERVE V). Both muscles work reflexively and bilaterally even if the sound only goes in one ear.

3. Inner ear: a bony structure which forms a snail-like shell and three semi-circular canals. It sends messages to the brain for hearing and balance. The vestibular mechanism allows a person to balance. The auditory mechanism is contained in the cochlea. It is filled with fluid in various sacks. When the cochlea is unwound it forms three tubes – the scala vestibuli contains perilymph as does the scala tympani while the scala media contains endolymph. The scala tympani ends in the round window while the scala vestibuli ends in the oval window. Between the scala media and the scala vestibuli is Reissner's membrane while the basilar membrane is between the scala media and the scala tympani. The organ of Corti is found in the basilar membrane.

See Denes and Pinson (1993); Kolb and Whishaw (1996); Tortora and Grabowski (2000).

eardrum *see* EAR (tympanic membrane).

Easytalk a small light-tech communication aid using DIGITISED SPEECH on four levels. It can be used with locations 1 to 40 and there are different models providing 4, 8 or 16 minutes of speech. It can be accessed using direct manual selection or switches. *See* Rumble and Larcher (1998); Appendix IV (Active).

EAT *see* EDINBURGH ARTICULATION TEST.

Echo4 a light-tech communication aid providing four messages from four integral switches although four larger switches can be attached to it. Each switch allows for 3–4 seconds of recorded messages to be stored. *See* Rumble and Larcher (1998); Appendix IV (Sandwell Special Projects).

echolalia a phenomenon found in many communication disorders where people repeat almost word for word what the therapist says to them. Delayed echolalia occurs when the repetition of the word, phrase or sentence is made after an interval of time has passed or after another person's utterances. *See* Eisenson (1984).

Eclipse a communication aid using DIGITISED SPEECH with 4 minutes (extended to 8 minutes) or 20 minutes (extended to 40 minutes) recording time depending on the model of device. It can be issued with overlays from 2–128 locations with up to 128 levels. Some models allow only direct manual selection while other models allow for SCANNING using one or two switches, joystick, multi-switch or optical headpointing. *See* Rumble and Larcher (1998); Appendix IV (Morphonics Ltd.).

ECochG *see* ELECTROCOCHLEOGRAPHY.

ECT *see* ELECTROCONVULSIVE THERAPY.

Edinburgh Articulation Test (EAT) devised by Anthony et al in 1971 (Appendix I), it is a standardised test of articulation which can be used with children of 3 to 6 years of age. It includes:

1. A quantitative score which provides a standard score and an articulatory age.
2. A qualitative profile based on the degree of immaturity of the articulatory realisations, together with the provision for noting atypical articulation.

The test is presented in the form of a picture-naming task, and phonetic transcription is made of the child's responses. *See* Antony et al (1971) in Appendix I; Beech et al (1993).

Edinburgh Functional Communication Profile (EFCP) a test for assessing someone's functional communication. There are 12 interaction situations, grouped into six communicative contexts: (1) greeting; (2) acknowledging; (3) responding; (4) requesting; (5) propositions; and (6) verbal problem-solving. It is designed to be used with elderly clients as well as aphasic clients who have difficulty in coping with aspects of daily communication. Rating is on a seven-point scale of carefully defined responses. Administration takes the form of observations either by therapist, spouse or medical staff. The profile looks at people's total communication including the use of signing, computers, etc., to help them communicate, for which they still receive credit. It can also discriminate between the non-language modes used by the person. *See* Skinner et al (1984) in Appendix I; Beech et al (1993).

Edinburgh Masker a device to help principally those with dysfluent speech. Earphones are linked into a control box which has a volume control on it. When switched on there is a white noise sound which blocks out dysfluent people's feedback systems, so that they cannot hear what they are saying. If such people cannot monitor their speech, then they can become more fluent. *See*

Adams and Lang (1992) (use with Parkinson's disease).

education of hearing-impaired children there are three main educational approaches to help the child who has a hearing loss:

1. The oral approach: the child is only allowed to use spoken communication which may include finger spelling or lip reading. Two approaches within the oral approach are:

   (a) acoupedic approach: the emphasis is placed totally on hearing for teaching speech and language. Its aim is to integrate those with a degree of hearing loss into the 'hearing' world. It was devised by Pollack.

   (b) multisensory approach: both hearing and visual stimuli are used. The child is encouraged to use lip reading but no sign languages or systems are allowed. When language is being taught it should be in a meaningful context. However, lip reading can be confusing as some sounds are very difficult to see while others are quite understandable. Its efficacy depends on the speaker making the sounds as clear as possible and the conversation must take place in good light. As it is not a language system, it is not a particularly good way for a child to develop language. The main aim is to prevent the child from becoming part of a 'deaf ghetto'.

2. The manual approach: the child can use sign languages such as British Sign Language or sign systems such as the Paget-Gorman sign system. Using sign language could result in the child being part of the 'deaf ghetto'. However, it can expand the child's communication capabilities as sign languages do have their own language systems. Many deaf parents ask for their children to be taught BSL as it is less ambiguous than lip reading.

3. Total communication: the child is encouraged to use aspects of both the oral and manual approaches to develop speech and language. No one approach is emphasised more than another. This approach may include other types of communication:
(a) Rochester Method: an oral approach used with finger spelling.
(b) CUED SPEECH.

See Northern and Downs (1991); Bench (1992).

educational audiology the testing of children so that those diagnosed as having a hearing loss will have suitable education and treatment given to them.

educational psychology an educational psychologist assesses and treats children in school who have learning problems (e.g. reading problems, DEVELOPMENTAL DYSLEXIA or emotional disorders (e.g. ELECTIVE MUTISM, AUTISM), or CONDUCT DISORDERS. Educational psychologists are also involved in special education. They counsel parents and teachers as well as other professionals about the causes of the child's problems at school. *See* Smith et al (2003).

EEG *see* ELECTROENCEPHALOGRAPHY.

EFCP *see* EDINBURGH FUNCTIONAL COMMUNICATION PROFILE.

ego *see* PERSONALITY.

egocentric speech *see* PREOPERATIONAL STAGE.

egocentricity *see* PREOPERATIONAL STAGE.

egressive airstream *see* AIRSTREAMS.

ejective a sound which is produced by a glottalic airstream (*see* AIRSTREAMS (3)). The sequence of movements required for producing an ejective is:

1. Close the glottis (compare lifting a heavy weight).
2. Make an obstruction in the mouth, e.g. at lips [p] or at the soft palate [k].
3. Move the larynx up (feel the air compressed in the mouth).
4. Release the closure.
5. If the obstruction is at the lips a voiceless ejective [p'] is produced

while if the obstruction is at the soft palate a voiceless ejective [k'] is produced.

See Catford (1989).

elective mutism a condition in which some children choose not to speak in certain situations, most commonly at school. However, although they may not speak at school, they may speak at home as well as to members of their class outside school but refuse to speak to the same friends when in school and elsewhere. The incidence is 8:10000 children, with the sexes being equally affected. There are several possible causes for this condition including SEPARATION ANXIETY, SIBLING RIVALRY, overprotective mothers, family history of mental disease, and severe NEUROSIS or DEPRESSION. It may also be caused by an articulation or phonological problem which children can have and for which they have been teased or mocked since they first spoke in school. Reinforcement can occur if other children or parents speak about the condition in front of the child to the teacher or therapist. It is an emotional disorder, which for some children may just take the form of shyness which can be overcome without many problems. However, in its severe form, it can become a lasting disorder revealing an abnormal temperament which appears as apathetic (*see* APATHY), morose, unprepossessing, withdrawn, timid, anxious or fearful. Since it results in a communication disorder, it can be treated by a speech therapist as long as it is recognised that there may be underlying psychological factors. PSYCHOTHERAPY in the form of BEHAVIOUR THERAPY or PSYCHOANALYSIS has been successful with such children. The child should be desensitised to the situation in which he or she does not speak. This can take some time but, following this, the child should be put in as many speaking situations as possible to gain confidence. Whispering should be allowed although the use of the child's normal voice should be encouraged as soon as possible. *See* Rutter (1975); Davison et al (2004).

electrocochleography (ECochG) an objective test to ascertain hearing threshold. Three electrodes are placed on the head – the active electrode is placed on the promontory in the middle ear (*see* EAR) which lies above the cochlea (*see* EAR), while another electrode is placed on the ear lobe and the earth is placed on the forehead. The active electrode picks up three potentials generated in the cochlea (*see* EAR) and auditory nerve. It is rapid; each ear can be tested individually and the state of the client is not affected. However, children may need to be anaesthetised. An ENT surgeon is required to place the electrode in the ear. It cannot test individual frequencies. *See* Graham and Martin (2001).

electroconvulsive therapy (ECT) a treatment procedure sometimes used with those who have DEPRESSION. Most clients are given a low electrical current to the non-dominant cerebral hemisphere (*see* DOMINANCE) which is intended to relieve any confused state after the treatment is finished. It is just as effective if given unilaterally or bilaterally. People are anaesthetised intravenously with succinylcholine or suxamethonium. After the session has ended, normal breathing has been restored and consciousness fully regained, the person cannot remember anything of the treatment although the memory of what occurred prior to treatment is intact. Treatments usually take place once or twice per week. PSYCHOTHERAPY is also required. It has been found that using both forms of treatment at the same time provides the most beneficial treatment programme. *See* Stafford-Clark and Bridges (1990); Kolb and Whishaw (1996); Smith et al (2003); Davison et al (2004).

electroencephalography (EEG) a technique for studying the electrical activity within the BRAIN. This emanates from the cerebral cortex. The waves are plotted on an electroencephalogram by an electroencephalograph. There are four types of wave which can appear on the printout:

1. Alpha waves appear at a frequency of 10–12 cycles per second and appear in most people while awake.
2. Beta waves appear between frequencies of 15 and 60 cycles per second and occur while the nervous system is functioning.
3. Theta waves appear at frequencies of 5–8 cycles per second and occur when the person is under emotional stress.
4. Delta waves appear at frequencies of 1–5 cycles per second and occur while the person is asleep. If they occur while the client is awake, this could indicate brain damage.

EEG is used in the diagnosis of EPILEPSY, TUMOURS OF THE CENTRAL NERVOUS SYSTEM, infectious diseases, such as MENINGITIS, and trauma. *See* Kolb and Whishaw (1996); Tortora and Grabowski (2000).

electrolarynx *see* ARTIFICIAL LARYNX.

elicitation the process of obtaining data, e.g. words, syllables, phrases, sentences, to form a sample of a person's use of language. In speech and language therapy, elicitation often takes the form of formal and informal assessments.

elision a process by which some words in contexts can lose a sound or syllable in certain environments, e.g. 'ladies an' gentlemen'. *See* Cruttenden (1994).

ellipsis the omission in context of elements of sentences. Responses to questions in English, for example, normally omit subjects and/or auxiliary verbs. For example:

A: What have you been doing?
B: Watching television.
In (B), the sentence lacks both a subject and an auxiliary verb. The full form would be:
B: I have been watching the television.

Many children use this form of sentence and so, during the assessment of language delay or language disorder, it is sometimes uncertain if the child is producing ellipsis and really knows the omitted part, or has produced what appears to be an elliptic sentence because he/she has not reached that stage of language acquisition to be able to produce complex sentences. *See* Lyons (1968).

embedding CLAUSES that are placed within a sentence are embedded sentences. The basic sentence is known as the matrix sentence. If a relative clause is placed within the utterance, it is central embedding.

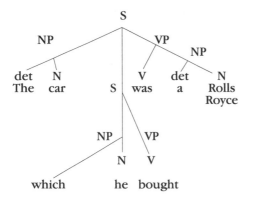

(1) The car which he bought was a Rolls Royce.

See Huddleston (1976).

embryo the developing human from fertilisation to the end of the second month of pregnancy. During this time, known as the embryonic period, the embryonic membranes form around the embryo. A specialised part of the membranes is the placenta, the function of which is to produce an oxygen and nutrient passage into the fetal blood from the mother and the passage of carbon dioxide and other products of metabolism back into the mother. The umbilical cord develops at this time and contains the fetal artery and veins which allow blood to flow between the fetus and placenta. After the second month, the developing human

becomes a fetus and from the third month, the time *in utero* is called the fetal period. *See* Haines and Mohiuddin (1972); Tortora and Grabowski (2000).

embryology the study of the developing human fertilised ovum from fertilisation to the end of the second month of pregnancy. *See* Haines and Mohiuddin (1972); Tortora and Grabowski (2000).

EMOS *see* ENHANCED MINSPEAK OPERATING SYSTEM.

emotional disorders found in children who have DEPRESSION or ANXIETY. Both these factors produce obsessional (*see* OBSESSIVE–COMPULSIVE DISORDER), phobic (*see* PHOBIAS) and psychosomatic symptoms. The prevalence rate is 2.5–5.5 per cent of all children, with an equal incidence between the sexes, although as children grow older there is a gradual increase in the number of female children affected. It is unlikely that there is one sole cause for emotional disorders but rather several intermingled such as SEPARATION ANXIETY, developmental fears and phobias (*see* FEARS AND PHOBIAS IN PRE-SCHOOL CHILDREN), developmental rituals (*see* AUTISM), etc., life events producing stress, e.g. loss, overwhelming traumatic events, family influences involving unconscious conflict and the use of DEFENCE MECHANISMS, e.g. id vs ego, SIB-LING RIVALRY, OEDIPUS COMPLEX, etc. PSY-CHOTHERAPY has been shown to be useful in treating these disorders. *See* Rutter (1975); Smith et al (2003); Davison et al (2004).

encephalitis the result of a viral infection which invades the CENTRAL NERVOUS SYS-TEM. The virus produces a fever, convulsions and coma. Treatment takes the form of antiviral agents, steroids and anticonvulsants. EEG is used as a means of diagnosis. *See* Gilroy and Holliday (1982); Kolb and Whishaw (1996); http://glaxocentre.merseyside.org/ence ph.html

encephalitis lethargica a type of ENCEPHALITIS due to an influenzal virus which was a cause of postencephalitic parkinsonism, found during the worldwide epidemic of 1917–1928. *See* Gilroy and Holliday (1982); Kolb and Whishaw (1996).

encoding in AUGMENTATIVE AND ALTERNATIVE COMMUNICATION (AAC), the way in which vocabulary is organised in low- and high-tech AAC systems so that the person using the systems can produce a desired message. This can include SALIENT LETTER ENCODING, letter-category encoding, alpha-numeric encoding, iconic encoding (e.g. MINSPEAK) and colour encoding. See Vanderheiden and Lloyd (1986); Glennen and DeCoste (1997); Beukelman and Mirenda (1998).

encopresis incontinence of faeces. This may be due to a failure to learn bowel control or a response to psychological stress. *See* Rutter (1975).

encounter groups a form of SENSITIVITY TRAINING used with those who lack social skills. The members of the group pair off and spend about one minute telling each other the most important facts about themselves, followed by two things of which they are proud and two things of which they are ashamed. *See* Trower at al (1978); Davison et al (2004).

endocrine system this system comprises glands which do not have ducts and secrete hormones directly into the bloodstream. The endocrine glands include the pituitary and thyroid glands, four parathyroids, two adrenal glands, two gonad glands and the pancreas which can function in both the endocrine and exocrine systems. The secretion by these glands is known as a hormone. *See* Green (1978); Smith et al (2003); Tortora and Grabowski (2000).

endocrine voice disorders some communication disorders are caused by a disorder of the endocrine system. Dysphonia is such a disorder:

1. Castrati voice.
2. Eunuchoid voice: responds to hormone treatment.
3. Incomplete vocal mutation: a failure of the voice to break at the normal time – it either breaks earlier or later

than average. The voice may become hoarse or weak, its range is very low and chest resonance is limited. The person will probably complain of vocal fatigue because of trying to lower the voice. The vocal folds show a varying degree of hyperaemia, congestion and irritation. The folds also show a 'mutational triangle' where they fail to adduct. Treatment takes the form of voice therapy, hormone treatment and PSYCHOTHERAPY.

4. Delayed maturation of pituitary gland of thyrogenic origin.
5. Puberphonia: the persistent falsetto voice in a male who has developed a larynx of normal adult proportions. It may be caused by psychological factors such as neuroses, a denial of adolescence, or a defect in the vocal folds resulting from habitual voice misuse or an endocrine imbalance. A person will possibly require both speech therapy to lower the voice and psychological intervention.
6. Precocious vocal mutation: the male shows true sexual precocity before 8 years of age.
7. Perverse mutation: occurs in females when the change from the infantile female voice to an abnormal male voice takes place by the excessive secretion of androgenic hormones.
8. Perello: after 6 months of pregnancy, there are physiological changes in breathing and a slight thickening of vocal folds which become oedematous. This can also happen when menstruation occurs.
9. Menopausal voice changes: the adrenocortical activity after the ovarian oestrogens have been reduced. This can produce a decrease in the fundamental frequency (Fo) (*see* ACOUSTIC PHONETICS), the glottal membrane becomes thicker, the mass of the vocal folds increases in size and there is a decrease in voice pitch.
10. Hermaphroditic voice: occurs in SCHIZOPHRENIA.

11. Voice disorders caused by thyroid disorder:

(a) cretinism: the person has a larynx similar to that of an infant. The voice is without intonationand has a very limited range of less than one octave.

(b) myxoedema: hypothyroidism produces voice loss. It could be referred to as hyperfunctional dysphonia. The person puts on weight, there is a decrease in the activity of the basal mechanism, the face becomes dry and puffy, there is a loss of hair and a bowing of the vocal folds.

(c) hyperthyroidism: slight weakness and huskiness in the voice but nothing really noteworthy.

All these causes can be treated by voice therapy and relaxation. *See* Greene and Mathieson (1989); Freeman and Fawcus (2001).

endogenous depression *see* DEPRESSION.

endolymph *see* EAR.

English Picture Vocabulary Test (EPVT) devised by Brimer and Dunn, this is a formal, standardised test to find out the extent of a child's 'listening vocabulary'. The child is asked to choose the correct picture from a selection of four and the resulting score measures what the child can understand semantically. *See* Brimer and Dunn (1962, 1973) in Appendix I.

Enhanced Minspeak Operating System (EMOS) this is an updated operating system for Touch Talkers and Light Talkers. It allows for text editing using left and right cursor keys and scrolling in both communication and storage modes. The conversation workspace expands from 40 characters to 255 characters and text and speech markers are maintained with written text in workspace. While those who use EMOS can still have 8-, 32- and 128-location overlays, they can also use any size and shape of location in a 128-location 'alternative' overlay. If an icon (symbol) is moved, all the vocabulary is moved with the icon and does not need to be reprogrammed. When the user reviews vocabulary in the device, the sequence and message appear on the same screen. The improved computer emulation allows the user to store emulator commands under 11 of the function keys. When storing an item of vocabulary, the programmer can stop storing, speak to someone or switch off the device and come back to it later and carry on in the middle of the storage procedure. *See* Appendix IV (Prentke Romich Company).

ENT (ear, nose and throat) *See* Pracy et al (1974).

environmental deprivation a possible cause of LANGUAGE DELAY. When taking a CASE HISTORY, the therapist should establish to what extent the mother plays with the child or takes time to talk with him or her about pictures and toys or how frequently she or his father tells the child stories. Unless the child has the experience of talking through play, then he or she may have difficulty in acquiring language. *See* Garvey (1990); Kolb and Whishaw (1996).

epenthesis a sound which is inserted in the middle of a word as a form of intrusion. It occurs a lot in historical linguistics and CONNECTED SPEECH.

epiglottis a structure at the top of the LARYNX and behind the hyoid bone (*see* MUSCLES OF MASTICATION). It is a leaf-shaped piece of cartilage which is attached to the thyroid cartilage (*see* LARYNX). The larger part opens and closes like a trap door. As the larynx moves up during swallowing, the epiglottis closes off the larynx, thus forcing the food to move down the OESOPHAGUS. *See* Tortora and Grabowski (2000).

epilepsy epilepsy is not a disease in itself but a symptom of a disease. While the symptoms last, there is an abnormal amount of electrical activity reaching the cerebral cortex from a focal site in the BRAIN. It occurs in the following diseases: CONGENITAL NEURONAL DYSFUNCTION, systemic metabolic disorder and STRUCTURAL BRAIN DISEASE. People who have epilepsy can have various types of seizure which in the past were described in terms of grand-mal and petit-mal epilepsy but there is a new classification which has been developed over the last few years.

1. Primary gerneralized seizures
   (a) Absence seizures – lasting for about 10–20 seconds, they occur between the ages of 4–14 years where the child stares into space but does not realize what is happening. Simple absence seizures are stares but in most absence seizures there is a change in muscle activity. The most common movements are eye blinks. There may also be hand movements and mouth movements. These complex seizures last for more than 10 seconds. Previously absence seizures were known as petit-mal seizures.
   (b) Atypical absence seizures – last 5–30 seconds (usually more than 10), they have a gradual beginning and ending and begin before the age of 6 years and can continue into adulthood. Similar to absence seizures, the child is responsive while staring. Eye blinking and mouth movements may occur.
   (c) Myoclonic seizures – very short jerky movements. There may just be one but at other times there will be many in a short space of time. These seizures usually cause abnormal bilateral movements of the body at the same time. They can appear in juvenile myoclonic epilepsy, Lennox-Gestaut syndrome, and progressive myoclonic epilepsy. Usually beginning in childhood, myoclonic seizures can occur at any age.
   (d) Atonic seizures – last less than 15 seconds, the person's muscles lose their tone or strength and the eyelids may droop, the head may nod and the person will drop things and often fall to the ground while remaining conscious. Hence, they are also known as 'drop attacks' or 'drop

seizures'. They begin in childhood and can continue into adulthood.
   (e) Tonic seizures – last less than 20 seconds, the person has increased tone in the muscles with the body, arms or legs making sudden stiffening movements while remaining conscious. They most often occur during sleep but if awake the person is likely to fall. They are particularly common in people who have Lennox-Gestaut syndrome.
   (f) Clonic seizures – while the length of time for these rare seizures varies, clonic seizures are rhythmic jerky movements of the arms and legs and sometimes both sides of the body.
   (g) Tonic-clonic seizures – formerly known as grand-mal seizures, they last between 1–3 minutes and are the combination of tonic and clonic seizures. The tonic phase comes first where all the muscles stiffen with air being pushed through the VOCAL CORDS producing a cry or groan and the person loses consciousness. The face may become blue. After the tonic phase comes the clonic phase where the arms and usually the legs begin to jerk quickly and rhythmically. After a few minutes the jerking slows and stops. Bladder and/or bowel control may be lost as the body relaxes. Consciousness returns slowly and the person may be drowsy, confused, agitated or depressed.
2. Partial seizures
   (a) Simple partial seizures – there can be different types of seizure: sensory seizures cause a change in a person's senses, e.g., hearing noises or smelling things which are not there; autonomic seizures cause changes in the nervous system producing strange or unpleasant feelings in the stomach, chest or head, change in heart rate or breathing; psychic seizures cause changes to the way a person thinks, feels or experiences things. They last for a varying length of time and can be controlled by medication.

(b) Complex partial seizures – last 30 seconds to 2 minutes, these seizures usually start in a small area of the temporal or frontal lobe of the brain. They affect alertness and awareness and it may seem the person is just daydreaming.

(c) Secondarily generalised seizures – start as a partial seizure but they spread very quickly to other parts of the brain becoming generalised. They occur in more than 30 per cent of people with partial epilepsy.

Status epilepticus is a severe form of tonic-clonic seizure and shows itself as a series of fits between which the person does not recover consciousness. It can last for hours and requires immediate treatment with drugs. Those with this form of epilepsy may have been removed suddenly from a drug regime or have removed themselves from it or may have STRUCTURAL BRAIN DISEASE.

In a review of the literature concerning language and epilepsy, Lebrun concludes that various types of language orientated activities, especially reading, can cause paroxysmal brain discharges. Epileptic fits may also interfere with verbal behaviour. The popular drug treatment for adults who have epilepsy is phenytoin, but it can produce facial hair, acne rash, thickness of facial features and may cause hypertrophy of the gums. Carbamazepine is given if phenytoin causes problems from its side effects. However, carbamazepine has a range of side effects particularly on the bone marrow and must be used with caution. Sodium valproate can reduce grand-mal and petit-mal seizures but it may cause an increase in weight and gastro-intestinal problems. Its side effects include drowsiness, headache, photophobia, dizziness, hiccoughs, bone marrow suppression and vomiting. Diazepam is given intravenously for those who have status epilepticus. The side effects of diazepam include somnolence, lightheadedness and increased muscle weakness. Surgery is offered to people who have epilepsy and are not responding to medication. Vagus nerve stimulation is another treatment designed to prevent seizures by sending regular, mild pulses of electrical energy to the brain via the vagus nerve. *See* Gilroy and Holliday (1982); Lebrun (1988); Kolb and Whishaw (1996); http://www.epilepsy.com; http://www.efa.org/index.cfm

epithelium epithelial cells form themselves into membranes which can be of one layer or several layers. The former is simple epithelium while the latter is stratified epithelium. The three types of epithelial cells which form themselves into these membranes are:

1. Squamous cells: cells that are flat and thickened at the nucleus.
2. Cuboidal cells: cells that are similar in height and width and are many sided.
3. Columnar cells: cells that are polygonal in shape, height is greater than width.

These three types differ in their appearance depending on whether they form simple or stratified epithelial membranes. *See* Leeson et al (1985); Tortora and Grabowski (2000).

EPVT *see* ENGLISH PICTURE VOCABULARY TEST.

ethmoid bone *see* NOSE.

Eustachian tube *see* EAR.

exceptional children children who are particularly talented and gifted. It is also used to describe children who have learning difficulties so that the stigma of being described as 'retarded' is removed.

Exeter Visual Training Device produced by Tudor and Selley (1974), it is a palatal training device designed to stimulate movement of the soft palate and thus treat hypernasality. The Exeter visual speech aid provides feedback about palatal movement.

exophora a term used to refer to a pronominal form in a construction which relies for its reference on the extra-linguistic context. Exophoric reference is usually contrasted with anaphoric pronominal reference, in which the referent is identified from a previous linguistic mention. *See* Allerton (1979).

expansion the rewrite rules used in CONSTITUENT ANALYSIS are also known as expansion rules since one constituent is expanded into a description of several constituents, e.g. NP = (det) + (adj) + N. *See* Lyons (1968).

experimental hypothesis *see* ALTERNATE HYPOTHESIS.

experimental psychology experimentation is used by many types of psychologist, especially behaviourist and cognitive psychologists. They use experiments to find out how people react to various types of stimuli, how they learn and how they use their memory, their emotional responses and how they are motivated to take action. *See* Smith et al (2003).

expressive aphasia *see* APHASIA (1).

expressive language communication by means of the spoken or written word. This is possible where COMPREHENSION is impaired, not the resulting language, although the resulting language is likely to be pragmatically inappropriate. Conversely, there can be a deficit of expressive language with normal comprehension. *See* Glennen and DeCoste (1997).

expressive-receptive aphasia *see* APHASIA.

Extended Standard Theory *see* TRANSFORMATIONAL GRAMMAR.

external auditory canal *see* EAR.

external carotid artery *see* CAROTID ARTERY.

extraneous movements movement which is inappropriate to the situation as in the case of some types of stammering where stereotyped movement of limbs accompanies efforts to speak. It also occurs as tics and choreiform movement in some neuropathological conditions. *See* Gilroy and Holliday (1982); Dalton (1983).

extrapyramidal system a system of fibres which operates outside the PYRAMIDAL (corticospinal) SYSTEM. Neurons originate in the BASAL GANGLIA. It modulates background for the motor system. *See* Barr (1988); Kolb and Whishaw (1996); Tortora and Grabowski (2000).

extrinsic muscles of the tongue there are three extrinsic muscles of the tongue:

1. Genioglossus muscle: it runs from the superior genial tubercle of the mandible and inserts itself under the tongue. It is supplied by the lingual artery, lingual vein and CRANIAL NERVE IX. This nerve supplies the surface of the posterior one-third of the tongue, the circumvallate papillae (*see* TASTE BUDS).

2. Styloglossus muscle: it runs from the STYLOID PROCESS to the tongue. It pulls the tongue backwards and upwards. It is supplied by the lingual nerve and CRANIAL NERVE VIII (*see* CRANIAL NERVES).

3. Hypoglossus muscle: it runs from the hyoid bone (*see* MUSCLES FOR SWALLOWING) to the tongue and pulls it backwards and downwards. It is supplied by the hypoglossal nerve (CRANIAL NERVE XII).

See Tortora and Grabowski (2000).

eye contact some people who have a stammer or a voice disorder are so embarrassed when they speak that they fail to look directly at the therapist or person to whom they are talking. It is an important part of deictic (*see* DEIXIS) communication. *See* Dalton (1983).

eye transfer communication systems these systems can be used to find out if a person can communicate, to train someone who may be given a more sophisticated communication aid in the future, or as a means for someone to communicate his needs. The system comprises a transparent panel to which any type of stimulus, e.g. symbols, pictures, words/phrases, etc., is attached on three fully adjustable standing bases. Those requiring this system use eye gaze with which to look at the symbols or words. Colour coding is often used for more complex systems. The base can either be mounted on wheels, a weighted base, or a clamp base which can be attached to any surface edge. *See* Glennen and DeCoste (1997); Beukelman and Mirenda (1998).

EZ keys a software system for use with specific communication aids. It uses word prediction, abbreviation expansion, a built-in reader for giving pres-entations and instant phrases organised in groups or topics of vocabulary. EZ keys for Windows allows for mouse emulation even if the person is just using the communication aid. All types of accessing are available including switches to infra-red input and touchscreen. It allows the person to control the environment through their environmental control, and a modem can also be used. There are versions to run in DOS or WINDOWS. *See* Glennen and DeCoste (1997); Beukelman and Mirenda (1998); Appendix IV (Words+).

facial nerve *see* CRANIAL NERVES.

facilitated communication an approach in AUGMENTATIVE AND ALTERNATIVE COMMUNICATION first used by Crossley in 1977 with her client Anne MacDonald, a young girl with cerebral palsy whose experiences during her rehabilitation are documented in the book *Annie's Coming Out*. Facilitated communication assumes competence in communication rather than impairment. It is also to be assumed by the facilitators that those with autism will produce a meaningful and even quite complex message. To facilitate the person's communication, the person's hand, arm or even finger is held over a keyboard. The keyboard, with letters or symbols, is gradually introduced to the person by direct questions e.g. 'show me the letter "t",' or 'show me the picture of the "house"' etc. Positive feedback is given when the correct letter or symbol is hit. The person is gradually asked to make more complex messages such as entering their name or following a cloze procedure exercise where the person has to fill in the blanks. The person is then encouraged to make longer and more complex statements using facilitation. The prompts are slowly removed although the physical support remains as long as the person wishes it. *See* Crossley (1988, 1997a, b); Jones (1995a); Adams (1997); Dockrell and Sterling (1997); Rosenbloom

(1997); Derbyshire (1997); Beukelman and Mirenda (1998).

facilitation the act of enabling a natural process. In speech and language therapy, facilitation is used with various client groups who have some degree of communication impairment to help them relearn or improve their communicative skills. The importance of facilitation in all types of communication disorder cannot be underestimated, not only with conditions such as APHASIA or childhood speech and language disorders but also in the use of augmentative communication where a person has to learn how to use their respective communication system. *See* Eisenson (1984) (facilitation for aphasia); Beukelman and Mirenda (1998).

facioscapulohumeral muscular dystrophy *see* DYSTROPHY.

factor analysis *see* TRAIT APPROACH.

failure to thrive a description of children who have poor physical development, usually caused by a failure to receive social and physical stimulation. *See* Kempe and Kempe (1978); Reber (1995).

false vocal folds ventricular folds. The superior part of the thyroarytenoid muscle lying above the VOCAL FOLDS. Their normal function is adduction when swallowing, but they function as vocal folds in some types of voice disorder, e.g. ventricular band voice. *See* Greene and Mathieson (1989); Tortora and Grabowski (2000).

falx cerebri a sickle-shaped structure within the BRAIN acting as a vertical partition along the longitudinal fissure of the CEREBRAL HEMISPHERES. Its dura is attached to the crista galli of the ethmoid bone at the front, to the midline of the vault as far back as the internal protuberance, and to the tentorium cerebelli. This midline fold of dura mater separates the two cerebral hemispheres. *See* Barr (1988); Tortora and Grabowski (2000).

family therapy the family goes regularly to see a therapist who observes how the family members interact with each other. Smith et al suggest 'the basic premise of family therapy is that the problem shown by the identified patient is that something is wrong with the entire family; the family system is not operating properly' (Smith et al 2003, p. 584). Each member of the family is directed in ways of how to improve their interaction with each other. The therapist may also go to the family's home for similar reasons. *See* Barker (1981); Smith et al (2003); Sauber et al (1993); Davison et al (2004).

fascia two types of fascia exist which form sheets of tough material to divide muscle groups:

1. Superficial fascia: loose CONNECTIVE TISSUE found deep in the skin that often contains a varying quantity of fat. If the tissue consists mainly of fat, it is called adipose or fatty tissue.
2. Deep fascia: dense connective tissue found in a continuous layer below the superficial fascia and formed in sheets. It can form part of a flat muscle which is then called an aponeurosis.

See Tortora and Grabowski (2000).

fasciculus a bundle or a group of nerve or muscle fibres, e.g. ARCUATE FASCICULUS. *See* Tortora and Grabowski (2000).

FAST *see* FRENCHAY APHASIA SCREENING TEST.

fauces *see* MOUTH.

FCP *see* FUNCTIONAL COMMUNICATION PROFILE.

fear thermometer *see* SYSTEMATIC DESENSITISATION.

fears and phobias in pre-school children EMOTIONAL DISORDERS which can affect young children. At the age of 2 years, children can be afraid of ghosts, witches and the supernatural which they hear about in fairy stories; at about 3 years of age, they have a fear of small animals, which may turn into a fear of any size of animal or anything furry, while at the age of 4 years, they often become self-conscious and have feelings which may make them frightened. They may also have the fear of losing someone close to them, e.g. a parent, especially after the death of one parent or close relative, or they may even fear that they themselves may die. Similarly after a divorce in the family, they may become very frightened that the other parent will disappear. If the family has to move house, the child may have a fear of leaving his friends and making new friends. All fears become phobias when they become extreme and begin to interfere with the everyday life of the child. For example, a phobia of the dark may arise because the child has been shut in the cupboard either accidentally or intentionally. As the child is so vulnerable at this early age to such events, his most fearful symptom, i.e. fear of the dark, becomes a phobia. Such phobias may even be reinforced by parents who agree with the phobia because they are frightened by the same stimulus.

Thus, children learn to be phobic because the parent is frightened by the same thing, e.g. mice. Children do have their own devices for dealing with fears and phobias. Some follow ritualistic routines, e.g. walking on the lines of the pavement, so that they will not be harmed, or they have favourite toys or objects, e.g. safety blanket, they believe will keep them safe. BEHAVIOUR THERAPY has been successfully used with such a disorder. *See* Rutter (1975); Smith et al (2003).

febrile convulsions fits that occur during a fever associated with an acute systemic infection. They are not caused by infection to the CENTRAL NERVOUS SYSTEM. Many children with this condition have a history of neurological or developmental abnormality. The movements during these convulsions are of the tonic and clonic (*see* EPILEPSY) type. If the child has only febrile convulsions as such, there is a good prognosis. When convulsions last for longer than 30 minutes, the brain is deprived of oxygen and scarring can produce a permanent focus for epilepsy in adulthood. Drug treatment is often not needed. Children should always be kept cool following a convulsion. It occurs in 3 per cent of all children, the highest incidence being between 10 months and 2 years of age. About 30 per cent have a family history. *See* Gilroy and Holliday (1982); http://www.parasolemt.com.au/Manual /febrileconvulsions.html

feedback

1. The means by which behaviour is monitored. Internal feedback provides information before and during the event; external feedback after the event. In relation to speech, auditory, visual, kinaesthetic and tactile feedback play an important part in communication. Many communication disorders are a result of poor monitoring by the speaker. Such disorders can include stammering (*see* STAMMER, DYSFLUENCY), DYSPHONIA, PHONOLOGICAL DISORDER and learning problems such as those encountered by children learning to read using the phonic approach. DELAYED AUDITORY FEEDBACK is used with those who speak at a very fast rate to try and slow down their speech in such conditions as stammering.

2. In the field of AUGMENTATIVE AND ALTERNATIVE COMMUNICATION (AAC), feedback refers to two processes – how the device indicates it has been accessed (i.e. activation feedback) and how the person using the AAC system receives information about the message they have produced (i.e. message feedback). Activation feedback is feedback which is of no real use to the communication partner. The feedback can be produced by a click or a beep when pressing keys, feeling different textures on each key, feeling the pressure required to press a switch or a key or a light flashing on and off to indicate a key has been pressed. Message feedback, on the other hand, can be provided in the form of auditory prompts where the name of this symbol is given before activation of a letter, word or phrase before being finally produced. With low-tech communication aids such as communication boards or books, the communication partner can read the letters, words or phrases as they are pointed to or name of the symbols. *See* Brosnahan and Malmberg (1976); Glennen and DeCoste (1997) (AAC); Beukelman and Mirenda (1998) (AAC).

3. The whistling heard in HEARING AIDS.

Feeding Checklist devised by Warner (1981), it takes the form of a series of questions relevant to the child's eating behaviour and is designed to improve it. It can be used by a caregiver or therapist. It comprises five sections: general; head and trunk control; food and feeding utensils; control of tongue and lips for feeding and drinking; and general features. Each of these sections has questions which are to be answered with a 'yes/no' response. *See* Warner (1981).

Feelix a solid, ergonomic table mounted on a wheelchair. The person using it can eat, drink, draw or play on it, but it is also an electronic communication aid. Symbols placed under a transparent plastic cover are accessed by placing a small magnet on the person's finger or on a pen and the message is spoken out. Feelix can also be accessed with a joystick and single or two switch scanning. *See* Appendix IV.

felicity conditions if a speech act, as a communicative activity, is to achieve its derived function then certain circumstances, known as felicity conditions, must pertain. So, for example, if the speech act is intended to assert the truth of the proposition expressed by the utterance, sincerity conditions, such as the speaker is not lying, should prevail. More crucially perhaps, in declarative speech acts such as those involved in christening, preparatory conditions ensure that the speaker has the requisite authority to perform the speech acts. *See* Clark and Clark (1977).

festinant gait *see* PARKINSON'S DISEASE.

fetal alcohol syndrome a condition first recognised by Lemoine and his colleagues in France in 1968 and confirmed by Jones and his colleagues in 1973. The child will have fetal alcohol syndrome if the mother has been drinking excess alcohol during pregnancy. It can produce learning disability and give the child a particular facial appearance – a small nose, slit eyes and a convex top lip. The child is often irritable, hypertonic (*see* HYPERTONIA) and has tremor and tonic seizures. *See* Gilroy and Holliday (1982); Jones (1997); Tortora and Grabowski (2000); http://www.nofas.org/main/index2.ht

fibreoptic laryngoscope a device made of a large number of glass fibres which are flexible and allow inspection of the recesses of the nose and throat. The person's nose is anaesthetised so that the tube can be passed along the floor of the nose, down the back of the nasopharynx, oropharynx and laryngopharynx (*see* PHARYNX) to the VELOPHARYNGEAL area where any muscle weakness or damage to the LARYNX is observed. *See* Edels (1984); Beech et al (1993).

fibrous meningiomas a type of meningioma (*see* TUMOURS OF THE CENTRAL NERVOUS SYSTEM) which results from CONNECTIVE TISSUE elements and consists of strands of intertwining spindle cells with long fibrils. *See* Gilroy and Holliday (1982).

field
1. In computer terms, part of a record which contains information. A database is made up of records all of which contain fields such as the person's name, address, date of birth, etc. *See* Bishop (1985).
2. *See* SEMANTIC FIELD.

figure and ground when a stimulus is presented with two or more distinct areas, e.g. a painting, part of it is perceived as figure while the rest is ground. Figure refers to the objects of interest and appears in front of the ground. This is the most basic form of perceptual organisation. *See* Smith et al (2003).

filiform *see* TASTE BUDS.

filled pause a gap between utterances which has been filled by a hesitation, e.g. 'er', 'ur', 'eh', etc. Otherwise these gaps would remain silent. *See* Clark and Clark (1977).

filter an electronic method of producing part of an acoustic analysis. It reduces the amplitude of a sound but at the same time allows others to pass through with little or no reduction in their amplitude. The frequencies which do pass through are called the bandwidth of the filter. *See* Fry (1979).

fingerspelling a form of communication used with those who have a hearing loss. Words are spelled out on the fingers, each finger formation forming one letter. It can be used in conjunction with British Sign Language for the Deaf where only one finger spelling is given to represent the initial letter of a word for which there may not be a sign or it may just be used as a shorthand form. It is sometimes called 'visible speech' or dactylology. Tactual reception of fingerspelling is also possible where the hand of the communication partner is placed over that of the person using fingerspelling (Jensema 1982; Mathy-Laikko et al 1987; Musselwhite and St. Louis 1988). A study showed that using a rate of approximately two syllables per second (about half the rate of speaking), people who are both deaf and blind and experienced in understanding fingerspelling, can receive key words in conversational sentences at roughly 80 per cent accuracy using tactual reception (Reed et al 1990). *See* Blackburn et al (1984); Wilson et al (1984); Reed et al (1990); Koehler et al (1994); Beukelman and Mirenda (1998).

First Word Language Programme developed by Gillham (1979), it is a language programme used with children who have language delay or disorder, those with learning difficulties and those who cannot produce speech for physical reasons. The child is taught using short structured sessions either once a day or more often. There is also the possibility of using informal settings for therapy where they occur. The therapist should keep records of the progress made by the children. *See* Gillham (1979).

first word stage a stage in a child's development of language. It lasts from about 1 to almost 2 years of age. A child's one-word utterances are sentences of one word which name objects, describe actions, make requests or, with correct intonation, express emotional states or surprise at seeing something unexpected. The sort of items used at this stage are:

1. Familiar things, objects: important people, e.g. dada, mama; animals; clothing; household items; body parts.
2. Actions/events: name of movers (agents); movables (objects affected by action); some children pay particular attention to names of objects while others to names of people.
3. Intonation used meaningfully (occurs later during this stage): recurrence; negation; location.

Although the child may not use these completely with meaning, the meaning can be taken from their use of gesture and the context of the utterance. *See* Cruttenden (1979).

'fis' phenomenon a common condition in language development. It occurs when a child does not accept the adult imitation of his own immature version of a word. The name derives from the observations of Berko and Brown (1960) in relation to the imitation of a child's realisation of /fɪʃ/ as /fɪs/. *See* Clark and Clark (1977).

fistula a hole or opening which remains after surgery, e.g. after surgery to close a cleft palate. *See* Watson et al (2001).

fit a layman's term for a seizure (*see* EPILEPSY).

Fitzgerald key a way of representing grammar using symbols from left to right using such categories as 'who', 'doing', 'modifiers', 'what', 'where', 'when' and so on. Letters or phrases which were used frequently would be placed along the top or bottom of the display. The aim was to make the word-by-word sentence construction easier going from left to right. *See* McDonald and Schultz (1973); Bruno (1989a); Goossens et al (1994); Beukelman and Mirenda (1998).

flaccid dysarthria *see* DYSARTHRIA (3).

flaccidity a description of a child or adult whose muscles are hypotonic, making it difficult for the individual to stand or sit upright. It may also produce dysarthric characteristics of speech (*see* DYSARTHRIA). See Tortora and Grabowski (2000).

flap *see* ARTICULATION.

flat a distinctive feature proposed by Jakobson and Halle to distinguish sounds produced with lip-rounding (*see* CARDINAL VOWEL SYSTEM) [+FLAT] from those which are produced with spread lips [−FLAT]. *See* Hyman (1975).

flattening of affect a phenomenon found in several conditions including SCHIZOPHRENIA in which the person fails to produce an emotional response to almost any stimulus. The person stares into empty space and has weakness in facial muscles (*see* MUSCLES OF FACIAL EXPRESSION). The voice shows no prosodic features (*see* PROSODY). *See* Davison et al (2004).

flexion a description of the forward movement of joints, e.g. head moving forward on neck, etc. *See* Tortora and Grabowski (2000).

flooding a therapeutic technique devised by Stamfl and Lewis (1967) used in

BEHAVIOUR THERAPY. The person is placed in the most feared situation for a long period of time without the possibility of escape. It is opposed to SYSTEMATIC DESENSITISATION. Some people can recover faster under flooding although it can be highly traumatic. *See* Purser (1982); Smith et al (2003).

fluency speech with little or no non-fluency or DYSFLUENCY. There may be hesitation while the speaker thinks of his next utterance, i.e. normal non-fluency. Fluency is the ultimate aim of all who stammer. *See* Dalton (1983).

fluent aphasia *see* APHASIA (2).

focal sites a specific part of the brain from where symptoms of diseases and disorders can occur. In APHASIA, for example, the focal sites could be Broca's and Wernicke's areas (*see* CEREBRAL HEMISPHERES), etc., or the site in the brain from which the electrical discharges emanate in EPILEPSY. *See* Gilroy and Holliday (1982); Kaye (1991).

font the typeface which appears on the monitor screen and is produced by different kinds of printer or printing processes depending on which fonts are installed in the computer. Dot matrix, bubble (ink) jet or laser printers can use different kinds of typeface direct from the computer as their print heads are made up of styluses or print heads. If daisywheel printers are used, the font for all characters will be the same, as they are all on the print wheel unless a wheel containing a different typeface is used. *See* Chandor et al (1985).

foramen a description of an opening or passage within the body. Several are called foramina. *See* Tortora and Grabowski (2000).

forced alternative a type of question which makes the person give a response to two or more alternatives, e.g. do you want tea or coffee? *See* Crystal et al (1989).

forebrain *see* DIENCEPHALON; Kolb and Whishaw (1996).

form in its most general sense, linguistic form is the patterning of elements that make up structure. Linguistic forms are patterns or structures themselves, e.g. SENTENCES, NOUN PHRASES, verbs. In this sense, form is contrasted to FUNCTION. *See* Lyons (1968).

formal assessments *see* ASSESSMENTS.

formal operations the final stage of cognitive development as proposed by PIAGET. It begins at about 11 years of age, when the child can understand abstract relationships and may begin to think in terms of possibilities. He will use hypothetico-deductive reasoning for working out these possibilities. This is probably the least controversial part of Piaget's theory as it is a familiar thought process for most people in everyday life. *See* Beard (1969); Boden (1994).

formant *see* SPECTROGRAPHY.

fortis a description of sounds which are produced with a strong egressive airstream (*see* AIRSTREAMS). They also require more muscle power to produce the sound. It is usually the voiceless consonants which are fortis, e.g. [f], while voiced ones are described as LENIS, e.g. [v]. *See* Cruttenden (1994).

FourTalk a light-tech communication aid for someone just starting to use high-tech devices. There are two models: the FourTalk 16 with one location with 16 seconds record time or two locations with 8 seconds or four channels with 4 seconds recording time in each location respectively. The FourTalk 32 has the same number of possible locations each with double the time of the FourTalk 16 for each location. It can be accessed by direct manual selection and single or double switch. *See* Rumble and Larcher (1998); Appendix IV (Active).

fourth ventricle a structure within the BRAIN which acts as a canal in the HINDBRAIN. It has a diamond-shaped floor while its roof is tent-like and covered by the CEREBELLUM. The floor is covered with symmetrical elevations caused by the grey matter of the CRANIAL NERVES. Dilatation of this ventricle by fluid produces HYDROCEPHALUS. *See* Barr (1988); Kolb and Whishaw (1996); Tortora and Grabowski (2000).

Fox a portable environmental control, it has unique coded radio signals, rechargeable batteries, two external switch sockets for single- or two-switch scanning and can be mounted on wheelchairs etc. It can scan from 0.75 to 5 seconds and has status indicators allowing the user to see what devices are on in any room. It can be used to control mains electricity, door opening, telephone and infra-red equipment. *See* Appendix IV (Hugh Steeper).

fragile X syndrome a sex-linked chromosome disorder (*see* CHROMOSOMES). It can produce varying degrees of learning disability with the facial appearance of large forehead, large mouth and ill-formed ears. Carriers can be affected. The child's expressive language is superior to comprehension while perseveration may also be found. *See* Tortora and Grabowski (2000); http://www.nfxf.org/home.htm

free association a part of PSYCHOANALYSIS. The person is encouraged to say everything which is in his mind however irrelevant, shameful or stupid it may seem. If the person stops or hesitates, it is assumed by the therapist that the person is hiding some sensitive information which is worth further investigation. It was first used by Freud (*see* PSYCHOANALYSIS; PERSONALITY). *See* Smith et al (2003).

free field audiometry an audiometric test for very young children who cannot use earphones. It usually takes place in two rooms. The person sits in one, equidistant from two loudspeakers. Live or pre-recorded voices are presented. However, the child's ears cannot be tested individually. It is part of speech audiometry.

free variation a phonological description of how one sound can be substituted by another without changing the meaning of the word. For example, the 'r' sounds found in some varieties of English are freely interchangeable in the word 'burns' which can be either [bʌrnz] or [bʌnz]. *See* Grunwell (1987).

Freeway a simple environmental controller with a large backlit scanning display using icons and auditory prompts for people with visual or cognitive problems. It can have up to seven menus programmed, each able to operate between one and 32 definable functions while basic pre-recorded phrases can be replayed to assist with basic communication. It uses infra-red to operate appliances such as beds, chairs, pagers, telephones, lights, curtains and door openers. *See* Appendix IV (Possum).

Frenchay Aphasia Screening Test (FAST) devised by Enderby and her colleagues in 1987 to establish the existence of APHASIA. It examines COMPREHENSION and EXPRESSIVE LANGUAGE as well as comprehension of reading and writing. Scores are compared with a cut-off score and results obtained determine if speech therapy is required. *See* Enderby et al (1987) in Appendix I; Beech et al (1993).

Frenchay Dysarthria Assessment devised by Enderby in 1980 (revised 1988), it is a formal standardised test which indicates the severity and type of DYSARTHRIA. The assessment covers eight sections: reflex, respiration, lips, jaw, palate, larynx, tongue and intelligibility. All eight sections are scored on a nine-point scale. The test takes about 30 minutes to administer. Enderby believes it has fulfilled six criteria: it is applicable to therapy; it can demonstrate changes in the person's speech; it is easy and short to administer; it has been standardised; no training is necessary for administering it; and the results are easy to understand both by speech therapists and other professionals. The computerised Frenchay Dysarthria Assessment runs on an Apple computer II, II Plus and IIe. *See* Enderby (1988) in Appendix I; Beech et al (1993).

frenulum *see* TONGUE.

Freud *see* PSYCHOANALYSIS; PERSONALITY.

fricative *see* ARTICULATION.

Friedreich's ataxia a degenerative disorder affecting the tracts of the SPINAL CORD. It occurs during adolescence and early adulthood. The condition is inherited as an autosomal recessive trait (*see* CHROMOSOMES). It produces dysarthric characteristics of speech (*see* DYSARTHRIA), spastic gait and INTENTION TREMOR. The CEREBROSPINAL FLUID is normal. It is progressive, those with the condition may not be able to walk 5 years after the symptoms have appeared, while death may occur 10–20 years later, usually due to respiration problems. *See* Gilroy and Holliday (1982); http://www.ataxia.org.uk/; http://www.frda.org/

fringe vocabulary when choosing vocabulary for either a low- or high-tech AAC system, there are two types of vocabulary – core and fringe vocabulary. The latter comprises words or phrases which are particular to the individual using the AAC system such as names of specific people, hobbies, places or dialectal variations for a particular region in which they live. *See* Beukelman and Mirenda (1998).

frontal lobe *see* CEREBRAL HEMISPHERES.

fronting in ARTICULATORY PHONETICS, sounds which are produced at the front of the mouth. This includes the front vowels in the CARDINAL VOWEL SYSTEM and the consonants made by the tip and the blade of the tongue. In generative phonology, these sounds are described as [+ANTERIOR] or [+CORONAL]. It describes also a phonological process proposed by David Stampe (*see* PHONOLOGICAL PROCESSES). *See* Grunwell (1987); Ladefoged (2001).

function when contrasted with FORM, function refers to the role which a linguistic element plays in a structure. So a NOUN PHRASE can function as a subject, an object or a complement in a clause structure. *See* Lyons (1968).

function words members of a closed class of grammatical categories such as determiner ('a', 'an', 'the'), auxiliary (e.g. 'may', 'could', 'have', 'should', etc.), conjunction ('and', 'but', 'if', etc.). The categories of which these words are members contain few members (hence 'closed class') and their role is largely grammatical rather than semantic. *See* Palmer (1976).

functional analysis *see* OPERANT CONDITIONING.

functional communication the social role of language in society. Specifically, it is the appropriateness with which language is used in various contexts. 'As language is used to establish interpersonal relationships, regulate the behaviour of others, satisfy material needs or desires, explore and organise environments and exchange messages and information (Halliday in Cole 1982), therapy for the language impaired also needs to focus upon such functions' (Green, 1984). Thus, the therapist should devise context-orientated therapy for these people. *See* Green (1984); Clinical Forum in *Aphasiology,* 6;1 (1992); Crockford and Lesser (1994) (functional communication and aphasia); Mirenda (1997) (AAC and functional communication); Beukelman and Mirenda (1998) (functional communication and aphasia).

Functional Communication Profile (FCP) a test of FUNCTIONAL COMMUNICATION, devised by Sarno in 1969 for all age groups. It tests five functions: movement, speaking, understanding, reading and other aspects of communication. The 45 items divided into these five functional categories have been selected according to what are considered functions of everyday urban life. The rating which is based on a nine-point scale is very subjective. Administration takes the form of an unstructured interview. It can be used for prognosis and is designed for all age groups. The profile describes residual skills rather than deficits, and yields a quantifiable measure of functional communication regardless of severity of impairment. It is a test primarily of language in a natural setting rather than all modes of communication. *See* Sarno (1969); Rosenbek et al (1989).

functional dysphonia a disorder of phonation to which no known organic cause can be directly attributed. There are different types of functional dysphonia:

1. Misuse and abuse of the person's voice which produces VOCAL NODULES, CONTACT ULCERS, etc.
2. Learned patterns of maladaptive behaviour.
3. Psychogenic causes: (a) in those with a psychiatric history, having psychosomatic symptoms and who are vulnerable to physical and mental stress; (b) in those with no history of psychiatric problems but who have prolonged life stress.

See Freeman and Fawcus (2001).

Functional Performance Record (FPR) devised by Mulhall in 1989, it is an assessment of behaviours of those people who have physical, social or psychological impairments. An assessment is made allowing the therapist to set goals and monitor progress. It has a numerical and descriptive means of giving information. It does not provide a diagnosis or reasons why people behave as they do nor does it provide an aetiology or any other type of classification.

There are three components:

1. The checklist: a 46-page booklet containing 777 items in 27 areas of functioning which can be assessed individually or in any combination. These areas of functioning include activity level, aggression, attention span, feeding, hearing, incontinence, memory, movement of limbs and trunk, reading skills, speech and language production, speech and language reception, toileting, etc.
2. The FPR software: individual client disk – an automated version of the checklist. A database can be made which performs all the functions of the individual client disk.
3. The handbook: contains information for using the FPR.

See Mulhall (1989) in Appendix I.

fundamental frequency *see* ACOUSTIC PHONETICS.

fungiform *see* TASTE BUDS.

G

galvanic skin response (GSR) change in the electrical activity of the skin when undergoing emotional stress. *See* Taylor et al (1982); Smith et al (2003); Davison et al (2004).

General Language Screen developed originally for use in the Cambridge Language and Speech Project (CLASP) (Burden et al 1996), the General Language Screen can be used as a screening assessment for children who are suspected of having speech and language disorders (*see* SPECIFIC LANGUAGE IMPAIRMENT). It comprises 12 questions, 11 of which concentrate on the child's receptive and expressive language while the 12th question concerns any worries the parent may have about the child's hearing. Each of the first eleven questions are put in such a way that a negative answer suggests a speech and language problem. *See* Burden et al (1996); Stott et al (2002).

generalisation *see* CARRY-OVER.

generative grammar a grammar consisting of a set of rules which define or generate all and only the grammatical sentences of a language. The term was introduced into linguistics by Noam Chomsky (*see* CHOMSKYAN LINGUISTICS) in his book *Syntactic Structures* (1957). For a natural language, Chomsky proposed that a generative grammar should not only define the set of grammatical sentences, but should assign structural descriptions to the sentences. While the goals of Chomskyan grammar have remained the same, their form has changed several times since 1957. The most novel and significant feature of early generative grammar was the notion of a transformational rule (*see* TRANSFORMATIONAL GRAMMAR), a device for formally linking related sentence types such as active and passive. In the most recent form of Chomskyan generative grammar, referred to as government and binding theory, transformations play a much more restricted role. *See* Huddleston (1976); Lyons (1991).

generative phonology a phonological theory in which phonological changes are used to describe sound changes in particular contexts or environments of the word. For example, the rule which allows vowels to be nasalised before nasal consonants would appear thus:

$$
\begin{bmatrix} + \text{voc} \\ - \text{cons} \end{bmatrix} \longrightarrow [+ \text{nas}] \Big/ - \begin{bmatrix} + \text{cons} \\ + \text{nas} \end{bmatrix}
$$

(Grunwell, 1987)

The terms used in square brackets are distinctive features. An explanation of this rule is: a sound that is voiced but is not a consonant (i.e. a vowel) becomes nasalised in the context preceding a nasalised consonant. Such rules can be useful for a speech therapist in that the child's representation of a sound can be

102

compared with the adult target sound by working out the differences of the features used by the child compared with the adult in particular contexts. The input side of the rule has the child's pronunciation described in the form of distinctive features while the output of the rule shows the adult's pronunciation, i.e. the one regarded as being normal. If the rule is context-sensitive, i.e. the error occurs in the same position of the word consistently, the therapist can find out if the child is making a consistent error in a particular part of the word. Grunwell gives an example where /f/ is pronounced as a homorganic affricate in word-initial position:

'feet'   [pfɪt]
'fence' [pfes̢]
'fish'   [pfeŋ]

The rule describing this error is:

$$\begin{bmatrix} +\text{cont} \\ +\text{ant} \\ -\text{cor} \\ +\text{strid} \\ -\text{voice} \end{bmatrix} \rightarrow \begin{bmatrix} -\text{cont} \\ +\text{del rel} \end{bmatrix} / - \begin{bmatrix} +\text{voc} \\ -\text{cons} \end{bmatrix}$$

An explanation of this rule is: a sound which is a fricative-type [+CONT], made towards the front of the mouth [+ANT], not made with the tongue tip [–COR], a strong sound [+STRID] and unvoiced [–VOICE] becomes a non-fricative sound [–CONT] and has a longer release time than a single consonant [+del rel] in the context of coming before a vowel. Generative phonology is quite widely used in analysing child speech and its applications to omissions, substitutions, distortions and transposition are:

- Change feature specifications (i.e. change segments).
- Delete segments, compare omission.
- Insert segments, compare additions.
- Interchange (reorder or permute) segments (i.e. metathesis), compare transpositions.
- Coalesce segments.

(Grunwell, 1987)

These phonological rules describe patterns of errors. Thus if the therapist decides to use rule-based therapy, then the generative framework for analysing a child's speech may well be useful. *See* Grunwell (1987).

geniculate ganglion found in CRANIAL NERVE VII, it houses the cells which pick up the sense of taste. It attaches to the lingual branch of the mandibular nerve, the fibres of which go to the taste buds on the front two-thirds of the tongue. *See* Barr (1988); Tortora and Grabowski (2000).

genioglossus muscle *see* EXTRINSIC MUSCLES OF THE TONGUE.

genital stage *see* PSYCHOSEXUAL STAGES OF DEVELOPMENT.

genitive the form of a word which represents possession. There are two forms for possession in English, the use of affixes and the use of the word 'of':

1. The man's car is brown.
2. The car of the man is brown.

See Lyons (1968).

genotype the particular set of genes carried by one organism. It contains all the hereditary factors which can be passed down through the generations. *See* Taylor et al (1982); Smith et al (2003).

gerontology the study of the ageing process. *See* AGEING.

Gerstmann's syndrome a disorder arising from a lesion in the left parietal lobe (*see* CEREBRAL HEMISPHERES) in the region of the ANGULAR GYRUS. The classic symptoms are: finger agnosia, PURE AGRAPHIA, ACAL-CULIA and right–left confusion. CONSTRUCTIONAL APRAXIA has also been reported. *See* Kolb and Whishaw (1996); http://www.citihealth.com/layout.cfm?HC=59 andbody=Articles/00004549

Gestalt psychology a particular school of psychology founded by Max Wertheimer in 1912. He and his followers were interested in groupings of visual stimuli and how they were perceived. FIGURE AND GROUND is one part of Gestalt psychology as is the way objects are grouped together where proximity (elements close to one another are grouped together) and closure (how elements are grouped together to complete figures with gaps) are important to the way we perceive these objects. *See* Reber (1995); Smith et al (2003); Davison et al (2004).

Gestural Reorganisation a therapeutic programme to improve the speech of people who have APHASIA by linking meaningful gestures with spoken words and phrases. *See* Rosenbek et al (1989).

gestures fine or gross body movement, facial expression, eye movements and postures used for communication. This can also be termed non-verbal communication. This type of communication can be systematised although many people who rely on non-verbal communication have their own system which is only known to family members or a few close friends. The gestures which are used can also be very similar and their meaning only changes because of the context in which they are used. It has been found that, with practice, people who have APHASIA can cope with gesture and use it effectively for communication, although some therapists dispute its efficacy. Those with aphasia who have a HEMIPLEGIA may have difficulty with using gesture. *See* Stuart-Smith and Wilks (1979); Beukelman and Mirenda (1998).

Getting Started with a Core Low Technology AAC Vocabulary devised by Robertson in 2000, Getting Started provides a core vocabulary of approximately 1000 words and phrases which are introduced in a very structured way to make teaching and learning easier. It provides vocabulary in 25 topics with a short quiz at the end of each to make sure the student has learnt the vocabulary. Since some of the inspiration for Getting Started comes from the author's young daughter, as she developed language, Getting Started can be used in a developmental way or if the therapist wants to decide on vocabulary for a particular topic in the student's

symbol board or book. There is also a record of spontaneous communication to record when a word or phrase was used spontaneously for the first time. *See* Robertson (2000).

GILCU *see* GRADUAL INCREASE IN LENGTH AND COMPLEXITY OF UTTERANCE.

Gilles de la Tourette syndrome an inheritable, metabolic disorder which produces tics. These tics begin in the face and, in time, increase and begin to affect the shoulders and upper limbs. As breathing becomes poor, the person's speech is affected. There are only minor neurological signs. The disease does not interfere with the person's life expectancy. Prognosis is good for those who are treated with haloperidol. It is also known as tic convulsif. This neurotic syndrome can take the form of obscene language, violent vocalisations and motor tics. These symptoms usually appear all at once. The condition begins before 12 years of age (75 per cent of cases) or before 20 years (96 per cent of cases). The incidence is 2:1 in favour of males. It can be a life-long illness although antipsychotic drugs, e.g. haloperidol, can suppress the obscene language and odd motor tics. *See* Kolb and Whishaw (1996); Davison et al (2004); http://www.umm.edu/ency/article/000733.htm.

Gilliam Autism Rating Scale (GARS) devised by Gilliam in 1995, GARS is a rapid behavioural checklist which helps to identify and diagnose autism. There are four subtests which can be administered by speech and language therapists, SENCOs and specialist teachers, the subtests being stereotyped behaviour, social interaction, communication and developmental disturbances. Scores have been standardised and percentiles are presented which determine the existence of AUTISM and the severity of the disorder. *See* Gilliam (1995) in Appendix I.

Glasgow Coma Scale an objective scale which is used in the assessment of those who have had a head injury. It gives a numerical value to the three most important responses which medical staff try to elicit from a head-injured patient – eye opening, the best verbal response and the best motor response. For eye opening, there is a scale of 1–4, for best verbal response there is a score of 1–5 while for best motor response there is a scale of 1–6. When calculated, a total score of 3–15 is produced. If the score is less than 8 a severe head injury exists, if the score is between 9 and 12, the head injury is moderate while a score of 13–15 indicates a minor head injury. *See* Kaye (1991); Kolb and Whishaw (1996).

glide when in transcription there are two symbols next to each other, phonologically, they are a part of the same phonological unit, e.g. diphthong. *See* Cruttenden (1994).

glioma the commonest type of intracerebral tumour. It can occur at any age, with increasing frequency up to 65 years of age. *See* Gilroy and Holliday (1982); Kolb and Whishaw (1996).

global aphasia *see* APHASIA (6); Mark et al (1992).

glossal a description of structures and disorders with tongue involvement.

glossectomy the surgical removal of part or all of the tongue due to disease, trauma or natural wasting. Resulting speech may be quite intelligible, although it may be produced at a slower rate. Exercises similar to those given in some types of DYSARTHRIA are useful. Counselling prior to surgery is very important. *See* Travis (1971);; Fox and Rau (2001) (AAC and glossectomy).

glossopharyngeal nerve *see* CRANIAL NERVES.

glottal constrictions total adduction of the glottis for producing EJECTIVES and IMPLOSIVES. It is a distinctive feature to mark place of articulation proposed by Chomsky and Halle. *See* Ladefoged (2001).

glottal stop the sound which occurs when the vocal folds come closely together and are opened suddenly during a period of silence. It is represented by [ʔ]. In some varieties of Scottish-English, a glottal stop is very prevalent. In Glasgow, for example, it appears in words such as 'butter', [bʌʔə] and 'bottle', [bɔʔl]. *See* Ladefoged (2001).

glottalic airstream *see* IMPLOSIVE; EJECTIVE.

glottis the space which appears when the VOCAL FOLDS open. The space alters in size and shape depending on the type of sound which is produced. When the sound is voiced the vocal folds are close together and vibrating whilst if it is voiceless the folds are open. Breathy voice is produced by opening the folds slightly, allowing the folds to vibrate while at the same time a lot of air rushes through the glottis. Creaky voice is produced by the folds vibrating only at one end while the other end is held together by the arytenoid cartilages (*see* ARYTENOIDS). This produces a low pitched sound. This type of voice can also be described as laryngealised. *See* Ladefoged (2001); Tortora and Grabowski (2000).

glue ear *see* OTITIS MEDIA (3).

Goldman-Fristoe Articulation Test this test is designed to discover which sounds a child has difficulty in producing. However, this test is different from the EDINBURGH ARTICULATION TEST in that the authors have put the emphasis on finding out in which part of the word the child makes an error. The results are scored in three columns headed word-initially, word-medially and word-finally. Not only are 'sounds-in-words' tested but also 'sounds-in-sentences'. In this subtest, the child has to listen and look at two sets of pictures while the therapist tells him the story. The child has to retell the story to the therapist producing as many of the words used by the therapist as he can recall. The scoring is carried out as in the first part of the test. *See* Goldman and Fristoe (1972) in Appendix I.

Goldman–Fristoe–Woodcock Auditory Skills Test Battery devised by Goldman and colleagues to diagnose an individual's ability to hear clearly under difficult conditions. It can be used with individuals between the ages of 3 and

105

85 years of age. There are 12 areas of measurement of auditory skills including: Auditory Selective Attention Test, Diagnostic Auditory Discrimination Test, various auditory memory tests and various sound symbol tests. *See* Goldman et al (1976) in Appendix I; Beech et al (1993).

Goodenough–Harris Drawing Test devised by Goodenough and Harris in 1963, this is a test in which the child is asked to draw a man or a woman or a picture of him/herself. Scoring is of 73 characteristics specified in the manual. The drawings can also be compared to 12 ranked drawings for each of the two scales of Man and Woman. The manual includes restandardisation data of the Goodenough Draw-a-Man Test, the Draw-a-Woman Scale and an experimental Self-Drawing Scale. It covers an age range of 3;0–15;0 years. The test offers a relatively quick method of assessing general and cognitive development. *See* Goodenough and Harris (1963) in Appendix I.

Gower's sign a symptom found in Duchenne muscular dystrophy (*see* DYSTROPHY). During this disease, the person can have difficulty in standing from either a sitting or a lying position. Gower's sign is the means used by the person to establish a standing position. The person rolls over and pulls himself onto his hands and knees, then pushes up until he has a firm base on his hands and feet. The last stage is to make his feet walk up towards his hands until he can stand upright. *See* Gilroy and Holliday (1982).

Graded Auditory Speech Perception Screen (GRASPS) devised by Parsloe and Morrell, GRASPS is a screening assessment of the acoustic cues used by the listener with hearing impairment to perceive speech by using MINIMAL PAIRS. It comprises 26 minimal pairs in picture and written form divided into two sections. The sections have been graded in terms of difficulty for a listener with a profound hearing loss taking into consideration the processes of temporal and frequency resolution. It is suitable for the age range of 5;00 to adult. *See* Parsloe and Morrell (1996) in Appendix I.

Graded Naming Test devised by McKenna and Warrington in 1983, it is an assessment for adults with naming problems as a result of brain damage. The person is required to name 30 black and white drawings which are arranged in a hierarchy of difficulty. Raw scores can be interpreted by comparing them to the pre-morbid vocabulary of the person. The test was standardised on both normal volunteers and clients aged between 20 and 76 years of age who have extracerebral disorders. *See* McKenna and Warrington (1983) in Appendix I; Beech et al (1993).

Gradual Increase in Length and Complexity of Utterance (GILCU) a structured programme to establish fluency in the MONTEREY FLUENCY PROGRAMME (MFP) for those who STAMMER. The therapist asks the person to say one word fluently and then extends this through the highly structured programme until the person can speak fluently in the three modes of the MFP. Fluent speech is reinforced by saying the word 'good'; for those under 12 years, coloured tokens are used for additional reinforcement. *See* MONTEREY FLUENCY PROGRAMME.

grand-mal epilepsy *see* EPILEPSY.

granulation tissue a granular formation which can occur during healing, for example, in the arytenoid region. *See* Tortora and Grabowski (2000).

grave a DISTINCTIVE FEATURE proposed by Jakobson and Halle to distinguish sounds made at the back of the mouth such as back vowels, velars and labials [+GRAVE] (*see* ARTICULATION) from those made at the front of the mouth [– GRAVE]. It is opposed to ACUTE. *See* Hyman (1975).

Great Ormond Street Speech Assessment devised by Sell and her colleagues, the Great Ormond Street Speech Assessment is designed to be a comprehensive screening procedure to describe the speech characteristics of children with cleft palate and/or velopharyngeal dysfunction. The assessment attempts to focus on all the features of speech associated with cleft palate and/or velopharyngeal inadequacy (including aetiological factors), and facilitates the process of systematic assessment, diagnosis and treatment planning. The assessment takes the form of a simple short interview and evaluates the following:

1. Nasal resonance is judged according to type (hyper, hypo, mixed hyper and hyponasality, cul-de-sac), severity and consistency. McWilliams et al (1990) stated 'cul-de-sac' resonance is really a variation of hypo- and denasality. It differs only in the place of obstruction and in the way the speech sounds.
2. Nasal emission and nasal turbulence
3. Nasal grimace is a facial apron that occurs when those with nasal emission try to inhibit abnormal nasal airflow.
4. Consonant production identifies any effects of the repaired cleft palate on articulation. A revised assessment was published in 1998 along with the Cleft Audit Protocol for Speech (CAPS) (Razzell 1996). The two protocols can be used independently but their results are comparable, while CAPS can be used for clinical audit. *See* Sell et al (1994, 1999); McWilliams et al (1990); Razzell et al (1996)

greater horn of hyoid *see* PHARYNX.
greater wing of sphenoid *see* MUSCLES OF MASTICATION.
Griffith's Test a test for developmental milestones devised by Griffiths, it involves four elements of the child's development which have to be closely observed:

1. Does the child kick vigorously?
2. Does the child enjoy the bath?
3. Does the child push the feet against the parent's hand?
4. Does the child have strong arm movements?

All children from 1 to 3 months of age may be assessed by this test. *See* Illingworth (1987).

groove a description of the TONGUE when it has a groove along the central longitudinal line of the tongue. It is used for some fricatives (*see* ARTICULATION) such as [s,z,ʃ,ʒ]. It is opposed to SLIT. *See* Catford (1989).

group design a design used for experiments. It is opposed to single case studies where statistical analysis attempts to show the effects of variables on single subjects. On the other hand, the group design is aimed at showing the effects of variables on groups of subjects which are either put into independent group designs, repeated measures or matched subjects design. *See* Miller (1984).

group therapy people can work out their problems with other people around them and find out how others in the group react to the way or ways those with the problem are given to overcome it. It can be used to supplement individual psychotherapy. It has many advantages:

1. People discover others with similar problems, thus creating support for one another.
2. Conversational situations can be created for context-oriented therapy so that the group can produce some functional communication.
3. More intensive therapy can be given.
4. Carry-over or maintenance is more likely.
5. A more stimulating environment is created, yet the patient is less tired than when given individual therapy since the burden of responding is spread around the group.
6. The person finds a social purpose.
7. The person becomes more involved in therapy.
8. A potentially more effective learning situation is created.

Group therapy is used mainly with those who stammer, or have an aphasia or dysarthria, as well as children who have phonological problems. *See* Fawcus (1989, 1992); Pachalska (1991a, b); Fawcus (1991); Aten (1991); Springer (1991); Loverso (1991); Repo (1991); Bollinger et al (1993) (group therapy in aphasia); Smith et al (2003); Davison et al (2004).

Guillain-Barré syndrome a condition produced by the ascending demyelination of the peripheral nerves. It is thought to be caused by a virus originally and may respond to steroids. It results in motor weakness with associated pains in the shoulders and back. Breathing can be affected and a tracheotomy should be undertaken. In very severe cases, there can be DYSARTHRIA, APHASIA and diplopia. The paralysis ascends through the body. *See* Gilroy and Holliday (1982); Beukelman and Mirenda (1998) (AAC); http://www.gbs.org.uk/

Guthrie test a test to screen newborn babies to check for such conditions as PHENYLKETONURIA. The heel is given a prick to remove some blood for examination. *See* Hosking (1982).

gyrus, gyri the CEREBRAL HEMISPHERES are covered in grooves due to folding of the CORTEX during development. The gyri are the elevated areas while the sulci (*see* SULCUS) are the fissures. *See* Barr (1988); Kolb and Whishaw (1996).

habilitation the process of therapy which aims to help the subject to recover to a level which allows him to function adequately within the community.

hallucination the person believes, by using his or her senses, that there is something in close proximity when there is no such stimulation close by. However, it has a quality for the person. Auditory hallucination occurs when the person believes he or she hears a sound when none exist. Hallucinations occur in SCHIZOPHRENIA when those with the condition believe they sense audible thoughts and voices arguing and commenting. *See* Kolb and Whishaw (1996); Smith et al (2003); Davison et al (2004).

hallux *see* PLANTAR RESPONSE.

hamulus *see* PHARYNX.

HandsOff an on-screen keyboard for Windows. There are ready-made grids for word processing, e-mail, web browsing and any communication software such as WINSPEAK. It can be accessed by scanning and can be used with most environmental control systems and can be configured to look however you want. *See* Appendix IV (Sensory Software International).

Hanen Approach a programme instigated with the founding of the Hanen Centre in 1977 to develop a more effective and family-centred approach to helping young children with a LANGUAGE DELAY. The philosophy behind the Hanen Approach is the involvement of parents and families in the remediation of their children's language problems and courses are provided to help families understand how they can adapt an everyday event and turn it into an opportunity for language learning. In this way, speech and language therapy extends beyond the formal therapy sessions. The Hanen Centre provides three courses for parents: It Takes Two to Talk – The Hanen program® for parents, More than Words – The Hanen program® for parents of children with AUTISTIC SPECTRUM DISORDER, and Target Word – The Hanen program ® for parents of children who are late talkers. The Centre also provides training for educators and childcare providers so that they can learn how to integrate everyday activities in a nursery or other centres into language learning. This course, Learning Language and Loving It – The Hanen program® for early childhood educators/teachers, focuses also on how the participants can promote children's social development, especially in relation to their interactions with their peers as well as to the development of early literacy skills. The Hanen Centre has certified speech and language pathologists who present the courses. *See* Sussman (1999); Ruiter (2000); http://www.hanen.org/Hanen2002/frames.htm

haptic perception a combination of tactile perception and proprioception concerned with an individual's sense of his body in relation to space. Some children and adults with certain types of language disorder, mainly of a dyspraxic nature, appear to be deficient in respect of perceptuomotor functioning.

hard copy information which is both printed out on paper as well as appearing on a monitor screen. It is opposed to soft copy. *See* Bishop (1985).

hard of hearing a description of a person whose hearing, though impaired, is used as a primary modality for auditory speech perception and language acquisition.

harmonic *see* ACOUSTIC PHONETICS.

harsh voice a type of DYSPHONIA with the essential feature being tension in the VOCAL FOLDS. The cause can be behavioural, such as excessive tension. Therapy is aimed at decreasing tension in the person generally, as well as particularly in the vocal folds. General relaxation or relaxation through suggestion can be used effectively so that the person can learn how to relax spontaneously when in stress-provoking situations. The YAWN/SIGH or chewing approach can be used to decrease tension in the vocal folds. *See* Freeman and Fawcus (2001).

Hawk II and III light-tech communication aids with vocabulary programmed in levels of eight locations – two levels in the Hawk II and three levels in the Hawk III. Hawk II allows for two minutes of recorded messages while the Hawk III allows for four minutes. It can be accessed by direct manual selection or by eight separate switches. *See* Rumble and Larcher (1998); Appendix IV (AdamLab).

head injury trauma to the BRAIN which can have widespread effects on the person's daily life. A closed head injury is caused by the brain being knocked against the skull. This is known as the contrecoup effect. In essence, the brain is a mass of tissue surrounded by fluid, so any heavy blow to the head, e.g. punch or hitting it on the ground from a fall, will result in it moving rapidly to the back or side of the skull. Such sudden movement can cause the blood vessels to rupture. The consequences are concussion and bruising, which cause haemorrhages and clots. Focal deficits produce HEMIPLEGIA, various degrees of APHASIA or DYSARTHRIA or acquired dyspraxia and problems as a result of damage to the CRANIAL NERVES. Global deficits produce loss of consciousness, disinhibition and memory deficits. Later complications can include postconcussion syndrome, HYDROCEPHALUS, DEMENTIA and fits. Medical treatment takes the form of steroids. The person with minor symptoms has a good prognosis but those severely impaired need a structured therapeutic programme, preferably in a rehabilitation unit. Those who have a head injury will probably require therapeutic intervention from various therapies such as OCCUPATIONAL THERAPY, PHYSIOTHERAPY and SPEECH AND LANGUAGE THERAPY. CLINICAL PSYCHOLOGY may also be involved. *See* Gilroy and Holliday (1982); Kaye (1991); Kolb and Whishaw (1996); http://www.headway.org.uk; http://hosting.texoma.net/business/biotech/thia-faq.htm

HeadMaster a mouse emulator system allowing those unable to use their hands to operate a computer. It does this by taking the place of the mouse. As those using HeadMaster move their heads, HeadMaster measures the rotation of the head and moves the cursor on the screen. Activating the puff switch or single switch makes a selection. On-screen keyboards such as WiViK allow for hands-free typing and other keyboard functions. HeadMaster can be used with an IBM PC or compatible in the Windows environment, mouse driven software or an Apple Mac. The same HeadMaster can be used for all computers and as a Remote HeadMaster by changing the configuration of three switches on the side of the control unit. The system comprises a control unit, a headset, a cable to link the control unit to the serial socket on the computer and another cable to link the headset to the control unit. A charging unit has to be attached to the control box at all times. The Remote HeadMaster allows the client to operate the computer without the cable linking the headset to the control unit, but it operates in the same way as the ordinary HeadMaster. *See* Appendix IV (Prentke Romich Company).

HeadMaster 2000 a small, lightweight mouse emulator which is operated by head movement. As the head is moved, the cursor moves on the screen and right and left button clicks are emulated by a sip-puff switch or an external switch. It is a remote system as there are no cables attached from the headset to the computer. A small infra-red sensor attaches to a headset or glasses sending a signal to an infra-red receiver. *See* Appendix IV (Prentke Romich Company).

HeadMouse a mouse emulator system allowing those unable to use their hands to operate a computer. There are no headset or cables required, only a small reusable sticker placed on the forehead, glasses, chin, finger or foot, etc.; the optical sensor tracks the person's head movements. It is used with an Apple Macintosh computer. *See* Appendix IV (Don Johnston Development Equipment Inc.).

hearing aid a device given to those who have a hearing loss. It works by taking in the sound vibrations from the air and converting them into electrical signals. There are two main types of hearing aid – analogue and digital. Analogue hearing aids pick up up sound through a microphone and convert it into small electrical signals. These signals are amplified and converted back to sound waves which are sent via the earmould to the ear. To allow this to happen, the hearing aid consists of a microphone (for picking up the sound and converting it to electrical signals), amplifier (makes the signal stronger), receiver

(receives the signal and converts it back to a sound signal, sending it through the tubing to the earmould in the auditory canal), battery (to power the aid) and the earmould (to make sure sound gets into ear). If the earmould does not fit in the canal correctly, sound leaks out causing feedback (a whistling sound). There are also buttons and dials used to control volume and an on/off switch – O = off, M = microphone (on), T = telecoil (to be used where there is a loop system). Digital hearing aids take the signal from the microphone and convert it into 'bits' of data which are manipulated by a very small computer in the hearing aid. This allows people to tailor and process sounds in a way to suit them. Many digital aids are designed to reduce steady kinds of background noise which can make listening more comfortable and some may have twin microphones allowing the person using the aid to switch between directional and all-around sound. In some aids feedback can be reduced or cancelled completely. Digital hearing aids, like analogue ones, come in behind-the-ear, in-the-ear or in-the-canal models. The main models of hearing aids are:

1. Body aids where the receiver is far from the microphone and amplifier. The sound signals are taken by a Y-cord to the earmoulds in each ear or through a single cord to the earmould.

2. Behind-the-ear aids have the microphone at the top of the body of the aid facing forward. These are relatively inconspicuous but feedback is more common than with body aids.

3. In-the-ear aids are most suitable for moderate to severe hearing losses. The components are built into a shell made from an impression of the client's ear.

4. CROS (contralateral routing of signals): this type of hearing aid is best suited for clients who have a rapidly

111

falling audiogram of the 'ski-slope' type (*see* PURE-TONE AUDIOMETRY). This is because it cuts out the low frequencies it receives but produces good amplification in the higher frequencies. The signal is carried by a cord from one side of the head to the other. Nowadays, there are cordless CROS hearing aids, in which sound is picked up on one side and activates a small radio transmitter on that side. The radio waves pass through the head and are picked up by a small radio receiver on the other side. The sound waves are amplified and sent to the receiver and the open delivery tube in the ear canal.

5. BICROS (bilateral contralateral routing of signals): hearing aids are similar to CROS hearing aids but use two microphones, one on each side of the head. These are connected to the same amplifier with a single receiver coupled to the better but impaired ear, using a closed earmould to avoid feedback.

6. IROS (ipsilateral routing of signals): IROS hearing aids are standard hearing aids with an open earmould on the same side. They can be used with ear-level aids with the tubing entering the ear canal. They are a very useful type of aid for those who have a mild to moderate, falling SENSORINEURAL HEARING LOSS and can be used binaurally. The only problem may be that feedback is more likely than with the CROS hearing aids.

7. Implantable hearing aids are of two types – one type excites the otic capsule and cochlea and so requires a functioning cochlea, while the second type of aid is attached to the ossicles when the hair cells of the cochlea have degenerated or are not functioning normally.

See Miller (1972); Lysons (1978); Katz (1985); Martin (2001); Tjellström (2001); http://www.rnis.org.uk/factsheets/hearing aids

Hearing Attitudes in Rehabilitation Questionnaires (HARQ) devised by Hallam, HARQ assesses three attitudes to hearing impairment and four attitudes to the provision of a hearing aid. They are designed to measure the following seven core factors: perceived self as distressed/inadequate in situations of auditory communication; perceived self as having reduced social status and perceiving others as having negative attitudes as a result of hearing impairment; minimising the importance of hearing impairment as a significant problem; perceiving an aid as stigmatising; perceiving self as not wanting/needing an aid if an aid is unhelpful; perceiving external pressure to be assessed for an aid; and having an over-positive expectation that an aid will restore normal hearing quickly. *See* Hallam (1997) in Appendix I.

hearing level the number of decibels above audiometric zero at which a person can just hear sound at a specific frequency. It is used in PURE-TONE AUDIOMETRY.

hearing loss a description of a person's hearing when the results of audiological assessment, e.g. PURE-TONE AUDIOMETRY, show that there is a varying degree of difficulty in receiving sound. There are several types of hearing loss such as CONDUCTIVE HEARING LOSS, SENSORINEURAL HEARING LOSS, mixed hearing loss, CENTRAL HEARING LOSS, CONGENITAL HEARING LOSS and ACQUIRED HEARING LOSS. *See* Katz (1985); Smith et al (2003); Plant (1993) (acquired hearing loss).

hearing threshold level (HTL) *see* HEARING LEVEL.

heart the heart is divided into four areas – the right and left atria and the right and left ventricles. The heart pumps blood around the body. Blood enters the heart by the inferior and superior vena cavae into the right atrium which contracts and pushes the blood through the tricuspid valve to the right ventricle. The ventricle pushes the blood through the pulmonary valve into the pulmonary artery from where it goes to the lung; here it picks up oxygen, turns bright red and returns to the heart via the pulmonary veins, entering the left atrium. When it contracts, the blood is pushed through the mitral valve into the left ventricle which in turn pushes the blood through the aortic valve into the aorta. As it goes along this artery, it passes into other arteries of the body, arterioles (smaller arteries) and the capillaries where it loses oxygen and becomes dark blue. From these different areas of the body, the blood flows back to the heart. When the heart muscle contracts, it is a period of systole, when it relaxes, it is known as a period of diastole. *See* Tortora and Grabowski (2000).

Hector speech aid an aid to help people who STAMMER to become more fluent speakers. It consists of a throat microphone placed against the LARYNX, a small amplifier and a control box which can be attached to a waist belt or put in a pocket. The microphone can be hidden under a high collar of a blouse, shirt or jumper. Its aim is to decrease the rate of the person's speech and hence allow the speaker to produce a type of PROLONGED SPEECH. If the speaker has a very fast rate of speech, it is picked up by the microphone and a tone is produced through the amplifier. The volume of the tone can be turned up or down so that it can blend into the background noise. It can be used for practice at home and during speech therapy sessions.

hemiplegia the result of trauma to the brain such as CEREBROVASCULAR ACCIDENT, HEAD INJURY or other trauma or disease which produces a focal lesion in the BRAIN. Two limbs are affected, usually the arm and leg on one side of the body. If the lesion occurs in the left cerebral hemisphere (*see* CEREBRAL HEMISPHERES), the hemiplegia will affect the person's right side. In such circumstances, anosognosia (*see* ASOMATOGNOSIA) can occur. PHYSIOTHERAPY is given to those with hemiplegia as well as OCCUPATIONAL THERAPY to increase upper limb function. *See* Kolb and Whishaw (1996).

herpes simplex usually a simple virus infection of the skin which is self-healing but may be recurrent, producing cold sores. Rarely it may cause ENCEPHALITIS. Both children and adults are affected, with an equal sex ratio. The person with encephalitis presents symptoms similar to those of flu, e.g. headache, fever, followed by irritation to the MENINGES, and becomes disoriented in space. Later, psychosis and memory problems can occur as well as APHASIA and monoparesis (one limb only is affected by weakness). The final stage is a coma. If a mother has this infection during pregnancy, it can cross the placenta and cause disorders to the fetus. It is part of the TORCH classification of infections which affect the fetus. *See* Gilroy and Holliday (1982); http://www.skinsite.com/info_herpes_simplex.htm

hertz (Hz) *see* ACOUSTIC PHONETICS.

hesitation periods of silence or FILLED PAUSES while the speaker either thinks of more information or reiterates and amplifies what has been said. Certain positions have been found in an utterance where hesitation occurs. These are at certain appropriate places in the grammar of the utterance, after other constituents and at the beginning of an utterance before the speaker has decided finally how to continue the utterance. *See* Clark and Clark (1977).

hierarchy a structure which starts with one unit at the top and has branches linking it to lower units. A TREE DIAGRAM is a type of hierarchical structure. The units above other units are called superordinate terms while the units below other units are subordinate terms. In the tree diagram, 'sentence' is superordinate to NOUN PHRASE and verb phrase (*see* CONSTITUENT ANALYSIS), while DETERMINER, ADJECTIVE, NOUN are subordinate to noun phrase. *See* Lyons (1968); Fromkin and Rodman (2003).

high a DISTINCTIVE FEATURE proposed by Chomsky and Halle to distinguish sounds produced with the tongue in a raised position of the mouth [+HIGH] from those produced with the tongue in a low position [–HIGH]. *See* Hyman (1975).

high frequency hearing loss the person who has this type of hearing loss is unable to perceive high frequencies such as some of the fricatives (*see* ARTICULATION) but can obtain a hearing device which allows high frequency sounds to be heard.

hindbrain part of the brain which comprises the PONS, MEDULLA OBLONGATA and the CEREBELLUM. It is found below the MIDBRAIN. *See* Barr (1988); Kolb and Whishaw (1996).

histogram a type of graph used in DESCRIPTIVE STATISTICS to analyse the results of an experiment. The measures are shown as a single block placed above the interval in which the measure is found. For example, if the 100m race was run with the following times being recorded: 9.1, 9.3, 9.4, 10.1, 10.3, the blocks would be placed above the interval of 9–10 and 10–11 respectively on the bottom axis of the graph. *See* Miller (1984).

hoarse voice a type of DYSPHONIA produced by the person straining to speak against the tension of the VOCAL FOLDS. Wilson (1979) described it as a 'combination of harshness and breathiness with harsh voice predominating in some cases and breathy elements in others'. *See* Freeman and Fawcus (2001).

homeostasis keeping the body's internal environment within certain physiological limits. *See* J.H. Green (1982); Smith et al (2003); Tortora and Grabowski (2000).

homonymy a phenomenon in SEMANTICS in which a lexical item can appear in different contexts with the same pronunciation but not necessarily the same spelling, and have at least two different meanings. Such words are homonyms. The form 'bear' has two meanings, one of which is a noun referring to a type of animal, and the other a verb which is a synonym of 'carry'. *See* Palmer (1976); Fromkin and Rodman (2003).

homophony a phenomenon in semantic theory in which two words pronounced

the same have a different meaning. Such words are called homophones. Examples are 'sun/son', 'boy/buoy', etc. *See* Palmer (1976); Fromkin and Rodman (2003).

homorganic a phenomenon where two articulations are made by the same articulators (*see* ARTICULATION). Thus, [p] and [b] can be described as homorganic sounds as they are both produced by two lips. *See* Ladefoged (2001).

hormones *see* ENDOCRINE SYSTEM.

HTL *see* HEARING THRESHOLD LEVEL.

Huntington's disease a rare autosomal dominant (*see* CHROMOSOMES) disease producing DEMENTIA. The onset of the disease occurs in middle age. The person's personality becomes psychopathic, violent and a dependence on alcohol may begin. The person shows a tremor at distal parts of the muscles and athetoid (*see* CEREBRAL PALSY) movement begins. Although there is no treatment available for this condition, L-dopa (*see* LEVODOPA) is given to stop the tremor. It is caused by problems in the caudate nucleus and BASAL GANGLIA. *See* Stafford-Clark and Bridges (1990); Kolb and Whishaw (1996); Smith et al (2003); Beukelman and Mirenda (1998) (AAC); Yorkston et al (1995); Klasner and Yorkston (2001) (AAC and Huntington's disease); http://www.hda.org.uk/

hydrocephalus a condition in which an abnormal volume of CEREBROSPINAL FLUID (CSF) is found in the skull. It can be caused by a tumour in close proximity to the FOURTH VENTRICLE with evidence of increased intracranial pressure. It can be treated by ventricular drainage. The incidence of infantile hydrocephalus is about 3–4 per 1000 and most children present with congenital abnormalities. The major clinical features in infants include: (1) FAILURE TO THRIVE; (2) failure to achieve milestones; (3) increased skull circumference; (4) tense anterior fontanelle; (5) a cracked pot sound on skull when hit; and (6) being able to see through the skull when a strong light is held against it. In severe cases, there are also the following clinical features: (1)

impaired conscious level and vomiting; (2) 'setting suns' appearance where the eyelids retract and the person cannot look upwards; and (3) thin scalp with dilated veins. The Arnold-Chiari malformation may also produce hydrocephalus. This malformation is produced by a disorder to the MEDULLA OBLONGATA and CEREBELLUM causing an obstruction for the cerebrospinal fluid. There are three types which differ mainly by severity. In adults, the major clinical features are headache, vomiting, papilloedema and deterioration of conscious state. *See* Gilroy and Holliday (1982); Kolb and Whishaw (1996); Kaye (1991); Tortora and Grabowski (2000); http://www.asbah.org/

hyoid bone *see* MUSCLES FOR SWALLOWING; Tortora and Grabowski (2000).

hyperkinetic dysarthria *see* DYSARTHRIA (1a).

hypernasality a condition caused by the failure of the soft palate (*see* MOUTH) to close when producing speech. This produces sounds which are both nasal and oral. This can be caused by large ADENOIDS.

hyperplasia excessive growth of a tissue or of certain cells. *See* Tortora and Grabowski (2000).

hypertonia an abnormal amount of power in limbs. It refers to increased muscle tone and is expressed in terms of spasticity (*see* CEREBRAL PALSY). There is a stiffness in the muscles and increase in tendon reflexes and rigidity. Rigidity is an increase in muscle tone which does not affect the reflexes. *See* Tortora and Grabowski (2000).

hypochondriasis a NEUROSIS in which a person's life becomes tortured by fears of having contracted some serious disease. In most cases, such people have ordinary illnesses which can be as minor as an irregular heartbeat, sweating, minor cough, etc. Men tend to have this condition more than women. It is very difficult to reassure them that their illness is not as serious as they believe.

The condition can be a symptom of depression. *See* Stafford-Clark and Bridges (1990); Davison et al (2004).

hypoglossal nerve *see* INTRINSIC MUSCLES OF THE TONGUE; CRANIAL NERVES.

hypoglossus muscle *see* EXTRINSIC MUSCLES OF THE TONGUE.

hypokinetic dysarthria *see* DYSARTHRIA (1b).

hypoplasia a description of an anatomical structure which has not developed as fully as it should. *See* Tortora and Grabowski (2000).

hypothalamus a small structure in the DIENCEPHALON found below the THALAMUS forming the floor and part of the lateral walls of the THIRD VENTRICLE. It is important for regulating sleep, thirst, hunger and temperature within the body. It affects the AUTONOMIC NERVOUS SYSTEM. *See* Barr (1988); Kolb and Whishaw (1996); Smith et al (2003); Tortora and Grabowski (2000).

hypotonia a description of flaccidity found in muscles. *See* Ginsbergh (1999); Tortora and Grabowski (2000).

hysteria a NEUROSIS in which stress becomes so overwhelming that, unconsciously, the person presents, and may even experience, symptoms of physical illness. Stress can also be shown by severe mental illness, e.g. DEPRESSION, SCHIZOPHRENIA. Minor hysteria causes a loss in or interference with the person's normal or sensory function. Such problems take the form of blindness, deafness, anaesthesia, PARAPHASIA and paralysis or disturbance of motor activity. The symptoms must be primarily physical. Treatment involves the removal of the underlying stress and/or depression. PSYCHOTHERAPY or hypnosis have also been used successfully to remove such symptoms. *See* Stafford-Clark and Bridges (1990); Davison et al (2004).

hysterical dysphonia *see* CONVERSION REACTION; Freeman and Fawcus (2001).

Hz (hertz) *see* ACOUSTIC PHONETICS.

IA (item and arrangement) *see* MORPH-
OLOGY.

icon

1. There are arbitrary conventions in
   semiotics. However, icons are fixed
   signs such as onomatopoeic words
   'splash', 'crack' and 'bang'. The form
   of these words can never change. *See*
   Robins (1971).
2. A symbol on a display. Instead of
   using the keyboard to operate the
   computer, icons can now be used for
   this purpose. When icons are called
   up, they appear in windows and the
   operator has to use a pointer to
   choose the appropriate icon. In
   some programs, the cursor keys can
   be used, others may require the use
   of a mouse, touchscreen or light pen.
3. Symbols used on high-tech electronic
   devices using MINSPEAK such as ALPHA
   TALKERS, TOUCHTALKERS, LIGHTTALKERS,
   DELTA TALKERS, INTRO TALKERS, the LIBER-
   ATOR COMMUNICATION AID, VANGUARD,
   PATHFINDER and SPRINGBOARD. *See*
   Beukelman and Mirenda (1998)
   (AAC/Minspeak).

iconicity the degree to which a symbol
relates to what it represents or its referent. At one end of the iconicity continuum there is the notion of transparency
where the meaning of the symbol can
be guessed if its referent were not present and at the other end is the notion
of a symbol being opaque where there
is no such relationship between the

symbol and its referent. In the middle is
the notion of translucency where there
may have to be some teaching of the
perceived link between the symbol and
its referent. *See* Fuller and Lloyd (1991);
Lloyd and Blischak (1992); Glennen
and DeCoste (1997); Beukelman and
Mirenda (1998).

IconSpeak is a symbol-based vocabulary
system designed for palm size PCs such
as Casio's Cassiopeia. It is accessed by
direct manual selection and vocabularies can be customised for any age
group. There can be a range from six
icons to 24 icons and messages per
page with a maximum of 100 pages.
Photographs can be scanned in to the
system. *See* Appendix IV (Bostock).

ICP *see* INTRACRANIAL PRESSURE.

ID *see* PERSONALITY.

ideal self *see* PHENOMENOLOGICAL APPROACH.

idiolect a term used for the individual linguistic system of a particular speaker –
his or her dialect. There are regional
dialects which have different variations
of the spoken language. However, there
are also differences of dialect between
people in that they have particular ways
of producing utterances which are different from other people. Idiolect continues to develop after a child has fully
acquired language as the child picks up
modifications from the language of his
or her family. Haas (1963) writes of a
child's phonological disorder as being
'a language of his own or idiolect'. In an
important passage, he writes why

speech therapists need to know about idiolect: 'It would seem speech therapy stands to gain in efficiency, if, to a greater extent than has been usual, it could take account of the underlying and interfering "idiolect" of the treated child' (Haas, 1963, p. 246). *See* Trudgill (1995); Fromkin and Rodman (2003).

idiom a phrase whose meaning is not given by analysing its constituent parts, e.g. 'kick the bucket', 'play the field'. *See* Lyons (1968); Fromkin and Rodman (2003).

idiopathic a disease which has no known cause.

IEP+ *see* INTERACTION, EDUCATION AND PLAY.

ill-formed a description of sentences which are ungrammatical in terms of a particular set of grammatical rules, i.e. they cannot be generated by the rule. It is found in discussions concerning GEN-ERATIVE GRAMMAR. If a sentence cannot be generated, it is ill-formed. *See* Huddleston (1976).

Illinois Test of Psycholinguistic Abilities (ITPA) devised by Kirk in 1969, ITPA is a formal, standardised assessment. It can be used with children aged 2–10 years old, although it is less useful for children below the chronological age of 4 years. It has 12 subtests: auditory reception; visual reception; visual sequential memory; auditory association; auditory sequential memory; visual association; visual closure; verbal expression; grammatical closure; manual expression; auditory closure; and sound blending. The raw scores from these subtests together produce a psycholinguistic age or separate scaled scores. These scores can be drawn on a graph to show each child's psycholinguistic abilities. *See* Kirk et al (1969) in Appendix I; Paraskevopoulus and Kirk (1985) in Appendix I; Beech et al (1993).

illocution a term used in speech act theories to denote the way in which a speaker intends his utterance to be taken. Examples are promising, requesting and regretting. In some types of language disorder, speakers are not able to convey their intention accurately. *See* Fromkin and Rodman (2003).

imitation

1. A process which has been proposed to explain the child's language acquisition as the imitation of sounds, words and sentences used by adults in his immediate environment. The realisation that children produced 'errors' never heard in their language environment, e.g. goed, camed, casts immediate doubt on the validity of imitation as a complete explanation. Imitation, however, is often used in language remediation by speech and language therapists. *See* Clark and Clark (1977); Fromkin and Rodman (2003).

2. A form of therapy given to those who have poor social skills. It is a difficult form of therapy as the instructor has to provide almost impeccable social skills for the person to try and copy exactly. *See* Trower et al (1978); Smith et al (2003).

IMPACT: Implementing Augmentative Communication Training a training programme to help those who work with people who use AAC to implement the devices more successfully. There are many factors which work together to develop augmented communication skills. If any of these fail or the significant others helping those who use AAC fail to realise something is wrong with the way they are trying to implement the augmented system, the system itself may fail and the person using the device or the device itself may be blamed. This programme tries to bring to the attention of those working with the device, what these factors are, how they may fail, and how they can put them right based on the experience of the author and his colleagues. The programme is divided into two parts – the first is a series of cartoons featuring the many situations in which AAC systems may fail while the second part has notes on each topic presented by the cartoons. *See* Jones (1995a).

impairment a disease or injury which causes people certain difficulties in functioning. For example, if a lesion in the BRAIN affects the motor co-ordination of the speech mechanism producing DYSARTHRIA, the person is said to have an impairment in the affected part of the brain.

impedance the opposition offered by an object to the transmission of sound or some acoustic energy. The greater the impedance, the less sound will be transmitted. It is opposed to compliance.

impedance audiometry the means of finding out about the status of the tympanic membrane and middle ear (*see* EAR) using tympanometry. There are three types of impedance measures:

1. The compliance peak shows that the air pressures in the ear canal and middle ear are equal and the tester can assume the Eustachian tube is functioning. Thus, the height of the compliance peak reflects mobility. Static compliance is the height of the tympanogram at its peak and is a measurement of system mobility.
2. Static impedance which is measured when the pressure in the external auditory canal equals the atmospheric pressure and the muscles of the middle ear (*see* EAR) are at rest.
3. Dynamic impedance is measured when the tympanic membrane (*see* EAR) is moved suddenly from its position at rest by the contraction of the stapedius (*see* EAR) muscle, i.e. it shows the amount of reflected energy as a function of change in the position of and stiffness of the tympanic membrane.

The impedance bridge or impedance audiometer comprises three small rubber tubes which are attached to a small metal probe. One is attached to a miniature microphone which picks up the sound in the canal, another to a loudspeaker which puts a pure tone (*see* PURE-TONE AUDIOMETRY) of 220 Hz into the ear, and the third is attached to an air pump which creates either a positive or a negative pressure in the canal. An air-tight seal is created when the probe is placed in the canal. The results from static compliance are not particularly useful for making a diagnosis while the results from dynamic impedance are important. If there is a stapedius reflex, it indicates hearing is normal, the middle ear is functioning normally (if obtained at normal hearing level), or there is a sensory hearing loss (if obtained at a low sensation level). If there is no stapedius reflex this indicates either a facial nerve (*see* CRANIAL NERVE VII) lesion is present on the side of the tested ear, or there is a problem with the ossicles (*see* EAR), or a CONDUCTIVE HEARING LOSS on the side of the earphone (i.e. sound is not loud enough in the ear to elicit reflex), or a severe to profound SENSORINEURAL HEARING LOSS in the earphone ear. The results from tympanometry are in the form of diagrams. Jerger found five types:

1. Type A – indicates normal middle ear function.
2. Type As (shallow) – indicates normal middle ear pressure and a partially immobilised stapes (possible OTOSCLEROSIS).
3. Type Ad (deep) – indicates malfunctioning of the ossicles (*see* EAR) producing high compliance.
4. Type B – a flat trace indicates that the middle ear is filled with fluid, which makes it impossible to find a point of maximum compliance. Type B tympanograms must be analysed along with the ear canal volumes. If there is normal ear canal volume, it usually means OTITIS MEDIA exists; small ear canal volume suggests the ear canal is filled with wax or that the immitance probe is pushing against the wall of the ear canal while a large ear canal volume suggests a perforation in the tympanic membrane
5. Type C – indicates negative pressure in the middle ear produced by a

blockage in the Eustachian tube (*see* EAR) causing serous otitis media (*see* OTITIS MEDIA (3)).

implosive a glottalic ingressive voiced stop. It is very difficult to produce voice with an ejective stop, while devoicing may be difficult with implosives. The sequence of movements for producing an implosive is:

1. Close the glottis.
2. Make a closure of the lips (e.g. [b]).
3. Move the larynx downward (compare taking a gulp).
4. Release the closure.
5. A voiced implosive [ɓ] is produced.

See Catford (1977).

imprinting a learning process usually referring to the type of learning used by young birds to form an attachment to their parents. It takes place at a critical period just after birth and ends when a parent model is learned. *See* Smith et al (2003).

INCH *see* INTERACTION CHECKLIST FOR AUGMENTATIVE COMMUNICATION.

independent group design an experimental design which gets together a group of subjects to take part in the experiment as a whole. The individuals are then divided up randomly into the two conditions with equal numbers being allocated to each experimental condition. *See* Miller (1984).

indirect object the term traditionally used for the syntactic relation obtained between the verb and either a prepositional phrase (to Nara), as in (1), or the first noun phrase (Nara), as in (2), with verbs like 'give' in English:

1. Joyce gave the book to Nara.
2. Joyce gave Nara the book.

See Lyons (1968).

industrial hearing loss *see* NOISE-INDUCED HEARING LOSS.

infantile autism *see* AUTISM.

infantile swallowing pattern a persisting immature pattern of swallowing involving anterior tongue thrust. It may be associated with dental malocclusion and with articulatory disorder.

inferential statistics a study of statistics in which statistical tests are used to show whether or not a significant difference exists between the control and experimental groups. It also allows the experimenter to generalise the result of one small group to other groups of people. The tests which can be used are divided into parametric and non-parametric tests (*see* PARAMETRIC TESTS). *See* Miller (1984).

informal assessments assessments which do not have a fixed format. They are evolved by the therapist to assess a person's difficulties, if the person is unable to cope with a formal assessment, or used during therapy to assess the efficacy of a therapy programme. Such tests allow more latitude which may, by giving cues, discover how much and what kind of help the person requires to succeed. Material used in such tests must be different from the material used in formal assessments so as not to invalidate the results used later in therapy.

information processing a model of language in which there are three main components involved – a receiver, whereby information is taken in, i.e. the sensory channels in the case of language; an integrator which is responsible for perception of the incoming stimuli and for their storage in memory and a response system.

infra- a description of the area below the structure to which the prefix is attached.

infraglottic a description of the whole area including the structures below the glottis.

Ingfield Dynamic Vocabularies (IDV) a vocabulary set which can be used with the CAMELEON family of high-tech communication aids. IDV uses colour-coded symbols in four levels. The sets increase in complexity through the addition of more symbols per page, an increase in the range of topics and the sophistication of the language available. The top page shows all the topics which, when accessed by the people using IDV, will take them to one or more pages of related vocabulary to the chosen topic. At all levels, there are 'sentence starters' or phrases accessed by one hit, an 'about me' page and a 'Quicktalk' page which offers useful complete sentences. Different colours represent different syntactic categories (e.g., adjectives have a blue background, verbs have a green background). The words are placed in a left to right order for natural sequencing of language. *See* Appendix IV (Ingfield Manor).

ingressive *see* AIRSTREAMS.

InGrid a mouse-controlled on-screen keyboard for Windows. It can be used by anyone who can use a mouse, trackball or any other pointing device to control the computer. InGrid can be used with any vocabulary grids for WINSPEAK or HANDSOFF and graphics can be scanned indirectly. *See* Appendix IV (Sensory Software International).

inhalation *see* OESOPHAGEAL VOICE.

initial interview the first session that a therapist or any other professional has with a client. This session is important for setting up a rapport with the client and any accompanying relatives and for taking a sufficient case history. The initial interview normally has six stages:

1. Introduction: often called 'meeting, greeting and seating' (Nelson-Jones 1982). It is important to make the client feel as comfortable as possible at this stage since therapy of any kind can be seen as a threat. There can also be a stigma attached to coming for therapy. On the other hand, some clients may have their hopes raised too high and expect therapists to be miracle workers.
2. Assessment of the presenting disorder: this can be either a formal assessment or an informal assessment (*see* ASSESSMENTS) to find out what the client can or cannot do. This should be explained to the client as some of the subtests can be very easy while others may be more difficult.
3. Exploration of presenting disorder: this is really the case history, finding out how the disorder occurred and how it affects family life and the relationships within the home.
4. Reconnaissance: the therapist tries to find out how the client views him/herself since the onset of the disorder and examines the history of the disorder.
5. Contracting: takes place when the therapist and client come to an agreement on the type of therapy which the client will begin to receive regularly.
6. Termination: the final stage where the therapist clears up any confusions which may have arisen from this initial interview and, most importantly, another appointment is made.

During these six stages, the therapist should have in mind the following four interrelated objectives:

1. Creating a 'working alliance', i.e. a good rapport with the client.
2. Forming a 'working model' of the client, i.e. client's feeling concerning change in lifestyle and aspirations for the future.
3. Forming 'working goals', i.e. treatment programme.
4. Deciding which therapy method to use.

See Nelson-Jones (1982).

injection *see* OESOPHAGEAL VOICE.

innateness a theory to explain how people learn. Noam Chomsky used this theory to explain the language ACQUISITION of children. He believes humans are born with several different areas in their brains for specific functions. Language is one of these areas. This innate knowledge of language has become known as the LANGUAGE ACQUISITION DEVICE. It is the LAD which sparks off the hypothetical language area in the child's brain. *See* Steinberg (1982); Smith et al (2003).

input devices hardware used to access software on a computer, particularly for people who do not have the fine motor control to use a regular keyboard or who develop such conditions as repetitive stress injury.

1. Alternative means of accessing a computer include specialised mice such as the Anir mouse, LIGHT PEN, CONCEPT KEYBOARD, TOUCHSCREEN and speech recognition systems such as dradon dicate or viavoice, devices which can be used by eye tracking such as the QUICK GLANCE EYE TRACKING SYSTEM or those which use head movements such as HEADMASTER, HEADMOUSE or smart-nav. These pieces of hardware would allow the use of on-screen keyboards such as WIVIK or those used in REACH INTERFACE AUTHOR.

2. Communication aids can be accessed by a variety of switches of shapes and colours which can be mounted onto a wheelchair in the best position for the person to activate them most reliably and not by accident, or using headpointer systems either like those discussed above or optical infra-red systems specific to certain communication aids. *See* Brookshear (1991); Glennen and DeCoste (1997); Beukelman and Mirenda (1998); Appendix IV (Applied Human Factors; Don Johnston; Prentke Romich Company).

insufflation *see* OESOPHAGEAL VOICE.

INTECOM devised by Jones in 1989, it is a programme to help develop the communication skills of clients with learning difficulties. It maximises functional communication, optimising a person's existing skills and communication opportunities. It is in two parts:

1. Programme planning package: it contains a rapid communication checklist, so that the therapist can plan a communication opportunities programme for each client.

2. Training package: speech and language therapists and psychologists can use this package to train carers and teachers how to develop communication skills through the use of the communication checklist and programme planner.

The programme planning package contains 10 communication checklists and a manual, while the training package contains training notes and other necessary materials to run training courses in basic communication theory. *See* Jones (1989) in Appendix I.

intelligence one of the most debated issues throughout the history of psychology where even providing a definition can show a preference for a particular theory about intelligence, so there follows a brief description of the various main theories of intelligence which have been proposed in the past and more recently. Certainly the early attempts to define intelligence were determined to a great extent on the beliefs of people such as Binet who designed INTELLIGENCE TESTS while others argued for three basic cognitive processes of abstraction, learning and dealing with novelty. Spearman in 1904 proposed the concept of factor analysis where everybody possesses a general intelligence factor known as 'g' while special factors, known as 's', are specific to particular abilities or tests. However in the last 20–30 years, this 'g' factor has been cast aside in favour of trying to explain intelligence in terms of the cognitive processes which people use when participating in intellectual activities. These theorists, therefore, look at the specific processes which individuals bring to a task and the speed and accuracy of those processes and measure the efficiency of each component of the process. Gardner (1993) proposed his theory of multiple intelligences to contradict the view that intelligence was about logical reasoning. Instead of considering intelligence having a 'g', he thought of there being seven intelligences – linguistic, musical, logical-mathematical, spatial, bodily-kinesthetic, intrapersonal and interpersonal. These seven intelligences existed because he had considered all the different skills and abilities which individuals need to survive in their own and different cultures so people can have different roles in society such as farmer, doctor, businessman and so on. However, a criticism levelled at Gardner's multiple intelligences is that a high level of ability in any of the seven intelligences is usually correlated with high ability in the others. Anderson proposes that changes to intellectual development and competence are explained by different mechanisms. His theory promotes the idea that differences to intelligence are produced by differences in the 'basic processing mechanism' which implements thinking and produces knowledge. This basic processing mechanism varies in speed from person to person. These mechanisms which provide universal capacities are known as 'modules', each of which functions independently of the other working out complex computations, and are unaffected by the basic processing mechanism as they are virtually automatic. Anderson has put forward the notion that it is the maturation of new modules which causes the increase in cognitive abilities during development. There are also two specific abilities to complete his theory on intelligence – propositional thought (language and mathematical expression) and visual/spatial functioning. Another modern theorist often cited for his ideas about intelligence is Sternberg and his triarchic theory. In this theory, he considers experience and context as well as basic information processing mechanisms. There are three parts to his theory: componential subtheory dealing with thought processes; the experiential subtheory dealing with the effects of experience on intelligence; and the contextual subtheory which takes account of the person's environment and culture. The criticism levelled at Sternberg's theory is that it is not coherent because there are too many parts to it, it does not show how problem solving occurs and it does not take into account the biological aspects of intelligence. Stephen Ceci has taken Sternberg's theory and tried to extend it but has put much more work into looking at context and how it affects problem solving and so he proposed his bioecological theory for intelligence. The basis for his theory is that while there are multiple intelligences, they are biologically based and limit mental processes, but the way in which they appear is determined by the challenges and opportunities which are presented to people depending on their environment or context. For Ceci 'context' relates to domains of knowledge as well as a person's personality, motivation and education. He believes that even if a person does not show high mental abilities for a particular activity, by giving them a more interesting and motivational approach the same person or group can show higher levels of performance. By taking all these theories into account, the study of intelligence has left behind theories for intelligence testing and instead is concentrating on the complex interaction between biological and environmental factors which has become the main focus in today's psychology or as Gardner wrote in 1999, 'The theory of multiple intelligences has helped break the psychometricians' century long stranglehold on the subject of intelligence'. *See* Gilman (2001); Smith et al (2003).

intelligence quotient (IQ) the score obtained from carrying out an intelligence test. It is calculated by using the formula:

$$IQ = MA/CA \times 100$$

This reads 'the client's IQ is his mental age (MA) divided by his chronological age (CA) multiplied by 100 and rounded to bring the result to a whole number'. *See* Kolb and Whishaw (1996); Smith et al (2003).

intelligence tests psychological tests aimed at finding out the ability of the child or adult to carry out various tasks presented to him usually without reference to previous learned material. Psychological testing tends to be controversial but there are safeguards built into most tests to make as sure as possible that the scores obtained are reliable and valid. The controversy surrounding the tests arises from a number of misconceptions. Some believe intelligence tests measure innate intelligence and that IQs are fixed and cannot be changed; they measure all one needs to know about the client's intelligence. IQs obtained from several tests are interchangeable and a battery of tests tells psychologists all they need to know to enable them to make judgements about a person's competence. All such beliefs can be countered by arguing that test results should not be taken at face value but that any interpretation put on them must take into account other factors such as case history information as well as any behaviour disorder which the client may have, his temperament, e.g. fatigue, language disorders, etc., at the time of testing. In certain parts of the country, it will be necessary to take into account the child's cultural background. It is, therefore, important to note the time of testing and the appropriateness of the test used. Intelligence tests which are most frequently used include: (1) STANFORD-BINET INTELLIGENCE SCALES; (2) BRITISH ABILITY SCALES; (3) WECHSLER INTELLIGENCE SCALE FOR CHILDREN – REVISED (WISC-R); (4) WECHSLER ADULT INTELLIGENCE SCALE – REVISED (WAIS-R); (5) MERRILL-PALMER PRE-SCHOOL INTELLIGENCE TEST; (6) RAVEN'S PROGRESSIVE MATRICES and vocabulary scales. *See* Kolb and Whishaw (1996); Smith et al (2003); Davison et al (2004).

intention tremor a tremor caused by a disorder to the CEREBELLUM. The person's limb produces an observable tremor when specific movements are made. *See* Gilroy and Holliday (1982).

Interaction Checklist for Augmentative Communication (INCH) a checklist devised in 1984 by Bolton and Dashiell so that a therapist can decide on the most important needs for people who use AAC to communicate with their facilitators and friends and family. It looks at strategies used in a communicative exchange. It distinguishes four types of strategy: initiation, facilitation, regulation and termination. INCH also examines the modes or means by which messages are communicated. It looks at five major types of modes using verbal and non-verbal communication: linguistic, paralinguistic, kinesic (non-verbal communication such as facial expression and body movement including eye contact, etc.), proxemic (distance between those communicating) and chronemic (timing of responses and rate at which communication takes place). Finally, INCH analyses the contexts in which a communication aid will be used, i.e. those who will use it (both the person using AAC and receiver) as well as the situations in which it will be used, e.g. at school, at home, in a restaurant or in hospital, etc. The authors have divided participants into four classes depending on the degree of familiarity or unfamiliarity with the person who is going to use the AAC system and on their competency with the person's communication aid. The four classes are: familiar-trained, familiar-untrained, unfamiliar-trained, unfamiliar-untrained. In general, by administering INCH, the authors hope to provide a 'systematic observation of interaction between augmentative system users and their receivers' (Bolton and Dashiell 1984, p. 14). *See* Bolton and Dashiell (1984).

Interaction, Education and Play (IEP+) devised by Bruno in 1988 and revised in 1990, IEP+ is a MINSPEAK APPLICATION PROGRAM (MAP) for children with a mental age of 3;6–9;0. The icon set and pre-stored vocabulary need to reflect the user's abilities, needs, experiences, interests and goals. The person using the system must be able to use a 128-location overlay with a cognitive/language performance at the 3;6 year level.

The prestored vocabulary takes into account the following speech acts: (1) greeting and social exchanges; (2) protests and negative comments; (3) requests and clarification; (4) information; and (5) requests. All these speech acts can be accessed by not more than two icon actuations. A single word lexicon is also available. A simple vocabulary can be accessed by using two icons. Commonly used words can be accessed so that the person using IEP+ can produce grammatically correct messages. A group of words can be accessed for classroom use. The system can also be used in play, accessing story books, rhymes and songs as well as high interest vocabulary items. *See* Bruno (1989a).

interdental *see* ARTICULATION.

interface the attachment of a central processor to various peripheral units. For example, when a printer or disk drive is linked to a computer, they are said to interface with the computer. This type of interface is sometimes called a master/slave interface because one machine, e.g. computer, has control over one or more machines, e.g. disk drive and printer. *See* Bishop (1985).

internal carotid artery *see* CAROTID ARTERY.

International Phonetic Alphabet (IPA) a system of symbols used in transcribing a person's speech. It was devised by the International Phonetic Association which was inaugurated in 1886 by a small group of language teachers in France who found phonetics useful in their work. The Association produced the IPA chart (1951, revised 1979, 1989, 1993 and 1996) which divides up the sounds into place and manner of articulation (*see* ARTICULATION) for consonants. It also shows the CARDINAL VOWEL SYSTEM as well as a list of the DIACRITICS which can be used in narrow transcriptions (*see* TRANSCRIPTION SYSTEMS). *See* Appendix III; Abercrombie (1967); Duckworth (1990); Fromkin and Rodman (2003); http://www2.arts.gla.ac.uk/IPA/ipa.html

intervocalic a consonantal sound which appears between two vowels, e.g. /t/ in 'butter' where the /t/ sound is intervocalic.

intonation *see* SUPRASEGMENTAL PHONOLOGY.

intracranial pressure (ICP) pressure within the cranium produced by the amount of CEREBROSPINAL FLUID, blood and size of brain. If the pressure varies slightly in one area, another area can compensate. Large lesions to a particular area may be so significant that no compensation can take place and the pressure is increased with resultant damage to other structures. *See* Hosking (1982); Kaye (1991).

intraoral a description of structures or disorders which appear in the mouth itself.

intraoral pressure the build-up of pressure in the MOUTH to allow a person to produce the sounds for speech. For those who have a CLEFT PALATE, this pressure is usually lacking.

intrinsic muscles of the tongue the TONGUE has three intrinsic muscles which, with the three extrinsic muscles (*see* EXTRINSIC MUSCLES OF THE TONGUE), control its movement. The intrinsic muscles are named longitudinal, transverse and vertical. They are supplied by the hypoglossal nerve (*see* CRANIAL NERVE XII). The vertical muscle fibres pull the sides of the tongue down while the transverse muscle fibres help lengthen the tongue. *See* Tortora and Grabowski (2000).

Intro Talker a high-tech communication aid with digitised speech output. It uses MINSPEAK to organise vocabulary to store into the device. The Intro Talker uses an 8- or 32-location overlay with Minspeak icons which can be used in sequences to produce the required utterances. It has a memory of one minute standard speech and two minutes extended speech. The Intro Talker has a rechargeable battery which should be recharged regularly. If the battery becomes low, the machine will produce its own message 'battery low' and the LED lamp will flash on and off. The machine remains on when programmed for a particular client. If it is switched off (the main on/off switch is inside the machine), the contents in the memory will be lost. There are two models of Intro Talker, POINT AND SCAN INTRO TALKER and REMOTE-SWITCH INTRO TALKER. *See* Glennen and DeCoste (1997); Appendix IV (Prentke Romich Company).

Intro Talker IEP+ devised by Cross in 1991, IT-IEP+ is a MINSPEAK APPLICATION PROGRAM (MAP) for use originally with the INTRO TALKER but can also be used with the ALPHA TALKER. It comprises a 32-location overlay with IEP+ icons which represent the interactive sentences from INTERACTION, EDUCATION AND PLAY. All the vocabulary can be stored into the Intro Talker without any extra memory modules if the device is switched into 'extended' speech. *See* Cross (1991).

introversion the process of turning in on oneself, becoming preoccupied with one's own thoughts and feelings. This can be 'normal' but when it becomes extreme it produces maladaptive behaviour, e.g. AUTISM. *See* Smith et al (2003).

intrusion sounds which do not appear in the written form of a language but do appear in some accents. A very common intrusive sound in English is the intrusive /r/ as in such phrases as /lɔr æn ɔrdə/. The first /r/ is intrusive as it does not appear when 'law and order' is written. *See* Cruttenden (1994).

intuition linguists use the native-speaker's intuition as to which sentences are acceptable or unacceptable as a guide to the validity of the set of rules they devise to generate the sentences of a language. Intuition thus becomes an important source of data in GENERATIVE GRAMMAR. *See* Lyons (1968).

inventory a gathering together of data concerning the sounds people use in different situations. There is no structure to this list. When an inventory, for example, of sounds has been collected, it is called that person's sound inventory.

IP (item and process) *see* MORPHOLOGY.

IPA see INTERNATIONAL PHONETIC ALPHABET.

ipsilateral a description of structures and nerves, etc. which are on the same side of the body. It is opposed to contralateral. *See* Tortora and Grabowski (2000).

IQ *see* INTELLIGENCE QUOTIENT.

irregular the form of words, phrases and sentences which do not follow the normal rules for these constructions. A very common example can be found in the use of plurals in English. The regular allomorphs (*see* MORPHOLOGY) used to show plurality in English are /s/, /z/, /ɪz/, e.g. 'dogs', 'trees', 'buses', while there are irregular plural forms in such plurals as 'mice', 'children', 'oxen', etc. *See* Matthews (1974).

isthmus of fauces *see* MOUTH.

item the different forms used in a language.

item and arrangement (IA) *see* MORPHOLOGY.

item and process (IP) *see* MORPHOLOGY.

ITPA *see* ILLINOIS TEST OF PSYCHOLINGUISTIC ABILITIES.

jack a place for fitting in a plug often found at the back of a computer or on a tape recorder or similar machine. It is also called a socket.

Jackson's syndrome first described by Hughlings Jackson. A condition in which there is unilateral paralysis of the soft palate and LARYNX and a hemiatrophy of the tongue leading to a peripheral dysarthria (*see* DYSARTHRIA (3).

Jacksonian seizure a tonic/clonic-type seizure (*see* EPILEPSY) which gradually spreads throughout the body, involving ipsilateral structures. The focal lesion is in the precentral gyrus of the brain. *See* Gilroy and Holliday (1982); Kolb and Whishaw (1996); http://www.medhelp.org/glossary/new/gls_2560.htm

Jakob-Creutzfeldt disease (*see* CREUTZFELDT-JAKOB DISEASE).

jargon aphasia Butterworth described jargon as a 'rare and spectacular manifestation of a dysphasic condition'. There are four types of jargon aphasia:

1. Undifferentiated jargon: a disorder of language where the person uses phonemically possible words, i.e. the structure of the words follows the rules for word formation in English. However, they do not come out as real words.
2. Phonemic jargon: the person does produce real words but sometimes substitutes non-words which are related phonologically to the target word.
3. Asemantic jargon: the person uses real words in possible syntactic contexts but the sequences produced do not make sense.
4. Neologistic jargon: the person uses non-words (unrelated to the target) placed in possible syntactic structures.

People who produce jargon are unaware they are not communicating satisfactorily. Jargon does not contain the hesitations, word-finding difficulties and self-corrections, etc. found with those who have APHASIA. *See* Butterworth (1984); Simmons and Buckingham (1992); Robson et al (1998, 2001).

Jelly Bean Switch a single plate switch for operating toys, communication aids or switch access software for computers. It can be mounted on table tops or wheelchairs using the slim Armstrong mount or the universal mount. *See* Glennen and DeCoste (1997); Appendix IV (AbleNet).

joystick an input device used with a computer especially in arcade games for moving objects around the screen. It may also be used with icon software (*see* ICON). A joystick is also referred to as a games paddle. A joystick can also be used to access a high-tech communication aid which has a scanning system. *See* Bishop (1985); Glennen and DeCoste (1997); Beukelman and Mirenda (1998).

jugular vein there are two types of jugular veins – the internal and external veins.

The right and left internal jugular veins receive blood from the face and neck while the right and left external jugular veins run down the neck outside the internal jugular veins. They drain blood from the parotid gland (see SALIVARY GLANDS), facial muscles, scalp and other superficial structures into subclavian veins. *See* Tortora and Grabowski (2000).

juncture the phonetic or syntactic boundaries between words, phrases and sentences. These boundaries are often marked by silence although they can also be marked by changes in intonation and stress patterns. *See* Clark and Clark (1977).

Jung Carl Gustav Jung (1875–1961) disagreed with Freud's emphasis on libido and examined the interpretation of symbols and dreams. He founded the schools of 'analytic psychology'. *See* Smith et al (2003).

justification the characters produced in word processing are aligned vertically either on the left or right or both margins.

Ke:nx an interface for the Apple Macintosh allowing those with physical or cognitive impairments to access their computers. The system has hardware and software components. Ke:nx (pronounced 'connects') allows for switches and other input systems to be linked up to the Mac. These include a touchscreen, various communication aids such as the Touch and Light Talkers, Liberator Communication Aid, Dynavox and other dedicated communication aids, an alternative keyboard which allows for squares or groups of squares to act like keys, mouse commands or voices. *See* Glennen and DeCoste (1997); Appendix IV (Don Johnston Development Equipment Inc.).

Kendal Toy Test a hearing test used with children from 2;6. Objects are placed on the table in front of the child. The tester checks that all the toys are known, then stands behind the child and names an object. The child must point to it. The test requires no verbal response from the child. The tester looks at the pattern of errors. For example, a confusion between 'duck' and 'bus', may indicate a high frequency hearing loss, as the high frequency sounds are missed. The tests consists of three sets of 15 toys.

keyboard the usual type of keyboard on a computer or communication aid is a QWERTY KEYBOARD. However, some people who do not have the fine motor skills for using an ordinary keyboard may require an expanded keyboard which has larger keys and may or may not be in the ordinary QWERTY layout. Two examples are the Tash PC Mini Keyboard and the Tash PC King Keyboard where, in the latter, the most frequently used keys are in the centre of the keyboard and are laid out so that the common words are easily spelt. *See* Glennen and DeCoste (1997).

keypad it is similar to a keyboard but smaller as it may contain only number keys or function keys. *See* Chandor et al (1985).

kinaesthesia awareness of the position of one's head in relation to the trunk. *See* Tortora and Grabowski (2000).

Klinefelter's syndrome one of the most common sex chromosome (*see* CHROMOSOMES) abnormalities, it was first described by Klinefelter and his colleagues in 1942. It affects about 1:500 males. Although not severe, it may be associated with LEARNING DISABILITY. Those who have this syndrome often have delayed speech and language development which may include degrees of anomia. Some may have an INTENTION TREMOR which may be severe enough to make drinking a glass of water difficult. There may also be behavioural problems. It is caused by the presence of two X chromosomes along with the Y chromosome. Males who are affected are eunuchoid, have gynaecomata, are infertile and are tall and thin with long legs and arms and small genitalia. *See* Salmon (1978); Jones (1997); Tortora and Grabowski (2000); http://www.klinefelter.org.uk

L-dopa *see* LEVODOPA.

label the name given to constituents in a CONSTITUENT ANALYSIS when represented by a TREE DIAGRAM or by BRACKETING. This occurs in GENERATIVE GRAMMAR. *See* Lyons (1968).

labial a description of where some sounds are made, as long as either one lip or both lips are moved to form the sound. Sounds in which one lip is moved are labio-dental (*see* ARTICULATION) while sounds in which both lips are moved are bilabial (*see* ARTICULATION). *See* Catford (1977).

LAD *See* LANGUAGE ACQUISITION DEVICE.

laddering *see* PERSONAL CONSTRUCT THEORY.

laminal a description of sounds made with the blade or lamina of the tongue. These include the alveolar (*see* ARTICULATION) sounds [t,d,s,z]. *See* Catford (1977).

Landau-Kleffner syndrome a possible symptom of those children who have a specific developmental language disorder. Such children have severe problems in comprehension, it is not just delayed. The errors they make are usually consistent and not found in unaffected children of the same age. These comprehension problems do not only occur with auditory stimuli but also with written and signed stimuli. Thus, it does not matter how the sentence is presented to them, they have equal difficulty. Their problem in comprehension could be because they fail to understand the hierarchy of struc-

tures used to form the utterances presented to them. The TEST FOR RECEPTION OF GRAMMAR has been used with such children as the hierarchy of structures is presented in progressively more difficult subtests. *See* Bishop (1982); Adams et al (1997); Vance (1991); Wing (1996); http://www.epilepsy.org.uk/info/landafr m.html; http://www.bobjanet.demon. co.uk/lks/fws.htm

language a term with several different senses. It can refer to a system of linguistic units, which, when put in the correct order, provide spoken or written utterances. This is the PERFORMANCE or PAROLE aspect of language. The underlying knowledge of a language is often referred to as the native's competence or langue. Dialects are regional variations of an established language while an IDIOLECT is a personal variation of language. *See* Lyons (1968); Kolb and Whishaw (1996); Fromkin and Rodman (2003).

language acquisition *see* ACQUISITION and Appendix II.

language acquisition device (LAD) part of a psycholinguistic theory proposed by Noam Chomsky (*see* CHOMSKYAN LINGUISTICS) to explain how children acquire language. He believes children's language acquisition is an innate process. Chomsky believes humans to be born with several areas in their brains which allow them to develop various skills. Language is one such skill and it is

LAD which sparks off this hypothetical language area in the child's mind. *See* Steinberg (1982).

Language Activity Monitor (LAM) an automated system for monitoring the language activity of people who use AAC. LAM allows for the connection and analysis of language samples in either structured or natural settings. The Language Monitor records anything which is said using a communication aid with a date and a time stamp. The samples can be transferred to a computer and analysed for SYNTAX, communication rate, use of vocabulary and so on. It is available as a stand-alone unit, or is built into some communication aids such as the PATHFINDER and VANGUARD and is also available to run on a PC using the Windows operating system. See Appendix IV (Prentke Romich Company).

Language Assessment, Remediation and Screening Procedure (LARSP) a procedure devised by David Crystal in 1976 (revised 1989) to analyse the results of informal-type assessments to find out how well the child has developed expressive language. It shows how the child organises language, the main stages of language acquisition reached by the child as well as the way the child interacts with the therapist. There are no rules for carrying out the assessment. The procedure is to have a 30-minute taped play session, discussion, picture description, free conversation or a combination of all these. The tape is analysed and the grammatical structures summarised in a single profile chart. Any delay in grammatical development of the child can be discovered and the missing structures can be taught to the child. A computerised version of LARSP has been produced by Dorothy Bishop for both the BBC and Apple microcomputers. The program has been written so that the child's utterances can be analysed into the word, phrase and clause structures of the original profile. Each part of the program runs automatically from one stage to another. A summary sheet is printed out following the same format as the non-computerised profile chart with all the calculations carried out by the computer. *See* Bishop (1984); Crystal et al (1989).

language delay a condition in which the child's language level reflects that of a younger child and will be less mature than is appropriate for his or her age. The child produces language of a much younger child, i.e. below his chronological age. The therapist uses assessments such as RDLS or DLS to find out how significant the delay is. Language delay may be associated with the following: (1) hearing loss; (2) mental handicap; (3) visual impairment; (4) severe emotional disorders; (5) gross neurological problems; and (6) environmental deprivation. This differentiates children who have SDLD who would not have any of the six causes given above.

language deviance this does not fit into a normal developmental sequence. There may be abnormal sound structure, syntactic and/or semantic manifestations. Gross deviance is frequently associated with pathology; it can also occur without any discernible cause. *See* Byers Brown (1976).

Language Imitation Test devised by Berry and Mittler in 1981. It assesses the expressive language of learning disabled children of 2;6–4;0, using six subtests: (1) sound imitation; (2) word imitation; (3,4) syntactic control (two subtests are used); (5) word organisation control; and (6) sentence completion. The child has to repeat words and sentences after the therapist has said them. The child's production is scored so that a numerical score can be obtained or a score which will reveal the child's strengths and weaknesses in this area of expressive language. *See* Berry and Mittler (1981) in Appendix I.

Language, Learning and Living (LLL) a MINSPEAK APPLICATION PROGRAM (MAP) devised by Jones in 1989, it is designed

131

for adolescent and adult individuals with developmental disabilities and associated learning difficulties. It uses a single word/phrase vocabulary with 11 parts of speech represented, including 57 classes of noun. As with all MINSPEAK programs, it uses Minspeak icons to represent different parts of grammar as well as functions. Spelling can also be used to increase literacy skills. In 1995, Tony Jones devised a 'beginners' vocabulary called 'Pathways' which uses the 128-location overlay but uses single word and sentence formats. There are six pathways to the full LLL program. Pathway 1 has 128 single-key-activated sentences which relate to the sentences and words in LLL; Pathway 2 has 128 single-key-activated words which relate to LLL; Pathway 3 combines the first two pathways with single-key-activated words and sentences started with the 'judge' icon as in LLL; Pathway 4 allows the user to activate the sentences as in Pathway 3 but all the single hit words of Pathway 2 start with the 'name' icon; Pathway 5 introduces sentence types where statements begin with the 'judge' icon, questions with the 'witch' icon, 'negations' with the 'knot' icon, past tenses with the 'big ed' icon and amusing, rude or emphatic sentences with the 'bottom' icon. The individual words used in Pathway 2 beginning with the 'name' icon are still available; Pathway 6 is a variation of Pathway 5. The words from Pathway 2 are available as a single activation except where the icon is used as a category icon in Pathway 5 ('witch', 'big ed', 'knot', 'bottom' and 'name'). In these instances, the word can be obtained by a double hit on the icon. The majority of words, therefore, are available as a single hit but all other forms require a two-icon activation. *See* Jones (1989, 1991, 1992, 1995b); Morris (1998, 1999, 2000a, b).

Language Master a machine which can be used in a similar fashion to a tape recorder. It uses different sizes of cards with a two-track magnetic tape running along the length at the bottom of the cards. The cards can have sounds, words, phrases or pictures on them with the auditory stimulus on one of the two tracks spoken by the therapist for the person to imitate on the second track of the tape. The person can find out by listening carefully the difference between the way the stimuli are said as compared to the correct version by the therapist. *See* Code and Müller (1989).

langue the grammatical system which each person has in his or her mind after having learned the language. It was proposed by de Saussure and is opposed to PAROLE. *See* Saussure (1916); Lyons (1968); Culler (1986).

LARSP *see* LANGUAGE ASSESSMENT, REMEDIATION AND SCREENING PROCEDURE.

laryngeal nerve palsies neuropathologies can produce a paralysis of one or both VOCAL FOLDS. Both the abduction and the adduction of the folds can be affected and paralysis can occur unilaterally or bilaterally. There are several types of laryngeal nerve palsies:

1. Unilateral adductor paralysis is caused by a disorder in the arytenoids which bring the vocal folds together.
2. Bilateral adductor paralysis, where both the vocal folds take up a paramedial position and remain open and cannot be closed.
3. Unilateral abductor paralysis produces temporary hoarseness as the affected fold is held in the midline of the LARYNX. A Teflon injection (*see* TEFLON INJECTION) is given to the vocal fold.
4. Bilateral abductor paralysis is perhaps the most serious condition as both folds remain closed at the midline of the glottis and cannot be opened. These patients require a tracheotomy to allow them to breathe. The person may also have to undergo an arytenoidectomy in which the arytenoids are removed.
5. Right recurrent laryngeal palsy is caused by a carcinoma in the oesophagus, thickening of the pleurae at the

apex of the right lung, aneurysm of the right subclavian artery or pneumonectomy, i.e. part of the lung removed. Symptoms include a very weak, breathy voice. Straining it to produce voice will make the person hoarse.

6. Left recurrent laryngeal palsy, commonly caused by an aortic aneurysm with similar symptoms as with the right recurrent laryngeal palsy.

See Freeman and Fawcus (2001).

laryngeal web most frequently a congenital condition in which a band of mucous membrane is stretched across the anterior part of the VOCAL FOLDS. It may produce hoarseness and a high pitched voice due to limited movement of the vocal folds. In severe cases, there will be inspiratory stridor, and surgical intervention will be necessary. The acquired type can occur following trauma or infective illnesses like diphtheria or tuberculosis.

laryngectomy it may be partial or total.

1. Partial:
(a) Hemilaryngectomy: this is a surgical procedure in which a vertical half of the LARYNX is resected. This usually involves removal of one VOCAL FOLD (CORDECTOMY), one of the false vocal folds and parts of the thyroid cartilage. Soft tissue is then rotated to provide a site against which the remaining vocal fold can vibrate. The resulting voice is hoarse and weak. Swallowing may also present a problem.
(b) Supraglottic laryngectomy: this involves removal of the EPIGLOTTIS, aryepiglottic fold and the false vocal folds and the hyoid bone. The larynx is then raised and anchored to the base of the tongue to preserve a patent airway and to assist swallowing. Swallowing does present severe problems as a completely new swallowing pattern has to be learned. Voice may well be hoarse despite the fact that the true vocal folds remain intact.

2. Total laryngectomy: this procedure is carried out when the malignancy is extensive. Depending on the size of the tumour, resection may include the hyoid, the whole of the larynx, part of the pharynx and trachea. The remaining part of the trachea is then sutured to an external stoma at the base of the neck anteriorly. Following surgery an alternative method of speech has to be acquired. This will be either by means of oesophageal (alaryngeal) production or through the use of an ARTIFICIAL LARYNX.

See Edels (1984); Fox and Rau (2001) (AAC and laryngectomy); http://www. origin8.nl/medical/ (voice rehabilitation after total laryngectomy).

laryngitis *see* ACUTE LARYNGITIS and CHRONIC NON-SPECIFIC LARYNGITIS.

laryngofissure the removal of one VOCAL FOLD which allows the other to compensate completely. *See* Freeman and Fawcus (2001).

laryngoscopy there are three types of laryngoscopy:

1. Indirect laryngoscopy: the first examination using a palatal mirror to view the relevant parts of the larynx. If there appears to be a growth, a direct laryngoscopy will be undertaken.
2. Direct laryngoscopy: after anaesthesia is administered, a rigid laryngoscope is placed along the floor of the mouth and down the back of the person's throat. A light system shows up the subglottic and supraglottic areas of the larynx. If any tumours are found, tissue can be taken for further analysis by using long-handled biopsy forceps.
3. Microlaryngoscopy: the process of removing small growths from the vocal folds without damaging the folds with the aid of an operating microscope.

See Edels (1984); Beech et al (1993).

larynx the organ of the voice. It contains the VOCAL FOLDS which produce voice. It extends from the back of the TONGUE to the TRACHEA. It is 4.5 cm long, 4 cm in transverse section and 3.5 cm from front to back. It is smaller in the female than in the male after puberty. It comprises cartilage held together by membrane and ligament. The hyoid bone (*see* MUSCLES FOR SWALLOWING) is at the top, the thyroid cartilage in the middle and the cricoid cartilage at the bottom. The thyroid cartilage is made up of two quadrilateral structures joined in the midline at the laryngeal prominence to which the vocal ligament is attached. The cricoid cartilage is like a ring. The arytenoid cartilage (*see* ARYTENOIDS) is attached to the lamina of the cricoid and has an apex and three roughly triangular surfaces. The larynx is controlled by the following muscles:

1. Cricothyroid muscle is formed by vertical and oblique fibres. The muscle tilts the cricoid up or thyroid down and tightens the vocal folds.
2. Arytenoid muscle: the transverse and oblique arytenoid muscles control the arytenoid cartilages and go up either side of the aryepiglottic folds.
3. Posterior cricoarytenoid muscle runs up to attach to the muscular process of the arytenoid. When it contracts, it abducts the vocal folds by rotating the arytenoid cartilage; when it pulls the arytenoid cartilages backwards, the vocal fold tenses.
4. Lateral cricoarytenoid muscle is attached to the superior border of the cricoid cartilage passing upwards and backwards and attached to the muscular process of the arytenoids. When it contracts, it adducts the vocal folds by rotating the arytenoid cartilage inwards.
5. Thyroarytenoid muscle is attached to the front of the inner surface of the laryngeal prominence. It passes backwards and upwards and becomes attached to the anterolateral surface of the arytenoid cartilage and its muscular process.
6. Vocalis muscle: part of the muscle is attached to the lateral aspect of the vocal ligament and some of its fibres run up to the aryepiglottic fold. When it contracts, the arytenoid cartilages rotate medially to adduct the vocal folds, while in pulling the arytenoid cartilage forward the vocal folds relax.
7. Thyrohyoid muscle leaves the thyroid cartilage and attaches to the greater cornu of the hyoid bone. It raises the thyroid cartilage and pushes down the hyoid bone.

See Tortora and Grabowski (2000).

latency *see* PSYCHOSEXUAL STAGES OF DEVELOPMENT.

lax a DISTINCTIVE FEATURE proposed by Jakobson and Halle to distinguish sounds made with little muscular effort [+LAX] from those which are produced with a stronger muscular effort [−LAX]. It is opposed to tense. *See* Hyman (1975).

learnability a term used in language acquisition to refer to problem areas for learners. A general problem for the normal acquisition of language is assumed to be the absence of negative evidence. Negative evidence would be explicit information from mature language users that a particular form used by the learner, e.g. over-regularised past tense, was not grammatical in the language being learned. Retreating from incorrect hypotheses about the structure of the language being learned, on the basis of positive evidence only (the 'correct' forms of a child's language environment) is a learnability problem for the child learning his language.

learning *see* CLASSICAL CONDITIONING; OPERANT CONDITIONING; INNATENESS.

learning disability the established term used in the UK to refer to 'mental handicap' defined as 'a condition of arrested or incomplete development of mind which is especially characterised by subnormality of intelligence' (World Health Organisation 1967). Those children and adults who have a learning disability can have difficulty in learning tasks, in communication, with motor skills and with sensory input. Such problems can be helped by different types of therapy such as occupational therapy, speech and language therapy, physiotherapy and clinical or educational psychology. Whatever therapy is required by the person, the respective programmes must be planned carefully and take into account the specific learning difficulties found in such clients. Research has found these difficulties are complicated by additional features such as:

1. Attention problems.
2. Inability to learn incidentally, so the person requires long and frequent exposure to the stimulus.
3. React badly under pressure.
4. Auditory information processed better than visual information.
5. Memory improved by using more than one modality.
6. Clang associations produce confusion.
7. Difficulty in generalising what has been learnt.
8. Concrete stimuli should be used as these are learnt better than abstract stimuli.
9. Verbalising helps improve memory during the task.

Clients who have a learning disability require a structured approach so that they can have a better chance of learning material as well as those without a learning disability. In a study in 1997, comparing three approaches to providing speech and language therapy for people who have learning disabilities, it was found that overall changes in communication occurred more significantly in a combination of the two approaches which had been looked at individually – namely, working directly on a one to one basis with the person and partner and working indirectly by providing teaching partners. See Shakespeare (1975); Clarke and Clarke (1974); Kolb and Whishaw (1996); Davison et al (2004); Money (1997).

LED *see* LIGHT EMITTING DIODE.

Leiter International Performance Scale a non-verbal cognitive assessment, designed by Leiter in 1969, which is particularly well adapted to the needs of hearing- or language-impaired children. It involves a series of progressively more complex matching tasks. The age range for administration is 2;0 years upwards. *See* Leiter (1969) in Appendix I.

length the period of time used to produce a sound or syllable. Length modifies the articulation and makes a difference between sounds. It is also known as duration and quality. *See* Catford (1977).

lenis a sound which has little air pressure in the airstream to produce the sound. There is also a reduction in muscle power required. It is opposed to fortis. *See* Cruttenden (1994).

lesser horn of hyoid *see* PHARYNX.

Let's Talk – Developing Prosocial Communication Skills a therapeutic programme for children and adolescents with a LEARNING DISABILITY, language disorder or HEARING LOSS or with those who are shy and find it difficult to communicate in social situations. *See* Wiig (1982a) in Appendix I.

Let's Talk – For Children a programme to involve children in real-life interaction, by using hundreds of activities divided into four communication functions – ritualising, informing, controlling and feeling. The 41 different skills are sequenced developmentally and organised in learning steps. *See* Wiig (1983) in Appendix I.

Let's Talk – Intermediate Level a therapeutic programme for adolescents and young adults with developmental delays or acquired language disorders as well as those with literacy problems. The teaching activities provide real-life situations for adolescents. *See* Wiig (1984) in Appendix I.

Let's Talk – Inventory for Adolescents an assessment for adolescents and preadolescents consisting of 40 items in a picture manual. The adolescent is given a short description of the context of the picture and is asked what the adolescent in the picture might say in the given situation. The assessment pinpoints communication problems. The results can show where therapy begins using the Let's Talk Intervention Programmes for Adolescents, Let's Talk – Developing Prosocial Communication Skills and Let's Talk – Intermediate Level. *See* Wiig (1982b) in Appendix I.

Let's Talk – Inventory for Children based on the Inventory for Adults, this assessment gives a standardised method of assessing speech acts within the communication functions of ritualising, informing, controlling and feeling. The 34 pictures give a different situation involving peer or adult interactions. *See* Wiig (1987) in Appendix I.

letter-by-letter reader *see* ACQUIRED DYSLEXIA.

levator anguli labii superioris *see* MUSCLES OF FACIAL EXPRESSION.

levodopa (L-dopa) a drug which provides dopamine to those who have an insufficiency of dopamine in the brain. It can be used with those who have PARKINSON'S DISEASE as it has a significant effect on bradykinesia (*see* PARKINSON'S DISEASE). However, it can produce nausea, depression and dyskinesia (*see* CEREBRAL PALSY). *See* Gilroy and Holliday (1982); Kolb and Whishaw (1996); Kaye (1991).

lexical syntactic deficit a term used by Rapin and Allen (1987) to describe a subtype of language disorder. The predominant difficulty is one of word finding. There appear to be two groups: those who have a sparsity of language with difficulty in retrieving lexical items and those with similar word-finding difficulties but who use a number of word fillers and circumlocutions in an effort to retrieve words. *See* Adams et al (1997).

Liberator Communication Aid a high-tech communication aid with synthetic voice output (DECTALK). It uses MINSPEAK to organise vocabulary to store into the device. It has a memory of 512K and can be accessed using direct manual selection, infra-red headpointing, single, dual or two-switch scanning as well as a joystick or multi-switch. Scanning and direct selection can be used on the same keyboard at the same time. It can be set up to use 8-, 32- or 128-location overlays. Other features include icon prediction, which shows by illuminating a light on a symbol which symbols have messages stored under them; predictive selection, which makes symbols with nothing stored under them inoperative when being used with direct manual selection or infra-red headpointing; while with scanning, the scanning light jumps the unused symbols. The Liberator Communication Aid also uses auditory prompts. This allows a person to hear the names of the symbols before they are activated. This feature can be used either with direct manual selection, infra-red headpointing or with switch access. The memory can be backed up on a computer. The Liberator can also be used for computer emulation and can be linked to the DIRECTOR, an environmental control. Other features include Notebooks which allow large amounts of text to be stored and spoken or printed out on the Liberator's internal printer. These may include songs, essays, different educational subjects and so on. A maximum of four unique programs can be loaded into one device simultaneously. Maths problems can be solved using either the Maths Scratch Pad or the four-function calculator. *See* Glennen and DeCoste (1997); Rumble and Larcher (1998); Appendix IV (Prentke Romich Company).

Lidcombe Programme of early stuttering intervention devised by Onslow et al, the Lidcombe Programme is a treatment for children who stutter. The authors offer this overview of what constitutes early stuttering: 'Stuttering is a speech disorder that begins mostly in the first few years of life. Stuttering can be mild to severe at onset. Onset can be rapid or gradual, with the appearance of multiple syllable repetitions that progress, either rapidly or gradually, to other speech perturbations such as sound blocks and prolongations. Early stuttering may cause significant distress to small children. Such distress may arise from attempts to communicate normally, from reactions of others to their problem, and – apparently – from novel, subjective feelings associated with an uncontrollably misfunctioning speech system. Parents often experience significant distress when their children begin to stutter, particularly in cases where there is a clear family history of the disorder, as is the case more often than not' (Onslow et al 1997a, p. 232). There are three parts to the programme: a procedure that parents can use to control stuttering which uses the principles of OPERANT CONDITIONING where stutter-free speech is praised and when a child stutters a parent is trained to respond appropriately to their particular child in that situation; regular speech measures within and beyond the clinic in that there are clinical procedures to measure the disorder and clinical procedures to control it. Such measures provide a means to clearly specify the targets of the programme, guide the clinician's management decisions during the programme, enable the clinician and parents to communicate about the child's progress and provide guidelines so that parents can respond to the variable nature of stuttering and hence be able to alter the format of the programme according to the child's speech on a daily basis. The final component is programmed maintenance where the clinic withdraws gradually from seeing the child over a 12 month period but the parents are encouraged to continue to monitor the speech of their child and give feedback as necessary. *See* Onslow et al (1997a, b); Cook and Rustin (1997); Hayhow (1997).

light emitting diode (LED) a light which illuminates when a machine is switched on to show that it is functioning. It is usually placed on control panels or the machine's surface. *See* Chandor et al (1985).

light for dates a light birth weight is defined as one third of the normal birth weight. The child is born near to full term. This condition is caused by placental insufficiency produced by toxaemia, multiple pregnancy or smoking, intrauterine infections, e.g. TORCH, and chromosomal abnormalities (*see* CHROMOSOMES). Babies are very alert, thin, wasted and have wrinkled skin and a poor response rate. There is fetal distress in labour and the baby passes meconium after the first day of delivery. If the child inhales meconium and starts poor breathing, producing meconium aspiration syndrome, this can cause brain damage and can lead to death. *See* Illingworth (1987).

light pen an input device to operate a computer instead of using the keyboard. The device looks like a pen but has a light-sensitive end. *See* Bishop (1985).

LightHawk a high-tech communication aid with DIGITISED SPEECH. There are three levels each of which can give access to eight locations. Up to 7.5 seconds of digitised speech are available on the first two levels while there are up to 15 seconds on the third level. It can be accessed by single switch and two-switch scanning. *See* Appendix IV (AdamLab).

LightTalker a high-tech communication aid with synthetic voice output (*see* DECTALK). It uses MINSPEAK to organise vocabulary to store into the device. It has about 40K of memory. It can only be accessed by optical headpointing, single, dual or two-switch scanning as well as joystick or multi-switch. The Light Talker has 25 different selection techniques which can be divided into three groups: 'direct selection' when using the optical headpointer or the Direct Selection Sensor for programming the device; 'switch scanning', either row/

column scanning in 32 and 128 locations or circular, linear or count when in eight locations; and 'joystick' or 'multi-switch'. The device can be set into 8, 32 or 128 locations and, if the Light Talker uses the ENHANCED MINSPEAK OPERATING SYSTEM (EMOS), it can also be set into the 'alternative' overlay. The memory can be backed up on a computer. It can also be used for computer emulation and can be linked to the DIRECTOR, an environmental control. *See* Glennen and DeCoste (1997); Appendix IV (Prentke Romich Company).

Lightwriters a range of high-tech communication aids with optional synthetic speech (*see* DECTALK). They have a double screen and a QWERTY or alphabetic keyboard. The message is typed onto the screens, one facing the person using the system while the other screen faces the 'listener'. The early model, Model SL4a, had a word store and a phrase store with 40 memories. It had a rechargeable battery which, when fully charged, lasted for a continuous six hours operation. A printing facility and speech synthesiser are also available. The SL1 and SL3 were the first of the smaller models. The latest models follow from these earlier ones. The SL5 has 2K memory with 36 memories while the SL30 is the same but allows for speech, a printout and 5K memory. The SL35 has three types of speech output: 'articulate', 'EuroTalk' (British speech) and 'DECtalk'. It has a memory of 32K with 2K of high-security memory as standard. It can be linked up to printers, remote displays, a giant keyboard, a remote control telephone and a plug-in scan module. It has an eight-function calculator among other functions. The SL86 uses both direct selection and scanning and the SL87 is integrated on a plastic plate with an integral carry handle and wheelchair mounting points in the base. The SL87 uses the latest version of software–version 5.7 which allows for increased memory capacity, scan-suspend, eight predictions for direct selec-

tion instead of just one and extended text allowing for different sizes of text. The SL87 model allows for both direct selection and scanning. This model also has eight predictions for direct selection as well as the option of different sizes of text on the screen. In all other respects it is similar to previous models as described above. *See* Glennen and DeCoste (1997); Rumble and Larcher (1998); Appendix IV (Toby Churchill).

lingual tonsil a structure formed by some lymphoid tissue at the back of the TONGUE. *See* Tortora and Grabowski (2000).

linguistic profiles assessment procedures proposed by Crystal in 1982. There are PROFILES OF PHONOLOGY (PROPH), PROFILES OF PROSODY (PROP) and PROFILES IN SEMANTICS (PRISM). LARSP is included as one of these procedures. The analyses are derived from a sample of speech obtained in free conversation, play sessions and picture description. *See* Crystal (1992).

linguistic variation *see* ACCENT; DIALECT; IDIOLECT.

linking a sound which appears in the spoken language but does not appear in the orthographic form of the language. An example is the intrusive /r/. *See* Cruttenden (1994).

LINKSicon a language application program designed for a 128-key MACAW communication aid. Key link allows for almost any number of keys to be combined to provide additional messages; four levels are used in this single-overlay application; 38 messages of digitised speech are available. LINKSicon uses a new semantically based method of key linking symbols and combines the alphabet, words, phrases and sentences on a single overlay. Almost all messages are coded as 'one-hit' or as a combination of two keys. *See* Appendix IV (Zygo).

lip reading a form of communication used with people who have a hearing loss. The person concentrates on lip movement alone to try to understand what is being said. However, only about one-third of sounds produced can be clearly seen, e.g. bilabials, labiodentals, inter-dentals, some alveolars (*see* ARTICULATION) and vowels (*see* CARDINAL VOWEL SYSTEM). Another difficulty is that many of these sounds can look the same, such as [p,b,m]. Speech reading is now preferred where the person takes into account not only lip movement but also facial expression and gesture, etc.

liquid a description of sounds such as [l] and [r]. *See* Ladefoged (2001).

LIS *see* LOCKED-IN-SYNDROME.

Listening Skills Test devised by Lloyd and his colleagues, this test is designed to assess the ability to evaluate language and monitor comprehension. It has four subtests including referent identification where ambiguities in messages with pictorial referents have to be detected; message appraisal where judgements have to be made about utterances concerning an illustrated event; comprehension of directions where following extended discourse is assessed; and verbal message evaluation where verbal statements without pictorial referents have to be evaluated. It has been developed in the UK and is fully standardised. It can be used with children in the age range of 3;06–6;11. *See* Lloyd et al (2001) in Appendix I.

literal paraphasia although the person's articulation is unaffected, syllables can be produced in the wrong order or wrong sounds are placed in a word producing confusion. *See* Goodglass and Kaplan (2000).

lithium a drug used to treat manic-depression. The level of the drug rises in the body as it is only effective in this manner; it will take a few days after therapy begins for it to take effect. It is used mainly for the maintenance of recovery from MANIC-DEPRESSION. *See* Stafford-Clark and Bridges (1990); Smith et al (2003); Davison et al (2004).

Living Language a remedial package, devised by Locke, for children who have a LANGUAGE DELAY, which can be used

from pre-school to 16 years of age. It is designed to help children to develop their use of expressive language normally. The package is divided into three parts: 'Before Words', 'First Words' and 'Putting Words Together'. 'Before Words' is used with children who have no use or comprehension of language. In this part of Living Language, the child is taught the basic skills required to acquire language, such as social-emotional development, play, listening and expressive language skills. The norms for such development are given in the manual. 'First Words' is used with children who are using single words but the level of vocabulary is not up to the child's age level and they do not have sufficient words to put two words together. This part of the programme contains 100 words which children first respond to or use – 58 nouns (e.g. toys, clothes, food, etc.), 30 verbs (e.g. describing concrete, easily identifiable actions, etc.) and 12 other words (e.g. early prepositions and adjectives). Picture cards are presented to the child by the teacher or therapist to assess the child's expressive language. 'Putting Words Together' is used with children who have a basic vocabulary and are beginning to put words together to form simple sentences. It comprises three parts: (1) a vocabulary of objects and events, including over 600 of the most familiar nouns and verbs; (2) a vocabulary of properties and relationships, including 200 adjectives, adverbs and prepositions used to describe objects and their relationships to each other, together with basic number words and more abstract vocabulary; and (3) a selection of syntactic features, including more than 200 grammatical constructions which children need to know to benefit from traditional teaching. Each of these three parts is divided into levels placed in developmental order. *See* Locke (1985).

LLL *see* LANGUAGE, LEARNING AND LIVING.

locationist theory proposed by a group of

aphasiologists known as the BOSTON SCHOOL. The theory itself dates from the 1860s when Paul Broca and Karl Wernicke and their contemporaries proposed groups of language disorders produced by lesions in certain parts of the brain producing specific aphasic characteristics (*see* APHASIA). *See* Eisenson (1984).

locked-in-syndrome (LIS) a condition often caused by a basal artery stroke, a tumour or trauma resulting in damage to the upper PONS or sometimes to the MID-BRAIN restricting the motor pathways to such an extent that in the complete state vertical movement of the eyes is the only movement possible. Sensory and cognitive function may be retained. Incomplete LIS allows some movement of the limbs but communication is anarthric and therefore restricted to almost unintelligible vocalisations. *See* Culp and Ladtkow (1992); Beukelman and Mirenda (1998); http://health.mcw. edu/article/921775038.html

logogen the British psychologist John Morton introduced this term to refer to a hypothetical memory unit which links together various aspects of a word such as its semantic, auditory, visual and pictorial properties. Morton suggested that individual 'logogens' (his name for word recognition units in the visual input lexicon) have variable thresholds. 'A logogen's threshold determines the amount of activity that must be present within it before it will "fire" and cause a word to be recognised' (Ellis 1993, p. 28). *See* Reber (1995); Ellis (1993).

logopaedics a name given to speech and language pathology in parts of Europe.

Logotron Logo software developed for use by children. It is designed to allow the child to operate a computer rather than allow the computer to control the child. Thus, it follows Piaget's beliefs that a child learns from experience. When the child enters the Logo program, he will find a small triangle on the screen called a turtle. By using a simple computer language, the child finds he can move the turtle forwards, backwards, sideways, diagonally, draw a white line, draw a coloured line or not draw a line at all. Thus, the child learns a form of language for moving the turtle. The graphics which the child produces in this way are called turtle graphics. It has been designed for the Apple computers in the USA and for the BBC computers in the UK. *See* Bishop (1985).

longitudinal method a research procedure using several subjects over a period of time.

longitudinal muscle *see* INTRINSIC MUSCLES OF THE TONGUE.

loop a process found in a computer program which allows instructions given to the computer to be repeated until a particular condition is satisfied. The types of loops may differ from computer to computer. The loops most often found in BASIC are for...next and repeat...until. *See* Bishop (1985).

loudness *see* AUDITORY PHONETICS.

low a DISTINCTIVE FEATURE proposed by Chomsky and Halle to distinguish sounds made by lowering the TONGUE in the MOUTH [+LOW] to produce open vowels (*see* CARDINAL VOWEL SYSTEM) from those made with the tongue raised in the mouth [−LOW]. It is opposed to high. *See* Hyman (1975).

lumbar puncture a technique for diagnosing such infections as MENINGITIS. A certain quantity, usually about 1 ml, of CEREBROSPINAL FLUID (CSF) is drawn off the MENINGES to check for infection. If the fluid is clouded by the presence of organisms and white cells, this may indicate the presence of meningitis. The pressure is also increased and the sugar decreased. Normal CSF fluid is clear. *See* Gilroy and Holliday (1982); Kaye (1991).

lungs there are two lungs in the thoracic cavity covered by a pleural lining. Air reaches the lungs by the TRACHEA and the BRONCHI which branch into the right and left lung. The right lung is divided into three lobes by an oblique fissure and transverse fissure. The left lung is divided into two lobes by an oblique fissure. Each lobe is supplied by a bronchus, an artery and a vein. They are necessary for respiration. The microscopic structure of the lungs is seen as a series of passageways. The bronchi divide into bronchioles which become respiratory bronchioles. These bronchioles divide into alveolar ducts, subdividing into alveolar saccules which produce alveoli at their ends. *See* Tortora and Grabowski (2000).

M

MA *see* MENTAL AGE.

Macaw a high-tech communication aid which uses digitised speech producing natural sounding speech to produce messages. There are three models: Macaw II, Macaw 3 and the Green Macaw. Macaw II has over 1 minute of high-quality recording as standard with optional memory modules producing up to 8.5 minutes of recording time. There are two models where one is direct-selection only while the second model is for both direct selection and scanning including auditory scanning. The Macaw 3 series has three models: Macaw 3 has 9 minutes of high-quality recording time, Macaw 3 + has 19 minutes of high-quality recording while the Big Blue Macaw 3 has an internal hard disk for 13 hours of recording time. All models include 32 levels and auditory scan with an earphone. Messages and setups are saved even when the device is turned off and there are no dead spaces on the keyboard. The Great Green Macaw has 19 minutes of recording time and its built-in hard drive can store over 13 hours of recording. It has a 128-key membrane keyboard with no dead spaces and can have as few as two enlarged keys to multi-levels of any key pattern in each level. Any number of keys may be combined for key-linked messages. This model of Macaw allows for both direct selection and scanning including auditory scanning as well as Morse code means of access. *See* Glennen and DeCoste (1997); Rumble and Larcher (1998); Appendix IV (Zygo).

macrocephaly an abnormally large head caused by an increased amount of tissue or fluid in the BRAIN. It is opposed to MICROCEPHALY.

macroglossia an abnormally large TONGUE. The condition may be congenital. It has been proposed that children who have DOWN SYNDROME have a longer tongue than those children who do not have this syndrome. However, the tongue may just seem very large because the child has a particularly small upper or lower jaw. Surgery can be used to reduce its size. Articulation disorders can occur. *See* Travis (1971).

magnetic resonance imaging (MRI) a diagnostic radiological technique using the magnetic properties of the body's hydrogen nuclei to produce pictures of cross-sections of the examined part of the body. The person is exposed to a uniform magnetic field which orientates some of the atomic nuclei in the body containing protons. When placed in a magnetic field some absorb this energy and move from a low to a high energy state, i.e. resonance effect. The images resemble CT scans and can be presented in colour or two- or three-dimensional images. MRI can be used as the guidance system for biopsy of tumours. It can also assess mental disorders, show changes in the brain in

PARKINSON'S DISEASE as well as show the causes of CEREBROVASCULAR ACCIDENTS, i.e. haematomas and infarction. MRI, formerly known as nuclear magnetic resonance, has the advantage of being non-invasive and does not use radiation. *See* Kaye (1991); Kolb and Whishaw (1996); Tortora and Grabowski (2000).

maintenance *see* CARRY-OVER.

major class feature a major grouping of Chomsky and Halle's DISTINCTIVE FEATURES. This group distinguishes sounds which are made with different degrees of openness in the VOCAL TRACT. This produces the distinctive features of sonorant/non-sonorant, vocalic/non-vocalic and consonantal/non-consonantal sounds. *See* Ladefoged (2001).

major depression *see* DEPRESSION.

Makaton a sign vocabulary system devised by Margaret Walker in 1977 for adults who were deaf and had severe learning difficulties. The core vocabulary contains about 470 concepts organised into nine developmental stages, and is the only sign system which follows closely the normal acquisition of vocabulary. Learning Makaton can increase the child's eye contact, attention, sociability, vocalisation and EXPRESSIVE LANGUAGE. Far from interfering with the child's ACQUISITION of speech and language, it can encourage it. It is sometimes used in therapeutic programmes for people who have various communication disorders including those with LEARNING DISABILITY and those with APHASIA who have WORD-FINDING DIFFICULTIES. By producing the sign, the person may find it easier to produce the word verbally. Makaton symbols, giving access to about 7000 concepts, are pictorial representations of the signs. They have been developed so that it will be easier for children to use and understand the original signs. Computer programs have also been written for use with Makaton. *See* Kiernan et al (1982); Peter and Barnes (1982); Grove and Walker (1990); www.Makaton.org/index.htm

Makaton symbols *see* MAKATON.

maladaptive behaviour *see* ABNORMAL BEHAVIOUR.

malignant a description of a tumour which can grow within different parts of the body destroying any neighbouring tissue. It is opposed to benign. See Tortora and Grabowski (2000).

malleus *see* EAR.

malocclusion *see* ORTHODONTICS.

Maltron keyboard a keyboard that has been designed to be more suitable than a regular QWERTY KEYBOARD for use because of its comfort and accuracy. The keyboard has been divided into two parts with two groupings of 26 switches on each side. The thumbs are left to operate 'space', 'return', 'e', '&', and full stop. The way the two groupings are set up takes away the strain on the wrists and keeps them straight. There is a single-handed keyboard for those who have a physical disability and cannot use even the standard Maltron. Maltron have also produced a keyboard which can be mounted on a stand and operated by a head or mouth stick if the patient cannot use any other limbs for operating the computer. *See* Appendix IV (Maltron).

management includes all the decisions which a therapist makes concerning a client, from the taking of a CASE HISTORY through to decisions concerning the best method of ASSESSMENT, the DIAGNOSIS, TREATMENT PROGRAMME and possible prognosis. *See* Byers Brown (1981).

mandible the lower jaw. It is used in the act of chewing or mastication and speaking. It has four muscles attached to various parts of its body – temporalis muscle, lateral pterygoid, medial pterygoid and masseter muscles (*see* MUSCLES OF MASTICATION). *See* Tortora and Grabowski (2000).

mandibular nerve the mandibular branch of the trigeminal nerve (*see* CRANIAL NERVE V). To distinguish this nerve from the other two which form the trigeminal nerve, the mandibular nerve is denoted as Viii. The sensory part of the nerve supplies the posterior two-thirds of the TONGUE, the MANDIBLE and lower teeth, and the mucous membrane of the floor of the mouth. See Tortora and Grabowski (2000).

manic-depression mania nearly always alternates with DEPRESSION to create a bipolar disorder; cf depression itself which is a unipolar disorder. Those who have attacks of mania appear in a happy and euphoric mood. While in this mood, people become overtalkative, overactive, suffer from sleeplessness, become very distractible, have sudden flights of ideas and can begin punning and rhyming. A severe case of mania causes physical collapse, incoherent thought processes and superficial moods. The treatment is by tricyclic antidepressant drugs (*see* ANTI-DEPRESSANT DRUGS), MONOAMINE OXIDASE INHIBITORS, LITHIUM, chlorpromazine (*see* PHENOTHIAZINES) and three to four sessions of ELECTROCONVULSIVE THERAPY. *See* Stafford-Clark and Bridges (1990); Davison et al (2004); http://www.depressionalliance.org/Contents/index.htm

Mann-Whitney test a non-parametric test (*see* PARAMETRIC TESTS) used in INFERENTIAL STATISTICS. It is used in experiments using the INDEPENDENT GROUP DESIGN and has its equivalent parametric test, the independent *t*-test (*see* *t*-TESTS). It is used for data which are arranged on a scale which makes no assumptions concerning the shape of the population distribution, e.g. two independent groups of subjects who are taught to read by different methods and subsequently rated on a scale of reading fluency from 1 to 10. The ratings are put on an ordinal scale, so the results of the experiment in this example could be ranked in order of fluency. Such scales do not allow for the calculation of mean scores and so the Mann-Whitney test cannot show differences of means between subjects. 'By finding the sum of the ranks of one of the samples, this test allows the tester to determine the probability that a given difference between the ranks of the two samples could have arisen by chance' (Miller 1984). *See* Miller (1984).

manner of articulation *see* ARTICULATION.

manual approach *see* EDUCATION OF HEARING-IMPAIRED CHILDREN.

MAOI *see* MONOAMINE OXIDASE INHIBITORS.

masking during audiometric tests such as PURE-TONE AUDIOMETRY, there is a possibility that the results will be contaminated by CROSS-HEARING. On such occasions, masking is necessary. Masking should be used when air conduction (*see* PURE-TONE AUDIOMETRY) thresholds in the test ear measure 40 dB or are poorer than bone conduction (*see* PURE-TONE AUDIOMETRY) in the non-test ear because sound is then loud enough to set the skull in vibration and stimulate the cochlea (*see* EAR) of the non-test ear. In bone-conduction testing, if the thresholds are better than air-conduction thresholds, masking should be used.

mass noun a noun which is not countable. An example of such a noun is 'butter' because 'one butter', 'two butters' cannot occur. *See* Palmer (1976).

masseter muscle *see* MUSCLES OF MASTICATION.

mastoid process *see* EAR.

matched group design an experimental design in which subjects are matched in pairs and those making up the pair are allocated randomly, one to each of the experimental conditions. Perhaps the commonest type of experiment using this design would be with identical twins but other experiments are possible. *See* Miller (1984).

matrix sentence the sentence that exists before embedding takes place or after the embedded sentences have been removed.

(1) The car which the man bought was a Rolls Royce.

In (1), the matrix sentence is 'the car was a Rolls Royce' while the embedded sentence is 'which the man bought'. *See* Allerton (1979).

maxilla the upper jaw. It is formed by the fusion of the palatal shelves during intrauterine growth. The maxilla comprises the hard palate (*see* MOUTH), the floor and sides of the nasal cavities, the floor of the orbits and the part of the nasolacrimal canal. The teeth in the top dentition are rooted in the maxilla. *See* Tortora and Grabowski (2000).

maxillary nerve a sensory nerve that supplies some of the skin of the scalp, part of the face, the lower eyelid, part of the inside cheek, the mucous membrane of the nasal cavity, palate and maxillary sinus, the upper teeth and gum. It is part of the trigeminal nerve (*see* CRANIAL NERVE V). To distinguish the maxillary nerve from the other two parts of the nerve, the maxillary nerve is denoted as Vii. *See* Tortora and Grabowski (2000).

mean *see* CENTRAL TENDENCY.

mean length of utterance (MLU) a theory used in language acquisition, proposed by Brown, which compares the child's age to the length of utterances measured in morphemes. They give a more precise idea of the complexity of the utterance than counting words. Brown put forward five stages of development of MLU:

Stage	MLU	Age (years)
I	1.75	1;6–2;3
II	2.25	1;9–2;6
III	2.75	1;11–3;1
IV	3.50	2;2–3;8
V	4.00	2;3–4;0

Age is not a good guide to development, as the rate of acquisition is so variable among children. However, MLU is a good guide to grammatical development especially until stage V. With children who have a language disorder, the MLU can show up mismatches between the child's language acquisition and the normal order. Age plus MLU is important as they can give indicators of the size of the delay which a child has. *See* Cruttenden (1979).

meconium aspiration syndrome *see* LIGHT FOR DATES.

medial pterygoid muscle *see* MUSCLES OF MASTICATION.

median *see* CENTRAL TENDENCY.

medulla oblongata part of the BRAINSTEM. It is about 3 cm long. The SPINAL CORD ends in the medulla. There are several tracts which it has in common with the PONS and MIDBRAIN. *See* Barr (1988); Tortora and Grabowski (2000).

megalencephaly a condition found in children who have an oversized head and overweight brain without neurological disorders. When these children are born, they have an abnormally large head and big bodies. Anatomical megalencephaly is inheritable as an autosomal dominant trait (*see* CHROMOSOMES) and can be familial. In a study in 1972, out of 18 children the incidence was 4:1 in favour of males and half of the children were familial cases. *See* De Meyer (1972); http://healthlink.mcw.edu/article/921440550.html

mellow a DISTINCTIVE FEATURE proposed by Jakobson and Halle to distinguish sounds which are made with a low frequency such as plosives and nasals (*see* ARTICULATION) [+MELLOW] from those made with a high frequency such as fricatives (*see* ARTICULATION) [–MELLOW]. It is opposed to STRIDENT. *See* Hyman (1975).

melodic intonation therapy (MIT) devised by Sparks et al (1974), Sparks and Holland (1976) and revised by Sparks (1981), it is a therapeutic technique originally devised for aphasic patients. It is based on a theory of right hemisphere dominance for music. The person is required to learn to intone propositional sentences in a manner which replicates their natural prosody and thus to facilitate verbal output. Some success is reported on its use with apraxic subjects. *See* Eisenson (1984).

membrane a layer or sheet of tissue that can surround cells and structures, line canals and separate structures. *See* Leeson et al (1985); Tortora and Grabowski (2000).

memory the many theories concerning memory mean it is difficult to provide one single definition but a description of the theories will show the way in which memory is considered. There are three major distinctions in memory theory. The first concerns three stages of memory, namely encoding (putting information into memory), storage (maintaining the information in memory) and retrieval (recovering the information from memory). The second distinction concerns storing the information for short or long periods of time. The third concerns using different memories to store different kinds of information, e.g., one system for facts and another for skills. Brain scans such as POSITRON EMISSION TOMOGRAPHY (PET) or functional MAGNETIC RESONANCE IMAGING (fMRI) where the activity in the brain is measured while the participants carry out certain activities show that during the encoding process most of the activated regions of the brain are in the left hemisphere whereas during the retrieval process the areas of the brain which are active are in the right hemisphere (*see* CEREBRAL HEMISPHERES). However, the three stages of memory do not work the same way in every situation. The memory processes are different if it is required to store information for less than one minute, for a matter of seconds or for a longer period from minutes to years. It has been suggested that information is placed first into a sensory store which has all the information from the environment gained from the sense organs; it is a transient store from which information is then put into the short term store. This short-term store has five characteristics: (1) it relates roughly to consciousness; (2) the information can be accessed quickly; (3) the information will begin to disappear after about 20 seconds; (4) to prevent it from disappearing it can be retained for longer if it is rehearsed sufficiently; and (5) the information can undergo other types of processing such as elaboration when it is transferred into the long-term store. Its size is unlimited and the information can be taken out of the long-term store and put back into the short-term store so that the activity the person is carrying out at a specific time

can be completed successfully. At one time it was thought that the same memory system could be used for all kinds of memories but more recent research has shown this not to be the case and there are different memories for different types of tasks. Explicit memory is where a person consciously recollects an event occurring in a particular time and place while implicit memory is where a person unconsciously remembers information of various sorts, e.g. how to ride a bike. *See* Smith et al (2003).

memory trace *see* CLASSICAL CONDITIONING.

meninges a membranous covering of the brain and the spinal cord. If it becomes infected, MENINGITIS occurs. *See* Barr (1988); Tortora and Grabowski (2000).

meningiomas *see* TUMOURS OF THE CENTRAL NERVOUS SYSTEM.

meningitis an infection of the lining membranes of the BRAIN and SPINAL CORD. Viruses are the most common cause. The symptoms are headaches, neck stiffness, fever and vomiting. Diagnosis has to be made from the CEREBROSPINAL FLUID which looks milky. The CSF is extracted by LUMBAR PUNCTURE. Treatment depends on the type of infection. There is no specific treatment for virus infections but antibiotics are used in bacterial infections. *See* Gilroy and Holliday (1982); Kolb and Whishaw (1996); Tortora and Grabowski (2000); http://www.meningitis.org/

meningothelial meningiomas a type of meningioma (*see* TUMOURS OF THE CENTRAL NERVOUS SYSTEM) coming from the arachnoid cap cells, consisting of sheets of cells which contain large, vascular nuclei. *See* Gilroy and Holliday (1982).

mental age (MA) an age-equivalent score which is obtained from INTELLIGENCE TESTS. It is used to calculate the IQ score by comparing it to the chronological age to find out if the child is below or above average compared with children of the same age. *See* Smith et al (2003).

mental handicap *see* LEARNING DISABILITY.

menu in computer terms, a list of options from which an operator can choose a particular function or part of a program to use. These may be a selection of games or operations in a business package. The option is automatically booted into the computer's memory. *See* Chandor et al (1985).

Merrill-Palmer Pre-School Intelligence Test an assessment to find out the learning abilities of children between the ages of 1;6 and 5;0 years. Devised in 1931, the scale has 19 verbal and performance subtests which test motor and language skills, manual dexterity and matching skills. Most of these subtests take the form of games so that children readily pay attention to them. The raw scores which are obtained can be converted to MENTAL AGE, intelligence quotients, percentile ranks and standard deviations. *See* Stutsman (1926–1931) in Appendix I.

Message Box a small portable AAC device with four locations and 80 seconds of DIGITISED SPEECH, each message being 20 seconds in length. It allows for only direct manual selection. *See* Appendix IV (Saltillo Corp.).

MessageMate a high-tech communication aid with digitised speech. It can be hand-held. There are several models all of which have similar features. Single keys can be made into larger keys. It can be accessed by direct manual selection or by linear and column–row scanning using one or two switches. The memory differs from model to model. It starts with the 20-20 model of 20 seconds up to the 20-120 model with 120 seconds. The MessageMate40 starts with the 40-60 model with 60 seconds and increases to the 40-240 model with 240 seconds. *See* Glennen and DeCoste (1997); Rumble and Larcher (1998); Appendix IV (Words+).

metalinguistics the study of knowledge of language, the way in which one thinks and knows about its properties. *See* Hjelmquist et al (1994).

Metaphon Resource Pack devised by Dean and her colleagues in 1985 (revised 1989) and published in 1990, it is a complete assessment and therapy programme for children with phonological

disorders. It is most effective with children up to 5;0 years but can be used for children of 7;0 years. The thrust of Metaphon is developing the child's knowledge of sounds and organisation of sound processing. It has four stages:

1. Screening: the child is asked to name pictures. The screening test assesses 13 systemic and structural simplifying processes in the child's phonological system, identifying areas for which the therapist should not expect the child to produce processes because of the age of the child.
2. Probing: a more in-depth assessment of the problem areas identified in the screening test. Responses are recorded on a quantitative and qualitative record form.
3. Intervention: the results of the probes will lead to appropriate strategies for treatment detailed in the manual.
4. Monitoring: the monitoring procedure happens regularly to assess the effectiveness of the treatment strategies.

See Dean et al (1990) in Appendix I; Beech et al (1993).

metastasis a malignant seeding of tumour which has come from a distant primary. Many tumours form metastases in the brain especially bronchial carcinomas. They develop in the CEREBRAL HEMISPHERES and can push the contents of the hemispheres across the midline. This is shown up on COMPUTED TOMOGRAPHY. The symptoms are headache and partial or generalised fits. Treatment is by corticosteroids with a possibility of radiotherapy for multiple tumours. *See* Gilroy and Holliday (1982); Kaye (1991); Tortora and Grabowski (2000).

microcephaly a condition marked by an abnormally small head and small BRAIN and low levels of intelligence. Microcephaly can be divided into primary microcephaly and secondary microcephaly. The former is inherited as an autosomal recessive trait (*see* CHROMOSOMES). It can occur as part of other conditions associated with chromosomal and non-chromosomal deficiencies such as Roberts' syndrome, Williams' syndrome and de Lange syndrome. Secondary microcephaly is produced by infection or other problems which may arise in the PERINATAL period. See Hosking (1982); Jones (1997); http://www.ayles.demon.co.uk/microcep.htm

microglossia an abnormally small tongue. The condition is relatively rare and is caused by the failure of the anterior two-thirds of the tongue to grow normally. It occurs in the prenatal stage. The person's speech can sound muffled. *See* Travis (1971).

micrognathia the failure of the mandible to develop normally.

midbrain part of the brain which is found above the PONS. It is the smallest of the three parts of the BRAIN – HINDBRAIN, forebrain (*see* DIENCEPHALON) and midbrain. It is about 12.5 cm long, 2.5 cm wide and 2 cm thick. There are ascending and descending tracts of cranial nerves III and IV (*see* CRANIAL NERVES). The floor of the THIRD VENTRICLE is formed at the front between the cerebral peduncles. The substantia nigra is situated in the midbrain. See Barr (1988); Kolb and Whishaw (1996).

Mind Express communication software which can be used on any PC using symbols so that people who use AAC can communicate about whatever they like as it can be customised. Mind Express uses the following symbol systems with which to encode vocabulary – BLISSYMBOLICS, REBUS, PICTURE COMMUNICATION SYMBOLS (PCS) as well as Beta, Picto's and Picture this. It can be accessed by various SCANNING techniques and allows the person who is using it to import photographs or drawings as well as record sounds and messages. *See* Appendix IV (Technology and Integration).

minimal pairs two words are said to have a different meaning if they differ by one sound in the same environment of the word. For example, 'pin' and 'bin' are minimal pairs because they differ by one sound, i.e. /p/ vs /b/, and thus the meaning is changed. A minimal pair can only exist if there is one difference in the sounds which occur in the same place in either word. This is also known as variation in sound. Minimal pairs have an important role in speech and language therapy, since they mark the fundamental difference between treatment programmes for phonological or articulation delay or disorder. In the former, the therapist teaches the child sound oppositions such as the difference between /tutər/ and /kukər/, while in the latter, the therapist teaches the child how to make particular sounds which the child has previously been incapable of making. *See* Grunwell (1987) .

Minnesota Test for the Differential Diagnosis of Aphasia (MTDDA) devised by Schuell in 1965 and revised in 1973, this is a formal assessment for testing the severity of a language disorder affecting those with APHASIA. Five modalities are tested: (1) auditory disturbance; (2) visual-reading; (3) speech/language; (4) visuomotor/ graphic; and (5) numeric/arithmetic functions. The 47 subtests in each section are arranged in ascending order of difficulty. There are 'easy' tests for examining residual skills in those who have a severe aphasia and 'hard' tests for those who have a mild aphasic impairment. The person's performance in the tests between these extremes allows the therapist to determine the level of breakdown in each language modality. The test is American but in some of the subtests British amendments have been made so it is possible to use the test more reliably in Britain. There are two rating scales to establish the functional ability of the person and the severity of his condition. The severity scale is from 0 (no impairment) to 4 (severe impairment). The five types of communicative behaviour are rated on a severity scale of 0–6. It has a prognostic potential. *See* Eisenson (1984); Beech et al (1993).

Minspeak the software system which operates ALPHA TALKERS, INTRO TALKERS, DELTA TALKERS, TOUCHTALKERS, LIGHTTALKERS, the LIBERATOR COMMUNICATION AID, PATHFINDER, VANGUARD AND SPRINGBOARD. It means 'minimum effort speech'. It uses multimeaning icons to access messages programmed into one of these devices. Bruce Baker, who developed Minspeak, started from the basis of semantic compaction in which one or two icons can have different meanings depending on the semantic context in which they are used. Thus, the icon of the 'sun' can mean 'sun', 'hot', 'fire', 'face', 'happy', 'orange', and the user may think of many more. When used in conjunction with another icon the meanings increase. Semantic compaction also allows a smaller number of graphics to represent a large number of semantic concepts, especially when the icons are combined together to produce messages. These messages can be accessed by fewer key actuations. Icons have three characteristics:

1. Transparent: the icons should be easily recognisable.
2. Multi-meaning: the icons should be able to represent several meanings.
3. Combinational potential: the icons should be able to be combined easily with other icons to produce new messages.

Although the icons produced by Bruce Baker are known as Minsymbols, they do not have to be used as any set of symbols can be used such as REBUS, BLISSYMBOLS or Makaton symbols (*see* MAKATON). Minspeak is the way the symbols interact with each other as long as they have the characteristics already given. Minspeak is reported to provide fast, effective communication in that as many characters as the user wishes can be represented by just two icons. It allows routine, frequent needs to be communicated using themes (*see* TOUCH TALKER) as well as

emergency needs. It allows conversational control for entering, initiating and controlling the conversation while the user can make formal presentations in class, at home or conferences. *See* Baker (1982); Bruno (1989b); Cross et al (1994); Glennen and DeCoste (1997); Beukelman and Mirenda (1998); Ferm et al (2001).

Minspeak Application Programs (MAPs) these programs have been designed by authors who are experts with a particular client-group. The programs apply the MINSPEAK principles for various client-groups. The aim is to produce fast, effective communication allowing the client to:

1. Communicate everyday needs.
2. Communicate needs in an emergency.
3. Enter and control a conversation.
4. Produce spontaneous and interactive dialogue.
5. Give lectures or speeches at conferences or social events, etc.

The Minspeak applications that have been designed in the past are: Power in Play; Stories and Strategies for Communication; Topics to Learn Communication; INTERACTION, EDUCATION AND PLAY; LANGUAGE, LEARNING AND LIVING; WORDS STRATEGY; and UNITY 128. There was also a MAP which combined BLISSYMBOLS and Words strategy known as Blissymbol Minspeak Words Strategy (BMW). However, these MAPs have been rationalised down to two – namely the UNITY series of MAPs and LANGUAGE, LEARNING AND LIVING (LLL). These programs, and adaptations to suit newer technology, can be loaded into the DELTA TALKER, TOUCHTALKER, LIGHTTALKER, LIBERATOR COMMUNICATION AID, PATHFINDER, VANGUARD and SPRINGBOARD. Each program can be customised for those using the devices. Rumble and Robertson, two speech and language therapists, have written a set of lesson plans for the MAPS Language, Learning and Living and Words Strategy. The starter module has 21 levels which, it is hoped, will produce a 400-word core vocabulary. Every fifth lesson there is a practice level to revise what the person has learnt in the previous four levels. Following this starter module, there are 40 topic modules covering a broad range of interests and communication needs such as food/drink, going on holiday, making telephone calls, art, sports and leisure and religion. Each of these modules will have five levels in the same format as the starter module. *See* Baker (1989); Rumble and Robertson (1995); Glennen and DeCoste (1997).

MIT *see* MELODIC INTONATION THERAPY.

mixed transcortical aphasia a particular syndrome used in the classification of APHASIA. The symptoms are non-fluent language, impaired comprehension and naming while repetition remains intact. *See* Eisenson (1984).

MLU *see* MEAN LENGTH OF UTTERANCE.

Möbius syndrome a CONGENITAL DISORDER which produces weakness of the facial muscles and the bilateral failure of the eyes to abduct. The syndrome may be caused by a congenital abnormality in the VI and VII cranial nerve nuclei in the BRAINSTEM. It is an IDIOPATHIC condition which can run in families. Other associated symptoms are syndactyly, club feet and LEARNING DISABILITY. *See* Gilroy and Holliday (1982); http://www.ciaccess.com/moebius/

mode *see* CENTRAL TENDENCY.

Model 1600 Voice Analyzer the voice analyser can be used in the clinic, home, hospital or school. It is designed to pick up fundamental frequency (Fo) and intensity level at the same time on the monitor. There are two lines which can be compared, the top one with the therapist's mode; and the lower one for the person's attempts. Both can be superimposed on the other for an easy comparison. The machine can be linked up to a printer so that the therapist can keep accurate records of assessments and progress during therapy.

modelling a therapeutic approach to

BEHAVIOUR THERAPY devised by Bandura in 1969. It is known also as vicarious conditioning since its aim is to provide a model participating successfully in the person's feared situation while being watched by the person. After each stage the person is encouraged to copy this behaviour. *See* Smith et al (2003).

modem a device for transmitting data over the telephone system from a computer. It stands for MOdulator/DEModulator. There are many on the market. They can be connected to the operator's telephone system, so that data can be transmitted over long distances to another computer or to access the internet and send and receive e-mails. *See* Bishop (1985); Brookshear (1991).

modification a change of a person's behaviour. Also a term used in BEHAVIOUR THERAPY.

monoamine oxidase inhibitors (MAOI) a form of drug used with those who have DEPRESSION. The three main MAOI drugs are phenelzine, isocarboxazid and tranylcypromine. The evidence of efficacy of these drugs on depression is poor but they can act as a mild anti-anxiety drug. There is also a possibility that they are effective in cases where phobias and irrational anxiety are prominent. Dizziness, dry mouth and fatigue are common side effects in the first few weeks of starting the drugs. These drugs interact with certain foods, e.g. cheese, broad beans and yeast, producing unbearable headaches and a swing to low blood pressure. They should not be mixed with tricyclic antidepressant drugs (*see* ANTIDEPRESSANT DRUGS) or ELECTROCONVULSIVE THERAPY. *See* Stafford-Clark and Bridges (1990); Kolb and Whishaw (1996); Davison et al (2004).

monozygotic twins identical twins who develop from a single fertilised egg, having the same genetic make-up. *See* Smith et al (2003); http://search.bellaonline.com/articles/art2778.asp

Monterey Fluency Programme devised by Ryan and Kirk in 1978 and based on the ideas of those who follow the SPEAK

MORE FLUENTLY approach to the treatment of those who have a STAMMER, it is a highly structured behaviour modification programme following the principles of OPERANT CONDITIONING. Its main aim is to establish complete fluency; an ACCEPTABLE STAMMER is not regarded as success. It begins with a fluency interview lasting 30 minutes during which the person is put into as many communication situations as possible. The next stage is a criterion test in which the person is asked to perform for five minutes in three modes – reading, monologue and conversation. If the stuttering rate is less than 0.5 stuttered words per minute in any of the three modes, the person is put through an establishment programme in a particular mode using two techniques, GILCU or DAF. Another criterion test follows; if the person stutters more than 0.5 stuttered words per minute, he progresses to the transfer programme while if less than 0.5 stuttered words per minute are produced, the person is recycled through the establishment programme. The third criterion test follows the transfer programme with similar requirements to the previous one. If the person succeeds, he or she is placed on a maintenance programme which can last several months. If the person maintains fluency over a period of 22 months, he can be discharged. *See* Dalton (1983).

morbid jealousy also known as delusional jealousy, the person becomes so jealous, he becomes fanatically preoccupied at finding out if his beliefs have any truth. For example, the person has a delusion that his wife is having an affair. He begins to follow her everywhere and may assault anyone with whom she stops to speak. If the wife gives a false admission about any man she knows, it could lead to murder. *See* Stafford-Clark and Bridges (1990); Davison et al (2004).

morphology the part of linguistics that deals with the formation of words. Morphology recognises processes of inflection and derivation in the construction of words. Inflection relates to regular, rule-governed grammatical processes such as plural or past tense in English. Derivation refers to semi- or partially productive processes of word-formation such as suffixation of -ness on to adjectives in English to provide nouns, e.g. happiness, sadness. These affixes are called morphemes – the smallest meaningful unit in any language. The realisation of morphemes, e.g. /s/, /z/, /ɪz/ for the plural morpheme is called an allomorph. Each individual unit, i.e. each of the allomorphs in the last example, is called a morph. There are two types of morpheme:

1. A bound morpheme is an affix which can be attached to a word to represent number and tense, etc.
2. A free morpheme is a whole word which stands on its own without affixes.

An example of both of these types of morpheme is the word:

anti - dis - establish - ment - arian - ism.

The bound morphemes are 'anti', 'dis', 'ment', 'arian', 'ism' while 'establish' is the free morpheme. There are three models discussed in morphology:

1. Item and arrangement (IA): this examines word structure and syntactic structures which follow particular, logical sequences in a linear way: (1) The men played cricket. The example in (1) is analysed in the form:

det + MAN + plural + PLAY + past + CRICKET.

Difficulties in explaining some morphological phenomena occur, such as 'mice' in the form 'MOUSE + plural'.

2. Item and process (IP): a process is a derivational procedure which accounts for the form 'mice' as a vowel change from 'mouse'.
3. Word and paradigm (WP): a morphological model which takes the root of

a word and fits it into a paradigm. The resulting words and structures are formed by rules such as Latin verb declensions, e.g. amo, amas, amat, amamus, amatis, amant.

See Matthews (1974); Fromkin and Rodman (2003).

morphophonology refers to the study of the phonological effects or consequences of morphological processes. In the regular plural in English, the exact form of a plural noun is affected by the phonological form of the final segment of that noun. If the noun ends in a voiced segment (except /z/), the plural form is /z/; if the noun ends in a voiceless segment (except /s/), the plural form is /s/; if the noun ends in /s/ or /z/, e.g. bus, haze, the plural form is /ɪz/. See Matthews (1974); Fromkin and Rodman (2003).

mother's depression abnormal moods which a mother has which may affect her child. These moods are associated with low self-esteem, loss of energy, poor sleep, poor appetite or compensatory overeating, anxiety, obsessional symptoms, increased use of drugs and alcohol and a loss of sexual desire and pleasure. Maternal depression can double the chance of disturbance in the child from 15 to 30 per cent. The moods have specific effects on the child. The mother's apathy produces decreased interaction and stimulation which causes speech and language delay and attention-seeking behaviour in the child. If the mother's use of discipline and management is inconsistent, this may produce behaviour problems of all sorts (e.g. temper tantrums, eating and sleeping problems). If the family is socially isolated, there may be a lack of peer contact for the child which could produce a failure to develop social skills and, possibly, speech and language problems. A mother's resentment and threats of abandonment can produce fearfulness and SEPARATION ANXIETY. Irritability in the mother may make her use excessive physical punishment against the child which produces fearfulness and/or aggressiveness between the child and his peers. The child's difficult behaviour in turn can worsen the mother's depression. When the mother comes to the clinic, she will probably present psychosomatic complaints or anxiety about the child. She may not openly admit she has depression. Depression affects 5 per cent of women and 2 per cent of men. It affects 30–50 per cent of women in the lower social classes. PSYCHOTHERAPY can be used in treating such conditions. See Rutter (1975).

motor aphasia see APHASIA (1).

motor area see BRAIN.

motor equivalence the general pattern of planning of a configuration of movement necessary to achieve a target. In relation to speech, it is the determination of the sequence of movement throughout the entire vocal tract which is necessary to deliver the message.

motor neurone disease also known as amyotrophic lateral sclerosis, this is a progressive disease which causes failure in the motor neurons in the SPINAL CORD, loss of motor neurons in the BRAINSTEM and a loss of Betz cells in the cerebral CORTEX. Only motor cells are affected. The cause is uncertain. There is complete loss of motor control which produces DYSARTHRIA, i.e. progressive deterioration in speech, as well as the onset of DYSPHAGIA, loss of hand function and mobility. There is neither sensory loss nor DEMENTIA. Treatment is aimed at making the person's life as comfortable as possible since the disease progresses steadily until death. Speech therapy for these patients consists of maintaining the intelligibility of speech for as long as possible. When speech worsens significantly, some form of AUGMENTATIVE AND ALTERNATIVE COMMUNICATION will have to be found. Treatment is also given for the person's swallow. Perry et al (2002) carried out a pilot study investigating the maximum height of the soft palate during speech and swallowing, expressing it as an angle of elevation so that they could compare the movement of the soft palate in speech and swallowing. There can be remission but this may be just for a few weeks or months. *See* Gilroy and Holliday (1982); Beukelman and Mirenda (1998) (amyotrophic lateral sclerosis and AAC); Murphy and Bloch (2002) (MND and AAC); Perry et al (2002); http://www.mndassociation.org/

mouse an INPUT DEVICE which can move the cursor about a screen. It can be used with icon software in which windows are produced on the screen with menus of one or more item. The mouse is used to move an arrow around the menus to choose which option the operator wishes to use. It can be held under the hand and requires the touch of only two or three buttons and lateral movement over a flat surface. *See* Bishop (1985); Brookshear (1991).

mouse emulation the means of operating a computer if the person has no or little hand movement and is unable to use an ordinary mouse. Some of the hardware systems available include HEADMASTER/ HEADMASTER 2000, HEADMOUSE, SMART NOW, QUICK GLANCE EYE TRACKING SYSTEM, and software includes SCANBUDDY and Switch Access for Windows. *See* Glennen and DeCoste (1997).

mouth often called the oral cavity. The mouth has a roof which is formed by the hard palate and soft palate towards the posterior of the mouth. This part of the mouth is supplied by the greater palatine and nasopalatine nerves, the fibres of which travel in the MAXILLARY NERVE. The floor of the mouth is formed by the tongue which is supplied by the lingual nerve (*see* TONGUE) while the walls of the mouth, i.e. the cheeks, are supplied by the buccal nerve; both of these are branches of the MANDIBULAR NERVE. In the posterior wall of the mouth is the fauces (fauces are arches) which is also known as the oropharyngeal passage. Between the arches, the uvula hangs. Behind the uvula is the palatine tonsil

or true tonsil. The palatopharyngeus muscle (*see* MUSCLES FOR SWALLOWING) runs to the palate behind this tonsil. The front wall is formed by the teeth which are set in the upper and lower dentitions or dental arches. The alveolar ridge is the bony ridge behind the upper dentition. *See* Tortora and Grabowski (2000).

mouth breathing a symptom of adenoidal problems. The child's mouth is affected as he will have a high arched maxilla. He will also have narrow nostrils and the pharyngeal tonsils will be enlarged. This will produce the typical 'look', i.e. ADENOIDAL FACIES, of a child who has adenoidal problems. The sense of smell will be affected and the child will lose taste, with a possible reduction in appetite. There could also be a CONDUCTIVE HEARING LOSS. *See* Travis (1971).

MRI *see* MAGNETIC RESONANCE IMAGING.

MTDDA *see* MINNESOTA TEST FOR THE DIFFERENTIAL DIAGNOSIS OF APHASIA.

mucous membrane a sheet of EPITHELIUM which is supported by a basal lamina made of CONNECTIVE TISSUE. It lines a cavity in the body which reaches the exterior, e.g. the respiratory tract. The layer of epithelium secretes mucus which keeps the cavities moist. The connective tissue binds the epithelial layer to the underlying structures. It keeps the blood vessels in place and protects muscles. *See* Tortora and Grabowski (2000).

multi-infarct dementia a type of dementia which may occur in people who have hypertension and diabetes in whose CEREBRAL HEMISPHERES and BRAINSTEM small lacunar infarcts appear. The development of these infarcts is irregular and so the progression of the dementia is irregular. Such people produce a gradual deterioration in intellectual functioning, including impairment in judgement and lack of insight; memory is impaired while there is also lability of mood and sudden crying associated with DEPRESSION. Associated problems which have gradual onset include DYSARTHRIA, DYSPHAGIA, HEMIPLEGIA, ataxia of gait and the type of loss of emotional control associated with those who have pseudobulbar palsy. *See* Gilroy and Holliday (1982); Stafford-Clark and Bridges (1990); Davison et al (2004).

multiple sclerosis a disease of unknown aetiology, the features of which are due to multiple areas of demyelination of the BRAIN and SPINAL CORD. It affects all the areas, especially around the ventricles, spinal cord and BRAINSTEM. The symptoms are optic neuritis, double vision, DYSARTHRIA, ataxia, spastic gait (*see* CEREBRAL PALSY), HEMIPLEGIA and, occasionally, DEMENTIA. The diagnosis is made following tests such as visual evoked responses and an examination of CEREBROSPINAL FLUID which should show evidence of lymphocyte infiltration. It can follow a remission-relapse course and is a progressive disease which produces dysarthria. The main dysarthric symptoms are poor volume, harsh voice and poor articulation. *See* Darley et al (1975); Gilroy and Holliday (1982); Glennen and DeCoste (1997); Beukelman and Mirenda (1998) (AAC and MS); Doyle and Phillips (2001) (AAC and ALS/MS); McNaughton et al (2001) (AAC and ALS/MS); http://www. nationalmssociety.org/

multisensory approaches *see* EDUCATION OF HEARING-IMPAIRED CHILDREN.

Munchausen syndrome named after Baron Munchausen who told very tall stories concerning how good a cavalry officer he was, this is a form of DEMENTIA. An example of someone who has this syndrome concerns the person who likes hospital operations so much that he will be admitted, followed by discharge. The person goes to another hospital and a similar procedure ensues. A person who had this syndrome requested speech therapy a few years ago. He complained his speech was dysarthric as most consonants were substituted by glottal stops and, although he claimed to suffer from multiple sclerosis, his speech had none of the typical characteristics associated

with MS. It seemed his speech disorder was functional. He was put on a treatment programme of having his speech taped followed by his listening to it. Having listened to it, he began using normal speech quickly. His response to such therapy was very similar to the response of those with functional dysphonia. *See* Kallen et al (1986); http:// www.munchausen.com/

muscles for swallowing four muscles are used for swallowing:

1. Mylohyoid muscle: stretching along the mylohyoid line of the mandible. It originates from the inner surface of the mandible and inserts into the body of the hyoid bone. It is supplied by the mandibular branch of the trigeminal nerve and elevates both the hyoid bone and floor of the mouth and depresses the mandible.

2. Digastric muscle has two parts:
   (a) posterior belly originates from the mastoid process of the temporal bone and is supplied by the facial nerve VII;
   (b) anterior belly originates from the inner side of the lower border of the mandible and is supplied by the mandibular nerve. Both parts insert into the body of the hyoid bone through an intermediate tendon. The digastric muscle elevates the hyoid bone and lowers the jaw as in opening the mouth.

3. Stylopharyngeus muscle: originating from the base of the styloid process, its fibres insert into the lateral aspects of the pharynx and thyroid cartilage. This muscle lifts up the larynx and expands the pharynx to allow the food bolus to descend to the oesophagus.

4. Palatopharyngeus muscle: originating at the soft palate, its fibres insert into the back of the thyroid cartilage and the side and back wall of the pharynx. It is supplied by the pharyngeal plexus. It lifts up both the larynx and the pharynx and closes the nasopharynx during the swallowing process.

Other muscles associated with the process of swallowing are described in the discussion concerning the PHARYNX. *See* Tortora and Grabowski (2000).

muscles of facial expression these muscles are supplied by cranial nerve VII (*see* CRANIAL NERVES). There are two types of muscle:

1. Sphincters which close off openings.
2. Dilators which cause structures to open.

They modify the expression of the face and/or meaning to what is being said. The orbicularis oculi surrounds each eye and can be used to screw up the eyes. The orbicularis oris muscle allows pouting of lips. The muscle is supplied by the buccal and mandibular branches of the facial nerve. The buccinator allows the person to smile while the levator anguli labii superioris and depressor anguli labii inferioris allow the person to elevate and lower the lips respectively. All these facial muscles are derived from the second pharyngeal arch. *See* Tortora and Grabowski (2000).

muscles of mastication four muscles control the function of chewing or mastication:

1. Temporalis muscle: fan-shape muscle, the fibres of which reach a tendon that is inserted on the coronoid process. The anterior and superior fibres raise the mandible. The muscle is supplied by the deep temporal nerves which are branches of the anterior division of the mandibular nerve.
2. Masseter muscle: originating at the ZYGOMATIC ARCH, the fibres go downwards and backwards and are attached to the lateral aspects of the ramus of the mandible. It is supplied by the mandibular nerve. Its function is to lift the mandible, which, as a result, covers the teeth during the process of chewing.
3. Medial pterygoid muscle: originating at the middle of the lateral pterygoid plate, its fibres go downwards, backwards and laterally and end in the middle of the angle of the mandible. It is supplied by the mandibular nerve and assists in raising the mandible.
4. Lateral pterygoid muscle: originating from two places – one being the infratemporal surface of the greater wing of sphenoid and the second being the surface of the lateral pterygoid plate. Fibres reach the front of the mandible neck and articular disc of the temperomandibular joint. It is supplied by the mandibular nerve. Its function is to pull forward the neck of the mandible by the articular disc as the mouth opens. It also causes the rotating action of chewing.

See Tortora and Grabowski (2000).

mutism an inability to speak or phonate. It may be organic as in profound deafness or non-organic as an extreme example of conversion behaviour. *See* Fay (1993).

'My Turn to Speak' designed as a package to help those working with people using a communication aid to develop a consistent and cohesive team approach to their training in school and at home. It comprises five 90-minute sessions which cover the main factors affecting the communication of those using any augmentative communication system, including positions in and accessing of the device, methods of communication, functions of communication and communication breakdown. The workshop also concentrates on the child's current skills and setting long-term aims. The workshop can be organised by speech and language therapists, occupational therapists, physiotherapists and teachers with a special interest in AAC. It can be used with teachers, classroom assistants, parents, managers and therapists. The pack consists of a tutor's manual, participant's manual and a video. *See* Pennington et al (1993).

myasthenia gravis a neuromuscular disorder. It is an autoimmune condition in which the person has a progressive muscle weakness during exertion but recovers after rest. There is a reduction in the number of acetycholine receptors in the neuromuscular joint. Thus, repetitive stimulation will result in the decrease of muscle fibres as there is receptor insufficiency in each neuromuscular joint. This is evidenced by progressive weakness. It is a rare disease with a prevalence of about 1 in 10000. It is more common in females than in males by 2:1. The mean age of onset is 26 years of age in females and 31 years of age in males. There is no significant familial occurrence. It can produce DYSARTHRIA which worsens as the amount of speech increases. The muscles used for speech become tired, hypernasality increases, articulation becomes worse and dysphonia sets in with the voice becoming quieter. *See* Darley et al (1975); Gilroy and Holliday (1982); Kolb and Whishaw (1996); Tortora and Grabowski (2000); http://www.mgauk.org/

myelography a diagnostic test to locate a lesion on or near to the SPINAL CORD. In this test, a radio-opaque material is instilled into the spinal cord and its movement up the canal is recorded by serial X-rays. *See* Kaye (1991); Tortora and Grabowski (2000).

myelomeningocele a form of SPINA BIFIDA. There is a flaccid paralysis of the legs as well as of the bladder and bowel. Abnormalities to the skin, SPINAL CORD,

vertebrae and MENINGES also occur. It is often associated with HYDROCEPHALUS. *See* Hosking (1982); Kaye (1991); http://www.pens.org/articles/henry-judy.htm

mylohyoid muscle *see* MUSCLES FOR SWALLOWING.

myoclonus a movement disorder characterised by sudden jerks. It can occur in the normal population while asleep but it becomes a disorder when associated with EPILEPSY. It is a symptom of acquired BRAINSTEM diseases such as CREUTZFELDT-JAKOB DISEASE which causes degeneration of the BASAL GANGLIA, hypoxic brain damage or drug dependency. *See* Gilroy and Holliday (1982); Kaye (1991); Kolb and Whishaw (1996); http://www.myoclonus.com/

myxoedema a metabolic disorder which results from under-secretion of the thyroid gland. There is a congenital form which if not diagnosed and treated at an early stage may lead to CRETINISM. Onset may also occur later in childhood as juvenile myxoedema. It is also sometimes a feature of senescence. In all cases, the predominating feature is change of pitch and voice quality. The voice becomes hoarse and pitch drops owing to thickening of the VOCAL FOLDS. *See* Greene and Mathieson (1989); Tortora and Grabowski (2000); http://www.nevdgp.org.au/Pattison/Thyroid/myxoedema.htm

N

naming a language function which is assessed and treated in those who have APHASIA. There are four stages of naming:

1. Picture recognition.
2. Retrieval of the semantic relation corresponding to the picture.
3. Accessing a phonological form using the semantic relation.
4. Producing the spoken word to name the picture.

If the person has an aphasia compounded either by AGNOSIA or by a difficulty in retrieving SEMANTICS, naming will be even more difficult. *See* Benson (1979); Rosenbek et al (1989).

narrow transcription *see* TRANSCRIPTION SYSTEMS (2).

nasal

1. A description of sounds which are produced by using the resonating nasal cavities. These sounds are /n,m,ŋ/. *See* Ladefoged (2001).
2. A description of any structure or disorder related to the NOSE. *See* Tortora and Grabowski (2000).

nasalisation a condition in which there is excessive nasal resonance throughout speech.

nasopalatine nerve *see* MOUTH.

nasopharynx *see* PHARYNX.

natural phonology a phonological theory proposed by David Stampe in the late 1970s. In essence, he believes a child will simplify sounds which cause difficulty. These simplifications are called PHONOLOGICAL PROCESSES. The thrust of his theory is that as these processes are INNATE, those sounds which are found difficult by the child will automatically be simplified by young children as they acquire speech and language. Thus, natural phonology becomes a suitable means for analysing children's speech as it is based on simplifying sound systems (*see* PHONOLOGY). By treating the child's simplifications the therapist is showing the complexity of sound production to the child and the sounds for which he is aiming. *See* Grunwell (1987).

natural process analysis devised by Shriberg and Kwiatowski in 1980 (Appendix I) to obtain a sample of SPONTANEOUS SPEECH for the therapist to discover which PHONOLOGICAL PROCESSES are used by the child when he produces sound changes. The elicited words are transcribed and then coded into stops, nasals/glides, fricatives/affricates (*see* ARTICULATION) and the information can be summarised. *See* Grunwell (1987).

negation the process of denial of the whole or part of an utterance. It is represented in English by the negative units 'no', 'n't' and 'not'. Negative affixes such as 'un-' and 'non-' can also be used. *See* Huddleston (1976).

neologisms *see* APHASIA.

neologistic jargon *see* JARGON APHASIA (4).

network a series of computers all linked together so that information can be transferred among them. This could be used in business such as the Stock Exchange where all the terminals will have the relevant data supplied from the main computer so that several stockbrokers can have the same information ready at hand. *See* Brookshear (1991).

neurilemmoma a benign tumour which affects cranial nerve VIII (*see* CRANIAL NERVES), the acoustic nerve. It produces TINNITUS, progressive HEARING LOSS and episodic vertigo. As it increases in size, it involves the other cranial nerves and structures of the BRAIN such as the CERE-BELLUM. Such interference can produce cerebellar ataxia (*see* CEREBRAL PALSY). Treatment is by surgery. *See* Gilroy and Holliday (1982).

neurofibroma *see* TUMOURS OF THE CENTRAL NERVOUS SYSTEM (3).

neurolinguistics the study of neurological programming for the comprehension and production of language and reasons for the breakdown in language or articulation. Research has come from clinical linguistics, to try to construct models to explain language breakdown in APHASIA, stammering (*see* STAMMER), DYSARTHRIA, etc., and hypotheses can be found to show how the brain can organise language. *See* Clark and Clark (1977).

neurons nerve cells which are responsible for passing nerve impulses to muscles, other neurons and glands. Most comprise three parts – cell bodies and two kinds of processes – DENDRITES and axons. Motor neurons receive information which makes movement possible. *See* Kolb and Whishaw (1996); Tortora and Grabowski (2000).

neuropsychological assessment there are several goals for making assessments in clinical neuropsychology including finding evidence of cortical damage or dysfunction and its location; facilitating rehabilitation and patient care; showing mild disturbances where other test results may be equivocal; and identifying unusual brain organisation

which may produce behavioural rather than organic problems. *See* Kolb and Whishaw (1996).

neurosis neurotic disorders are those which affect emotional and intellectual functioning without losing reality. Such disorders include ANXIETY, STRESS, OBSESSIVE–COMPULSIVE DISORDERS, DEPRESSION and MANIC-DEPRESSION. *See* Stafford-Clark and Bridges (1990); Davison et al (2004).

neutral a vowel sound which is described as being produced not at the front or back of the mouth or high or low but in a central position. This is shown clearly in the diagram of the CARDINAL VOWEL SYSTEM. The vowel in question is known as SCHWA or shwa /ə/. *See* Cruttenden (1994).

neutralisation a phenomenon which describes sounds which can be interchangeable in certain contexts with other sounds because they lose their distinction. For example, /p,t,k/ and /b,d,g/ can be distinguished from each other by the opposition of voicing (*see* ARTICULATION) and ASPIRATION. In the former set of sounds, aspiration is present, e.g. 'pin/bin', 'pit/bit', etc., while in the second set of sounds there is no aspiration present. However, when these sounds follow /s/, e.g. 'skate', 'spate', 'steak', they do not require the distinction because /b,d,g/ in similar positions do not exist, e.g. *sgate, *sbate, *sdeak. Thus, the distinction between these two sets of phonemes (*see* PHONOLOGY) is lost in the context following /s/, i.e. s_V where 'V' = vowel. *See* Cruttenden (1994); Fromkin and Rodman (2003).

NMR (nuclear magnetic resonance) *see* MAGNETIC RESONANCE IMAGING.

noise-induced hearing loss when exposed to a loud noise for any length of time, a person may eventually have a noise-induced hearing loss which is sensorineural (*see* SENSORINEURAL HEARING LOSS) in character. The degree of loss depends on how long the person has been exposed to the sound and its intensity. If an elevated threshold goes back to normal after a few hours, it is called temporary threshold shift (TTS) but if the exposure is for a longer time, it can become a permanent threshold shift (PTS). PTS can also occur if there is a sudden burst of noise – known as acoustic trauma and found on an audiogram (*see* PURE-TONE AUDIOMETRY) by a dip at 4000 Hz and a recovery at 8000 Hz. The loss is sensorineural. *See* Katz (1985); Coles (2001).

non-fluent aphasia *see* APHASIA (1).

non-word *see* NONSENSE WORD.

nonsense word a word that follows the PHONOTACTIC structure of a true word in English but does not have any meaning, e.g. dup, sep, mib, etc. *See* Fromkin and Rodman (2003).

normal distribution while the measures of CENTRAL TENDENCY may vary from study to study, there is a recurring shape of the distributions of different types of data. The shape shows a symmetrical distribution of scores with most values falling in the central part of the curve close to the mean. The curve is bell-shaped and because it is symmetrical the mean, median and mode will all have the same value. *See* Miller (1984).

normal pressure hydrocephalus a condition which can produce DEMENTIA. The features are a clumsy gait, urgency of micturition and eventual incontinence. The person's unsteadiness is due to a mixture of ataxia, spasticity (*see* CEREBRAL PALSY) and dyspraxia of gait. It can be reversed by placing a shunt in the ventricles of the brain to drain the excess CEREBROSPINAL FLUID. *See* Stafford-Clark and Bridges (1990); Davison et al (2004).

norms the explicit or implicit rules in a culture, society or other groups which dictate acceptable behaviour. Any behaviour which does not follow such rules significantly is considered abnormal. *See* Smith et al (2003); Davison et al (2004).

Northwestern Syntax Screening Test devised by Lee in 1969, it is a SCREENING TEST which can measure independently levels of verbal comprehension and expressive language in children between the ages of 3;0 and 7;0 years. The comprehension section requires a picture-pointing response to verbally presented stimulus sentences and the expressive section involves sentence repetition. *See* Lee (1969) in Appendix I.

nose the front part of the nose has two U-shaped cartilages forming the nostrils. At the posterior of the nose, there is an opening to the nasopharynx (*see* PHARYNX). The nasal cavity is formed by a roof, floor and wall. The floor is the top surface of the hard palate and the roof is divided into three parts – the anterior part is the slope or bridge of the nose, the middle part is the ethmoid or cribiform plate, while the posterior part is formed by the anterior and inferior surfaces of the cribiform plate. The cavity is divided by the nasal septum. The lateral walls are formed by the superior, middle and inferior conchae or folds. Between these folds are the superior, middle and inferior meati. Around the middle meatus, there are four openings of the frontal sinus, the anterior ethmoid sinus, the maxillary sinus and the middle ethmoid sinus. At the lower edge of the cavity, just above the floor, is the naso-lacrimal duct. This structure draws tears from the eyes down the nose through a flap in the nose. When the nose is blown, it stops material being blown upwards. If the flap does not shut and the nose is blown, bubbles may appear at the side of the eyes. Blood supply is by the ophthalmic, maxillary and facial arteries while the nerve supply comes from the ophthalmic, maxillary and facial nerves. *See* Tortora and Grabowski (2000).

noun in traditional grammar, a noun was said to be the name of a person, place or object. However, this definition was inappropriate for modern linguists, who preferred to define nouns and other grammatical categories in terms of their formal syntactic behaviour. Nouns, then, are elements which can only be placed in particular positions in the sentence and to which plural affixes can be attached. *See* Lyons (1968); Fromkin and Rodman (2003).

noun phrase a noun phrase is a constituent (*see* CONSTITUENT ANALYSIS) in GENERATIVE GRAMMAR and is generated by a head noun with optional premodification and/or postmodification. *See* Lyons (1968); Fromkin and Rodman (2003).

nuclear magnetic imaging *see* MAGNETIC RESONANCE IMAGING.

nucleus *see* SUPRASEGMENTAL PHONOLOGY.

Nuffield Dyspraxia Programme devised by Connery and colleagues, it is a complete articulation programme comprising an assessment and a detailed therapeutic programme. The required therapy is based on the scores of the assessment which assesses oral-motor skills and sound-sequencing abilities of speech in isolation, single words with differing phonotactic structures and sentences using picture material and imitation. It concentrates on improvement of speed and accuracy of articulatory movement. *See* Connery et al (1985).

null hypothesis this hypothesis is tested by statistical analysis. When using statistical hypothesis testing the investigator sets up a null hypothesis and an alternative hypothesis. It is normally assumed with the null hypothesis that nothing has changed while with the alternative hypothesis that a change has taken place or taken place in a particular statistical direction. If the difference between the means of the samples is among those that can occur rarely by chance, when the null hypothesis is true, the null hypothesis is rejected and the investigation can conclude the results are statistically significant. *See* Miller (1984); Porkess (1988).

numeric keypad a grouping of numbered keys usually 0–9 on a keyboard although they can form their own unit. Many computer keyboards have such a grouping with arithmetical functions on a separate section of the keyboard.

nystagmus an involuntary rhythmical movement of the eyes which can occur at rest or during eye movement. It can happen to both eyes or just to one and is caused by a disorder of the CEREBELLUM. The involuntary movement of the eyes can be horizontal, vertical, oblique or circular. Nystagmus can also be pendular where the eyes swing from side-to-side in a regular action or jerk where one phase of eye movement is faster than the other. This type of nystagmus may be caused by a loss of central vision. *See* Gilroy and Holliday (1982); Kolb and Whishaw (1996); Tortora and Grabowski (2000).

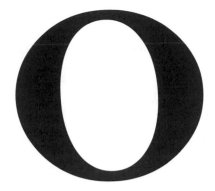

object *see* DIRECT OBJECT; INDIRECT OBJECT.

object permanence the awareness that an object continues to exist even when it is not present. This is part of the SENSORI-MOTOR STAGE of the child's cognitive development proposed by Piaget. He argued that if a child is presented with a toy which he is allowed to play with or handle, and it is then hidden under a box or cloth, the child will not make any effort to find or look for it. This stage is present until 5–6 months of age. According to Piaget, this shows the child's egocentricity (*see* PREOPERA-TIONAL STAGE), i.e. the child is only concerned with his own world and cannot take into account changes in the environment. The critics put forward the argument that it was how the object was hidden which was important. Thus, if the object was hidden gradually, the child might try and find it but, if hidden suddenly, then the child would not try to look for it. *See* Donaldson (1987); Smith et al (2003); Boden (1994).

objects of reference originally used to develop the communication of people who had dual hearing and visual impairments devised by van Dijk (McLarty 1997), objects of reference are used increasingly with people who have PRO-FOUND AND MULTIPLE LEARNING DIFFICULTIES (PMLD). Objects of reference can represent activities, places or people and can be used to aid understanding, memory or communication (Ockleford, 1994) while Rowland and Stremell-Campbell (1987) described them as 'everyday objects' which are used consistently to provide specific information. However, other authors believe that objects should be specific to an individual so that they meet the particular preferences and needs of the individual with PMLD (Rowland and Schweigert 1989; Ockleford 1994; McLarty 1995, 1997). In 1995, McLarty asserted that objects should be used in an activity while Park (1997) divided objects into indices, icons and symbols. Indices are objects used in an activity while icons are related by physical resemblance and symbols have an arbitrary relationship with the denoted item. Rowland and Schweigert (1989) argued that objects of reference allow individuals to progress from non-symbolic to symbolic levels of communication. *See* Rowland and Schweigert (1989); Ockleford (1994); McLarty (1995, 1997); Park (1997); Jones et al (2002).

observation an informal technique for assessing a person's behaviour. It is important for the therapist to decide the target behaviour to be aimed for and the stages through which the person has to pass to reach this behaviour. It is possible by observation to see changes in behaviour patterns from a baseline (found in initial assessment). If two therapists are observing the one person, they must have a common language which they can use to express

161

their findings. This language must be objective so that the biases and wishes of the therapists are not reflected in their reported findings. There are two main types of observation:

1. Direct observation: the researcher watches the types of behaviour presented by a client in particular environments or in a laboratory.
2. Indirect observation: the researcher uses interviews or questionnaires to find out how people feel about particular issues such as political affiliations, preferences for particular products, etc. The researchers have to be trained to use the questionnaire, the questionnaire itself has to be carefully assessed before use, a sample of people has to be chosen and appropriate methods of data analysis have to be used to make sure the results are interpreted correctly.

See Smith et al (2003).

obsessive–compulsive disorder a neurosis present in 0.5 per cent of the population at any one time. Those who have obsessions or compulsions about something, e.g. keeping clean, will spend their life carrying out such activities as are required to fulfil their obsession. For example, if a person has a compulsion concerning cleanliness, there could be extensive handwashing, washing utensils several times before using them, washing sink surrounds before using them to wash in, as well as keeping soap, cloths and towels in receptacles for cleanliness. Compulsive rituals are carried out a certain number of times which becomes a magical figure. If the ritual is repeated more often than the magical number of times the ritual starts all over again. Repetitive, unwelcomed and resisted thoughts become strengthened, i.e. ruminations. People's lives can be ruined by this disorder. PSYCHOTHERAPY such as BEHAVIOUR THERAPY or PSYCHO-ANALYSIS can be used successfully. *See* Stafford-Clark and Bridges (1990); Davison et al (2004).

obstruent a sound which is produced by an obstruction in the mouth made by the articulators such as plosives, fricatives, affricates (*see* ARTICULATION). It is also a DISTINCTIVE FEATURE proposed by Chomsky and Halle to distinguish such sounds from those produced without such an obstruction. It is opposed to SONORANT. *See* Fromkin and Rodman (2003); Ladefoged (2001).

obturator in relation to speech, a palatal device used to improve resonance and intraoral pressure as, for example, in the case of cleft palate where there is a residual fissure.

occlusion in relation to articulation:

1. The degree of closure necessary for the production of different consonants.
2. The relationship between the maxilla and mandible.

A malocclusion (*see* ORTHODONTICS) may contribute to articulatory defects. Angle's classification delineates the different types of occlusion. *See* Tortora and Grabowski (2000).

occupational therapy an occupational therapist works with people who have difficulty in coping at home on their own due to physical disability resulting from neurological incidents, e.g. CVA, head injury, progressive degenerative diseases, orthopaedic operations or problems with their upper limbs, especially hands. The therapist may have to help the person with dressing, eye/hand co-ordination and general cognitive skills. They will carry out home visits before the person is discharged from hospital to find out if the person will require particular adaptations for the house such as hand rails, an extra bannister, widening of doors if the person uses a wheelchair and hoists to allow the person to get in and out of a bath. They use assessments to assess the person's abilities. Treatment consists of using microcomputers, making objects in a workshop and working in the kitchen. The latter allows the therapist to assess the person's independence in the kitchen and gives the person help to cope in that environment. All these types of treatment have the aims of improving the person's performance in communication skills, initiative and decision-making, concentration, confidence and self-esteem. As with most therapies, motivating the person to capitalise on their strengths and compensate for their weaknesses is paramount. *See* Hopkins and Smith (1993).

Oedipus complex at about 5–6 years of age a boy forms sexual impulses towards his mother or a substitute, e.g. foster mother, and this leads him to consider his father as a rival to his mother's affection. This affection is produced by an emotional tie between the boy and the mother. Thus, the boy finds difficulties in life when separated from his mother (*see* SEPARATION ANXIETY). He is faced with a terrible dilemma: on the one hand he is jealous of his father as a rival, while on the other hand he knows he depends on his father emotionally in the family circle. Such frustrations lead to feelings of aggression against the father which the boy has to suppress because of the love and respect he has for his father. As the boy is still very young, he cannot speak about these feelings towards his father. He is in conflict over his emotional feelings towards his father. The Oedipus complex was first proposed by Freud, who suggested it was a possible cause of various neuroses which some people have. *See* Stafford-Clark and Bridges (1990); Smith et al (2003); Davison et al (2004).

oesophageal voice a laryngeal phonation. A method whereby, following a complete LARYNGECTOMY, PHONATION is achieved by intake of air through the mouth which, by combined compression of the pharyngo-oesophageal sphincter and intraorally, is driven into the OESOPHAGUS. There are three methods of sound production – by injection of air, by inhalation of air and by swallowing air. The last method is not generally recommended. *See* Edels (1984); Max et al (1997).

oesophagus a structure used in swallowing that is 25 cm long, and starts at the level of the sixth cervical vertebra and ends about the thoracic level of the 11th vertebra where it enters the stomach. It narrows at the PHARYNX, where it passes through the diaphragm and at the bottom of the thorax. It has an inner circular layer of muscles and an outer longitudinal layer of muscles. The top part of the oesophagus is covered with STRIATED MUSCLE while the bottom is covered with SMOOTH MUSCLE. It is possible to use the upper part for producing oesophageal voice as it has striated muscle. It runs behind the TRACHEA. *See* Tortora and Grabowski (2000).

off-/on-glide a description of movements of articulators (*see* ARTICULATION) which occur in the production of contiguous sounds. An off-glide occurs after the production of one sound when the articulators are beginning to take up the position of the next sound, while an on-glide occurs as the articulators are taking up the position for the intended sound from a previous sound or from rest. *See* Cruttenden (1994).

olfaction the sense of smell. The receptors are found in the epithelium in the roof of the NOSE on either side of the nasal septum. The free end of each olfactory cell contains a dendrite which ends in the olfactory vesicle from which six to eight microscopic hairs extend. These hairs react to the odours in the air, which then stimulate the olfactory cells, producing an olfactory reaction. *See* Kolb and Whishaw (1996); Smith et al (2003); Tortora and Grabowski (2000).

olfactory *see* CRANIAL NERVES.

oligodendrogliomas *see* TUMOURS OF THE CENTRAL NERVOUS SYSTEM.

on/off phenomenon *see* PARKINSON'S DISEASE.

on-screen keyboards software which produces a keyboard on the monitor screen which can be accessed by using the ordinary mouse or other INPUT DEVICES. Such software includes REACH

INTERFACE AUTHOR and WIVIK. *See* Glennen and DeCoste (1997).

one- and two-tail tests a statistical interpretation of any parametric or non-parametric test (*see* PARAMETRIC TESTS). Assumptions are made about the experiment before it is carried out. It is a rule in statistical hypothesis testing that a NULL HYPOTHESIS is set up and it is tested against an alternative hypothesis which will mean one of two things occurs – the null hypothesis is rejected or it is rejected in a particular direction. The former will require a two-tail test while the latter will require a one-tail test. Basically, the null hypothesis will show no difference in the means against a non-directional alternative hypothesis that there is a difference in the means. However, it may be necessary to show the expected direction of the difference between the means. By using a one-tail test, there will only be a significant difference at one end of the distribution (the tail of one end of the bell-shaped normal distribution curve) while by using a two-tail test the significant difference may be at either end. So, if the significant difference is shown at the 5 per cent end using a one-tail test, the significant difference for a two-tail test is shown at the 2.5 per cent value at both ends. See Miller (1984); Clarke and Cooke (1992).

One Step Communicator a light-tech communication aid which allows for one message of up to 20 seconds to be recorded into it. It can be accessed by direct manual selection or by a single switch attached to it. The One Step can also have a battery-operated toy or gadget attached to it to provide reinforcement of cause and effect. *See* Rumble and Larcher (1998); Appendix IV (AbleNet).

open bite an orthodontic condition in which the upper anterior teeth do not align with the lower teeth leaving a gap. Sometimes associated with tongue thrust and with an immature swallowing pattern.

open class word *see* PIVOT GRAMMAR.

open syllable a syllable ending in a vowel. In speech pathology, this refers to incomplete articulation of a word by omission of the final consonant. Also known as final syllable deletion. *See* Renfrew (1966).

open vowel see CARDINAL VOWEL SYSTEM.

operant conditioning a learning process used in BEHAVIOUR THERAPY. It is also known as radical behaviourism and was put forward by B.F. Skinner. He developed his reasons for operant conditioning by experimenting with rats in boxes known as Skinner boxes. These boxes had a bar in them which, when pressed, released a pellet of food. Thus, the rats were conditioned to press the bar because they learnt they would receive food. Those who undertake such behaviour modification believe that the reaction of a person to his environment causes the person's maladaptive behaviour. Such therapists see all maladaptive behaviour as a learnt response received through environmental reinforcement. To combat this, a suitable reinforcement conditioning programme has to be evolved. First of all, a functional analysis is developed to provide a set of possible sources in the environment of the reinforcement of the present maladaptive behaviour. Sometimes such behaviour can be caused by the acceptance of it by others thus allowing the person to continue living in a comforting situation and so they give the person an indirect reward. The functional analysis must detail the maladaptive behaviours of the individual, showing the number of occurrences and the particular environments in which these behaviours take place. A target behaviour pattern is then developed and various interventions decided on to try and establish a more acceptable behaviour pattern. These treatment plans are specific to each individual person. Such therapeutic interventions are individual conditioning paradigms which attempt to identify the source of the reinforcement of the maladaptive behaviour and try to remove it either by physical removal or aversive reinforcement. TOKEN ECONOMIES are also used in this form of therapy. *See* Smith et al (2003); Davison et al (2004).

operating system the software which enables a computer to perform different functions within itself to operate other pieces of hardware, computer programs and data.

Probably the most popular operating system is Microsoft's Windows which has appeared in various versions over the last few years starting with Windows 3.1 followed by Windows 95, 98, 2000, Millennium, ME and most recently Windows XP. However, other computer companies such as Apple have produced their own operating systems for their own computers. Again there are many versions which are revised with the latest being OSX2.3. Finally, the latest operating system to appear on the market is Linux. These operating systems use a system of icons and pull-down menus on the screen which can be accessed using the keyboard, mouse or other INPUT DEVICES. *See* Bishop (1985); Brookshear (1991).

optic nerve *see* CRANIAL NERVES.

Optimist a pen-tablet PC using Windows® 95 which can have any communication software compatible with Windows such as WINSPEAK, INGFIELD DYNAMIC VOCABULARIES and so on. It can be accessed by direct selection using the pen in conjunction with the built-in keyboard, switches, joystick, trackball or adapted mouse, an adaptive keyboard or voice recognition. A back panel has been built on to it which provides an amplifier and speaker, a carry handle and a folding stand. A jack has been added for switch input to the serial port. Since it is basically a 100MHz 586 PC, it can be used to log on to the internet or send e-mails, send or receive faxes and with the right software be used for communication and controlling appliances by infra-red. *See* Appendix IV (Ability Net)

Orac a high-tech communication aid with digitised speech and synthetic voice (ORATALK or DECTALK) systems which can be used independently of one another. It can be accessed by direct manual selection, single and two- switches, joysticks and concept keyboards. There can be various sizes of overlay from 2 to 128 squares. When using digitised speech, over 7 minutes can be stored. Word prediction can also be used to increase spelling rate. Prestored items can be combined with spelling messages. There is a disk drive which allows for rapid saving and loading of information. It can be mounted onto a wheelchair. *See* Rumble and Larcher (1998); Appendix IV (Morphonics).

oral approach *see* EDUCATION OF HEARING-IMPAIRED CHILDREN.

oral apraxia *see* APRAXIA.

Oral-Motor/Feeding Rating Scale devised by Jelm, this scale can be used to analyse lip/cheek movement, tongue movement and jaw movement while the person being assessed is eating an ordinary meal. It can be used in the age range from 1 year to adulthood. *See* Jelm (1990) in Appendix I.

oral sounds those sounds which have no nasal quality in their production. As suggested by the name, these sounds are produced in the oral cavity which produces the difference between them and nasal sounds made in the nasal cavities. *See* Ladefoged (2001).

oral stage *see* PSYCHOSEXUAL STAGES OF DEVELOPMENT.

Orator a tablet PC which can be used as a standard WINDOWS PC and a communication aid. It has a 30cm (12 inch) colour TFT touchscreen and a 600Mhz processor. It can be accessed by single or dual switch and MOUSE EMULATION such as a headpointer. It is pre-installed with Windows® 2000 and VOCAB+. The synthetic speech is DECTALK. *See* Appendix IV.

orbicularis oculi *see* MUSCLES OF FACIAL EXPRESSION.

orbicularis oris *see* MUSCLES OF FACIAL EXPRESSION.

orthodontics the study of teeth formation and other structures in the MOUTH which require treatment by the placement of various prostheses (*see* PROSTHESIS) to realign the dental arches if they are deformed. There are three descriptions of teeth formation:

1. Class I: the teeth are well related to each other as are the two dental arches, i.e. top teeth at front cover one-third or half the bottom teeth when clenched.
2. Class II (division 1): top teeth are protruding away from the bottom teeth by more than 2–4mm.
   Class II (division 2): an increase in overbite where the lower incisors are completely covered.
3. Class III: lower teeth completely cover over the top teeth when clenched.

Classes II–III are known as malocclusion. Orthodontists can also be involved with the treatment of children with cleft palate as the teeth may be formed in a haphazard formation. *See* Watson et al (2001).

ossicles *see* EAR.

otitis media a condition produced by an infection in the middle ear often found in children. There are different types:

1. Acute otitis media: often produced by respiratory infection entering the Eustachian tube (*see* EAR). The resulting HEARING LOSS is usually of a conductive nature. The hearing loss will clear up when the middle ear is ventilated. Antibiotics may be required to clear the infection completely.
2. Chronic otitis media: there are different causes for this type of otitis media. It may be the stage following an unresolved otitis media where the organisms contained in the infection damage the eardrum with a resulting perforation. It may also be the result of a long-lasting low-grade infection. The size and site of the perforation will determine the degree of hearing loss which the person has. If the perforation is small but above the round window, the hearing loss will be greater than with a larger perforation sited elsewhere. Perforations can be closed by a tympanoplasty. Incus necrosis and ossicular damage are other possible causes and are produced by subacute infection. Even with an unaffected eardrum, damage to the ossicles can cause a hearing loss up to 60dB. The eardrum perforation can be small or perhaps repaired, but the client can still have a significant CONDUCTIVE HEARING LOSS produced by large cartilage-like masses of plaques grouping in the middle ear involving the ossicles. This is known as tympanosclerosis. An audiometric assessment will show an air–bone gap, low compliance and absent stapes reflexes on immitance measures.
3. Serous otitis media: one of the most common causes of conductive hearing loss in children. This form of otitis media is usually caused by an infection or allergy although there can be other causes. It is presumed the middle ear fails to function correctly because of some form of disorder in the Eustachian tube. The pressure in the middle ear is thus negative, so the tympanic membrane is pressed inwards, reducing the efficacy of the conducting mechanism and producing a conductive hearing loss. This can be worse in the low frequencies. If this is not resolved, fluid can collect in the middle ear, producing a conductive loss in the high frequencies. To overcome this problem, a myringotomy is undertaken in which a tube is inserted to ventilate the middle ear. This action should bring the child's hearing back to normal.

On initial audiological assessment, the curve will show a greater loss in the low frequencies spreading to the high frequencies as time goes on. Tympanometry (*see* IMPEDANCE AUDIOMETRY) may show the presence of fluid in the middle ear even when it cannot be found under physical observation through otoscopy.

See Pracy et al (1974); Ginsberg and White (1985); Tortora and Grabowski (2000); Williamson and Sheridan (1994) (a test of hearing reception in otitis media); http://www.medinfo.co.uk/conditions/otitismedia.html

otorhinolaryngology a name used in the UK and other countries to refer to the study of the ear, nose and throat.

otosclerosis a disease which begins in the bony labyrinth of the inner ear (*see* EAR) and produces a bony growth in the inner ear. It has been found to occur twice as often in women as in men, with TINNITUS occurring approximately 50 per cent of the time. Hearing loss is noticed at an average age of 36 years. If it reaches the middle ear, the footplate of the stapes (*see* EAR) becomes stuck to the oval window. The hearing loss progresses slowly and, in most cases, it is conductive. The audiogram shows a low-frequency conductive loss with an air–bone gap (*see* PURE-TONE AUDIOMETRY) during the early stages, followed by CARHART'S NOTCH, and in a later stage, a flat loss. The hearing loss may become sensorineural when the structures in the bony labyrinth are affected. Treatment takes the form of removing the stapes and replacing it with a piston-type structure which acts in its place. *See* Pracy et al (1974); Katz (1985).

oval window *see* EAR.

overextension at the two-word stage of language acquisition, overextensions may occur. A child learns a new word, but may only recognise some particular aspect of it, e.g. shape, movement, size, sound, texture and, sometimes, taste, so that every time he sees a similar object, he uses the same name. For example, the child may call all four-legged animals with a tail 'dog', as the first time he saw such an animal, it was a dog. *See* Clark and Clark (1977).

overgeneralisation a stage of language acquisition. It occurs as a child learns how to use syntactic functions, e.g. past tense, singular vs plural, etc. The regular way to form the past tense is to add 'd' or 'ed'. However, there are irregular ways of making the past tense, e.g. 'went', 'gone', 'ran', etc. Once the child has learnt how to use the regular form of the past tense, he may overgeneralise its use to irregular forms, e.g. 'wented/goed', 'ranned/runned', etc. *See* Cruttenden (1979); Fromkin and Rodman (2003).

overlapping a description in phonology of sounds which are mutually exclusive. In other words, if the sound /k/ is to exist by itself and not be realised by /f/ from time to time, there must be certain contexts in which /k/ appears and not /f/ and vice versa. If this were not the case, the two sounds would overlap and lose their contrasting qualities. Such contrasts are sometimes lost in phonological delay/disorder and the making up of rules becomes almost impossible. *See* also NEUTRALISATION and MINIMAL PAIRS. *See* Grunwell (1987).

PACE *see* PROMOTING APHASICS' COMMUNICA-TIVE EFFECTIVENESS.

PACS *see* PHONOLOGICAL ASSESSMENT OF CHILD SPEECH.

PACS Pictures: Language Elicitation devised by Grunwell in 1987 for use with children with speech disorders. When the elicited speech is analysed, the therapist will have a complete description of the child's sound system (*see* PHONOLOGY) with several examples of each sound. It can be used as a screening test with a sample of 100 words including 41 words from the EAT while the basic assessment allows the same sample to be analysed with various techniques including PACS and the full assessment elicits a sample of 200 words allowing for more detailed phonological and grammatical analysis. *See* Grunwell (1987).

PACS Toys Screening Assessment devised by Grunwell and Harding in 1995, the PACS Toys Screening Assessment is a rapid screening procedure for assessing both speech and pre-speech vocalisation. It provides a descriptive and qualitative assessment using appropriate play items in a flexible and interactive way. Sixty words are targeted which can be elicited using any toys of any shape or colour as the test has not been standardised. It is suggested that this test can be used to monitor the phonetic development of young children between the ages of two and three years, to monitor the phonetic development in pre-verbal vocalisations, to screen children's speech patterns to determine if a more in-depth assessment is required using PACS PICTURES or PHONOLOGICAL ASSESSMENT OF CHILD SPEECH (PACS) or as an outcome measure. *See* Grunwell (1995) in Appendix I.

paediatric audiology part of audiology in which hearing tests are carried out on children to find out the severity and type of HEARING LOSS which a child may have. The audiologist has to counsel the child's parents as to the effects of a hearing loss both in the short term and the long term.

Paget-Gorman Sign System (PGSS) one of the earliest sign systems to have been developed. Designed by Paget in the 1930s and developed into the 1950s, by which time he and his colleagues had made up a 3000-word sign vocabulary. When Paget died, his work was carried on by Pierre Gorman and Paget's widow. The original signs were revised and the system named 'A Systematic Sign Language'. In 1971, Lady Paget changed the name to 'The Paget-Gorman Sign System' in recognition of Gorman's help in its development. The sign system has one sign corresponding to one word and has a sign for each morphological (*see* MORPHOLOGY) ending in English, e.g. plurals, tense endings, etc. The system has 21 standard hand positions and 37 basic signs used in different combinations. The

Box 1	DET	N	V	PREP	DET	N
	His	mouse	lay	in	the	cage
	That	dog	barked	from	his	kennel
	My	friend	sat	on	the	seat

basic signs represent groups of words with a common concept, e.g. time, position, animal life, and so on. One hand gives the concept, while the other hand is used to modify the concept to make the required communication clear. *See* Kiernan et al (1982).

PAL *see* PREDICTIVE ADAPTIVE LEXICON.

palatal lift *see* PROSTHESIS.

palatal shelves *see* PIERRE ROBIN SYNDROME.

palatalisation the process of raising the front of the tongue towards the hard palate. It is an example of secondary articulation and occurs also in phonological delay/disorder when a child produces a non-palatal sound with a palatal quality.

palatine tonsil *see* MOUTH.

palatopharyngeus muscle *see* MUSCLES FOR SWALLOWING.

palilalia a type of acceleration rhythmic disorder. It takes the form of increasingly rapid reiteration of an utterance with diminishing loudness and reduced intelligibility. It is associated with extrapyramidal pathology.

PALPA *see* PSYCHOLINGUISTIC ASSESSMENTS OF LANGUAGE PROCESSING IN APHASIA.

Panje voice button made of silicon with two flanges, the Panje voice button is used to help people who have had a LARYNGECTOMY to produce a voice. It is placed in the tracheo-oesophageal wall. The operation is reversible but the person for whom the voice button is suitable is limited by the diameter of the stoma, dexterity of the client and thickness of the tracheo-oesophageal wall. Placement is completed by out-patient surgery and no special instruments are required. The button is self-contained

in the tracheostoma. *See* Edels (1984).

papillae *see* TONGUE.

papillomata little bunches of pinkish growths, papillomata are benign neoplasms appearing on the VOCAL FOLDS, and also in the TRACHEA which can produce dyspnoea, i.e. difficulty with breathing. Juvenile papillomata are the most common laryngeal tumours in children, occurring most frequently between the ages of 4;0 and 6;0 years. They can be removed by various surgical techniques and also by drug therapy but there is a strong tendency for them to recur. *See* Greene and Mathieson (1989); Freeman and Fawcus (2001).

paradigm a base form from which other forms are made by adding affixes. *See* Matthews (1974).

paradigmatic relationships between elements of a grammatical category. They refer to subgroups of linguistic units, the subgroups being determiners, adjectives, nouns, etc. For an example see Box 1 above. The sentence analysed in this way is seen as a number of slots. Each slot can only be filled once by one of the units. A sentence such as that shown in Box 2 below is unacceptable as there are two units in the determiner slot. A different sentence analysis examines the syntagmatic relationships of units in a sentence. *See* Lyons (1968).

Parakeet 15 a high-tech communication aid with 15 keys with each message area allows for eight seconds of recording time for a total of two minutes. The device retains its memory even if the battery becomes flat. *See* Appendix IV (Zygo).

Box 2	DET	N	V	PREP	DET	N
	my the	book	is	on	the	table

paralanguage *see* SUPRASEGMENTAL PHONOLOGY.

parallel interface an interface where there is a parallel exchange of information between the central processor and other peripheral units. Most interfaces between computers and printers are parallel interfaces. It is opposed to serial interface.

parametric tests one of two types of test which are used in INFERENTIAL STATISTICS. Parametric tests are perhaps the most powerful tests from a statistical point of view and are very rigorous in their assumptions which are three in number:

1. The data must fall into a NORMAL DISTRIBUTION.
2. The STANDARD DEVIATION and variation must be relatively equal producing homogeneity of variation.
3. The data must be on an interval-ratio scale. An interval scale does not only take into account the characteristic being measured but also the relative separation of items in the scale. A ratio scale is where there is a separation of items as well as an interval between them.

Two parametric tests used to a large extent in statistics are the independent *t*-test (*see* *t*-TESTS) using an INDEPENDENT GROUP DESIGN and the related *t*-test (*see* *t*-TESTS) with a REPEATED MEASURES DESIGN. These tests take account of all the data which are collected by the assessment or whichever method is used to gather it. If the data do not conform to a normal distribution curve, a non-parametric test must be used. These tests are less powerful and do not use all the available data. Two such tests are the MANN-WHITNEY TEST for independent group design and the WILCOXON TEST for repeated measures design. These tests compare the results by ranking the results of the two groups. As a result of the ranking system of scores used in this type of test, they become less powerful than

parametric tests. *See* Miller (1984); Clarke and Cooke (1992).

paraphasia an error usually found in the language of those with APHASIA, where they substitute a word, sound or morpheme for another in the spoken as well as the written form of language. This condition is produced in aphasic people by the degeneration of the BRAIN while with others these errors may be caused by stress, fatigue or lack of attention. In the subtests of the expressive language section of the BOSTON DIAGNOSTIC APHASIA EXAMINATION, it is possible to score the type of paraphasic error produced. *See* Eisenson (1984).

parasympathetic nervous system part of the AUTONOMIC NERVOUS SYSTEM which produces the opposite effect to the sympathetic nervous system. It operates at its maximum potential during sleep, slowing down the heart. It is used to innervate the muscles controlling the digestive system as well as defecation and micturition. *See* J.H. Green (1982); Tortora and Grabowski (2000).

parental speech *see* BABY TALK.

parents and children together (PACT) devised by Bowen and Cupples, PACT is a collaborative approach to phonological therapy where phonological disorders are treated using the normal developmental route in solving children's intelligibility problems with parents and significant others taking an active role in management. It takes into account Stoel-Gammon and Dunn's (1985) proposal of four basic interacting components: auditory perception, cognitive, phonological and neuromotor for the model of a normal phonological development. In 1993, Stackhouse and Wells criticised the limitations of existing categories for developmental speech disorders such as 'dyspraxia' or 'phonological disorder'. They argued that a better model would be a psycholinguistic-based one which viewed children's speech difficulties in terms of three levels of breakdown: input processing (decoding the speech signal);

internal representations of linguistic items stored in memory; and output processing (encoding and articulating speech). The therapy model was constructed to include the interaction of five dynamic constituents: family education, metalinguistics tasks (e.g., ear training, phoneme–grapheme correspondences, activities involving phoneme segmentation for onset matching, activities to increase rhyme awareness among others), phonetic production procedures, multiple exemplar techniques (using minimal contrasts activities and auditory bombardment where the child is exposed to a particular sound in a specific word context or in a minimally contrasted word pair) and homework included in therapy according to the individual needs of particular children and their families. PACT takes into account linguistic, motoric and developmental factors. *See* Bowen and Cupples (1999a, b); Fey (1999); Ingram and Ingram (1999); Grundy (1999).

Parkinson's disease caused by disorders to the BASAL GANGLIA. The main areas of the BRAIN affected are the caudate nucleus and the substantia nigra (*see* MIDBRAIN). The disease itself can be caused by viruses, e.g. encephalitis lethargica, drugs given for other diseases, e.g. chlorpromazine, and poisons, e.g. manganese, producing a neural loss in the basal ganglia, CEREBELLUM and substantia nigra. There are three main symptoms:

1. Tremor which is the least disabling but, perhaps, most embarrassing as it can produce pill rolling (finger/thumb movements which are similar to rolling a pill between the finger and thumb). It may disappear but, during anxiety, can become worse.
2. Rigidity of the so-called cog-wheel type. There is also loss of facial expression.
3. Bradykinesia produces a slowness in carrying out purposeful movements.

The typical posture is a hunched forward appearance with head down against the chest, shoulders pushed forward with the arms hanging loosely at the side. Forward movement produces a festinant gait, i.e. a faster and faster progression. Speech is also affected producing the following characteristics:

1. Monotonous pitch and reduced stress.
2. Imprecise articulation.
3. Inappropriate silences and occasional repetitions of syllables and phonemes.
4. Speech is produced in short bursts with variable rate.
5. Breathy voice.

Although this may seem like DYSARTHRIA, it is not strictly speaking a dysarthria but rather what Scott and Caird (1981, quoted in Scott et al 1985, p.11) call a 'dysprosody'. The person also starts to produce micrographia, i.e. very small writing. The medical condition is treated with drugs such as LEVODOPA which is used to control the tremor as is bromocriptine. Speech problems are treated with exercises to maintain intelligible speech for as long as possible. If the voice becomes very weak so that it is almost impossible to hear what is being said, a PERSONAL SPEECH AMPLIFIER such as the Voicette, the Easi-talk or Porta-amp may be recommended. If speech becomes significantly unintelligible, a form of AUGMENTATIVE AND ALTERNATIVE COMMUNICATION may be prescribed. *See* Darley et al (1975) (communication problem); Gilroy and Holliday (1982) (medical); Scott et al (1985) (communication problem); Le Dorze et al (1992) (effects of therapy); Adams and Lang (1992) (use of masking on speech); Kolb and Whishaw (1996); Beukelman and Mirenda (1998) (AAC); Armstrong et al (2000) (AAC); Davison et al (2004); http://www.parkinsons.org.uk/

parole the act of using the internalised LANGUE which everyone has in their mind. It was proposed as a linguistic description by de SAUSSURE in 1913. He regarded parole as the way in which a speaker combines linguistic units to give meaning to their utterances and how the movements which are required to produce the utterance are made. *See* Saussure (1916); Culler (1986).

parotid duct/glands *see* SALIVARY GLANDS.

Parrot a high-tech communication aid which produces stored spoken messages produced by digitised speech. Its vocabulary is limited but can be highly functional. The memory can hold 16 single messages, so it can be used with users who have limited communication needs, to start users off with a small communication aid before being given a more advanced system or for immediate needs, e.g. in intensive care or during treatment. It gives 32 seconds of uninterrupted speech which can be extended to 64 seconds although the speech quality may be reduced. *See* Glennen and DeCoste (1997); Rumble and Larcher (1998); Appendix IV (Zygo).

passive usually contrasted with active, it refers to a grammatical construction in which the patient or theme of a verb is highlighted by appearing in subject position. This is accompanied by passive verb morphology and sometimes also by the appearance of the agent as a prepositional phrase following the verb. The 'short' or 'agentless' passive is illustrated in (1) and the 'agent' passive in (2):

1. The man was killed.
2. The man was killed by his neighbour.

See Lyons (1968); Fromkin and Rodman (2003).

Pathfinder a high-tech communication aid which uses both synthetic and digitised speech and is the first communication aid which uses both a static keyboard and a touchscreen on the one device. It encodes vocabulary using MINSPEAK on the static keyboard and specially drawn graphics which can appear on the Activity Row of the touchscreen. For example, while people using the Pathfinder can still use the regular Minspeak icon sequence, they can also hit an icon such as 'cups' for 'drinks' and pictures of the real drinks may also appear on the Activity Row on the touchscreen. The person using the Pathfinder can import their own graphics to use on the Activity Row. It has 15 minutes digitised speech and 20 Mb of memory. There are 32, 64 and 128-location overlays which can be accessed by direct manual selection, single/dual switching, infra-red headpointing or joystick. It can also be used as an environmental controller as it can learn infra-red signals to operate televisions, videos, hi-fis and so on. It can also be used as a computer keyboard emulator as it has its own computer mode which allows the person not only to write into any word processor but open applications and pull-down menus. By using serial keys in either Windows or Macintosh, the Pathfinder can emulate into either operating system. When using spell mode, the person can also use the word prediction feature. There are versions of Unity 128 and Language, Learning and Living (LLL) available for the Pathfinder. *See* Appendix IV (Prentke Romich Company); Morris (2000a) (LLL for Pathfinder)

Pausaid a small machine which makes the person's speech more intelligible. It has a throat microphone which will detect continuous phonation and prompt the client by an audible signal and make regular stops in speech. The therapist can alter phonation, length of pause and the machine's sensitivity level.

pausing *see* PROLONGED SPEECH.

Pavlov *see* CLASSICAL CONDITIONING.

PC abbreviation for PERSONAL COMPUTER, e.g. IBM PC. PCs are particularly manufactured by IBM, and IBM compatible computers are manufactured by other companies.

Peabody Picture Vocabulary Test (Revised) (PPVT-R) devised by Dunn (revised 1981), it is a formal standardised assessment to test the child's rate of vocabulary acquisition. It can be used with children between 2;6 and 18;0 years. The revised version has 175 pictorial plates, each with four pictures. The child has to choose the correct picture from the four at the request of the therapist. *See* Dunn (1969) in Appendix I; Aiken (1988).

peak experience *see* PHENOMENOLOGICAL APPROACH.

perceived self *see* PHENOMENOLOGICAL APPROACH.

percentile score a score or rank which shows how many subjects belonging to the norm will fall below the raw score in question. For example, if a person is given a percentile score of 79, this means there are 79 per cent of the norm group below the person's score with the same age range. *See* Aiken (1988).

Perceptions of Stuttering Inventory (PSI) devised by Wolff in 1967, it is a personality inventory used to discover situations in which those with a stammer expect to stammer or produce struggling behaviour, and which they try to avoid. There are five reasons for carrying out this inventory:

1. To describe what the stammerer does.
2. To give greater understanding of why the person stammers.
3. To give insight into the person's emotional state.
4. To give a check on progress.
5. To provide a profile for working out goals and expectations.

See Dalton and Hardcastle (1989).

performance the deployment of the speaker's competence in producing utterances. It is opposed to COMPETENCE. Both have been proposed by Chomsky. *See* Chomsky (1965); Lyons (1968).

performative specific speech acts in which the act is performed by the particular sentence uttered, with the verb in the sentence being crucial. For example:

1. I hereby name this ship HMS Fortress.
2. I promise to pay the bearer on demand.... (British £5 pound notes)
3. I apologise for the delay.
4. I congratulate you on your recent success.

All the verbs in (1)–(4) and other verbs which can be used in a similar way, e.g. advise, order, thank, announce, etc., are performative verbs. Huddleston writes: 'A performative verb identifies a particular kind of speech act that can be performed by virtue of uttering a sentence containing the verb...' (Huddleston 1976, p.134). *See* Huddleston (1976); Clark and Clark (1977); Fromkin and Rodman (2003).

perinatal period the period from the 28th week of gestation to the 28th day after birth. At this time, there are several factors which can produce a delay in the child's future development. Among these are birth asphyxia, birth trauma, preterm babies and those who are LIGHT FOR DATES. *See* Illingworth (1987).

peripheral unit any device which can be connected to a computer and, hence, controlled by it. These include disk drives, printers, visual display units, modems and all types of input, output and storage devices. *See* Bishop (1985).

peristalsis *see* SWALLOWING.

perlocution a term used in speech act theories to denote the effect that a speech act has on the hearer. In certain types of language disorder, in particular those where prosody is affected, the dysprosody may convey an interpretation different from that intended.

perseveration the persistence of an abnormal or incorrect response made by a brain-damaged or dysfluent (*see* DYSFLUENCY) person even when the stimulus which induced the initial response has been removed. It may take the form of continuous repetition or blocking, where the person makes repeated efforts to make a sound. *See* Eisenson (1984).

Persona an integrated system which can control the environment and a wheelchair and can be used as a small communicator. It has a large display screen with word or symbol representation and choice of text/symbol and up to 50 different selection screens. It can be accessed by switches using various scanning methods. As a communicator, it has five minutes of DIGITISED SPEECH, text to synthetic speech and word processing. *See* Appendix IV (Steeper).

personal aid for communication an electronic box divided into squares with a light above each. Overlays are placed into the box and by pressing a switch, the person can switch on the light above the appropriate picture, word or phrase. The standard PAC unit can take eight stimuli while the PAC 6, which is operated in a similar fashion, can take six stimuli.

Personal Communication Plan devised by Hitchings and Spence in 1991, PCP aids in the assessment of communication skills of those over 16 years of age who have mild to severe learning disabilities. It involves all relevant people in the person's life, takes full account of the communication environment and provides a practical framework for joint action planning. There are five parts which can be used interchangeably concerning: background information, speech and language profile, social communication skills, the person's environment, and shared action planning. *See* Hitchings and Spence (1991) in Appendix I.

personal computer (PC) a microcomputer which has sufficient memory to carry out business applications, word processing and spreadsheets. *See* Bishop (1985).

personal construct theory (PCT) a psychological theory proposed by Kelly in 1955. The Centre for Personal Construct Psychology in London practises PCT. The basis of the theory is put into the form of a fundamental postulate. According to Kelly, this refers to the way in which a person views the world and this depends on how much experience the person has of the world and what the experience has taught him. Human personality does not stand still but is an ongoing process which goes forward from construct to construct. Constructs are always being revised, validated, invalidated, discarded,

added to and so on. It is anticipated that constructs will allow a person to foresee his own behaviour and the reactions of others. 'Yet constructs themselves undergo change. And it is in the transitions from theme to theme that most of life's puzzling problems arise' (Kelly 1955). In therapy, the therapist has to discover how clients view the world from their experience, i.e. what constructs they use. If the therapist deems that these constructs require revision, then therapy will be given. Assessment techniques used in PCT are REPERTORY GRIDS, laddering and SELF-CHARACTERISATION. *See* Dalton (1983, 1994).

personal speech amplifiers devices given to those who have a weak voice either as a result of a LARYNGECTOMY or a medical condition such as PARKINSON'S DISEASE or MULTIPLE SCLEROSIS. There are different types:

1. Voicette: an amplifier which can be carried over the shoulder. The microphone is hand-held and attaches to the amplifier directly. It is particularly suited for teachers or others who have to speak to groups.

2. Porta-amp portable public address system: similar to the Voicette, the amplifier is in a case which can be placed on a flat surface or carried over the shoulder. A hand-held microphone attaches directly to the amplifier.

3. Easi-talk: an ear piece is placed behind the ear which allows an arm with the microphone to be placed in front of the mouth. The microphone is attached to an amplifier which can be clipped to a pocket or waistband. It can be operated by battery or recharged regularly. Since it has an ear attachment, users can use their hands while wearing it.

4. Jedcom speech amplifier: the system comprises a control box, a lightweight amplifier which can be carried in a jacket pocket, placed on a table top or hand-held, and a headset or throat microphone. The control

box has an on/off switch and volume control.

See Beukelman and Mirenda (1998).

personality Freud proposed PSYCHOANALYSIS to describe the development of personality. It consists of three parts – the id, ego, and superego. The id is present at birth and works at the unconscious level. The child's personality at this stage requires immediate gratification. The overriding need is pleasure and so the id is often known as a primary process. If the child is going to develop from this stage, the 'ego' must develop. Unlike the 'id', the 'ego' works at a conscious level. It produces the reality principle which makes children react to what is happening around them. Fantasies occur rarely as the child's personality is guided by the secondary process. Just as the 'id' produces the biological self, the 'ego' produces the psychological self. The 'superego' operates on the social and moral functioning of the person. These three parts of the development of personality can be summed up as: 'The id seeks pleasure, the ego tests reality and the superego strives for perfection'. *See* Smith et al (2003).

personality profile *see* TRAIT APPROACH.

pervasive developmental disorders a name given in the USA to try to avoid confusion with childhood schizophrenia (*see* CHILDHOOD PSYCHOSES). It was proposed in DSM-III and is supported by many mental health professionals in the USA. The condition differs from SCHIZOPHRENIA in that it does not include DELUSIONS, HALLUCINATIONS or THOUGHT DISORDERS as symptoms. However, children who are diagnosed as having it show difficulties in forming social relationships and produce odd facets to their behaviour. In DSM-IV five disorders are identified under the category of pervasive developmental disorder: AUTISM, RETT'S SYNDROME, CHILDHOOD DIS-INTEGRATIVE DISORDER, ASPERGER'S SYN-DROME, and pervasive developmental disorder not otherwise stated where children either do not fully meet the criteria of symptoms clinicians use to diagnose any of the four specific types of pervasive developmental disorder or do not have the degree of impairment described in any of the four specific types. See Davison et al (2004); http://www.ncihcy.org/pubs/factshe/fs2 0txt.htm

petit-mal epilepsy *see* EPILEPSY.

PGSS *see* PAGET-GORMAN SIGN SYSTEM.

phallic stage *see* PSYCHOSEXUAL STAGES OF DEVELOPMENT.

pharyngeal tonsil *see* TONSIL.

pharyngoplasty a surgical procedure in which the posterior wall of the PHARYNX is advanced so as to improve nasopharyngeal competency. Sometimes combined with the insertion of a pharyngeal flap in which the free end of a band of muscular tissue dissected from the pharynx is inserted into the upper (nasal) surface of the soft palate.

pharynx an anatomical structure which begins at the base of the skull and stretches downwards to the sixth cervical vertebra where it becomes continuous with the OESOPHAGUS. The pharynx is divided into three parts:

1. Nasopharynx: starts at the posterior openings of the nose and ends above the posterior opening of the MOUTH. The ADENOIDS are found in the nasopharynx.
2. Oropharynx: continues from the end of the nasopharynx, passes the posterior opening of the mouth and ends close to the LARYNX. The tonsil can be found in the oropharynx.
3. Laryngopharynx: continues from the end of the oropharynx to the top of the oesophagus.

The pharynx consists of three muscles:

1. Superior constrictor muscle: fibres leave the hamulus, pterygomandibular ligament and, from the MANDIBLE, the upper fibres end at the pharyngeal tubercle while the lower fibres mingle with the middle constrictor

muscle and attach themselves to the posterior wall of the pharynx.

2. Middle constrictor muscle: fibres leave the stylohyoid ligament, the lesser and greater horns of hyoid and attach themselves to the posterior wall of the pharynx.

3. Inferior constrictor muscle: fibres leave the oblique line, the side of the cricoid cartilage (*see* LARYNX) and insert themselves into the posterior wall of the pharynx.

Cranial nerve IX (*see* CRANIAL NERVES) provides the sensory nerve input to the pharynx while cranial nerve X provides motor nerve input. The pharyngobasilar fascia is a membrane which runs down the vertebrae. As the person swallows, all these muscles lift up together. The salpingopharyngeus muscle leaves the auditory tube and inserts itself into some of the fibres of the palatopharyngeus muscle (*see* MUSCLES FOR SWALLOWING). This muscle raises the top part of the side wall of the pharynx and opens the auditory tube. *See* Tortora and Grabowski (2000).

phases of stuttering a description of how stuttering (*see* STAMMER) can develop from a mild problem to a very severe problem interfering in the person's daily life. Four phases were described by Bloodstein:

1. Mild repetitive stammering which becomes worse in communicative stress.

2. Stammering at school where the disorder becomes chronic and blocking behaviour becomes more common.

3. Continual blocking produces secondary symptoms.

4. Full-blown pattern of stammering found in adolescents and adults with the ensuing avoidance of speaking situations, e.g. speaking to boss, using the telephone, speaking in front of groups, etc.

See Dalton and Hardcastle (1989).

phenomenological approach an approach often considered to be a reaction against PSYCHOANALYSIS. It was developed by Carl Rogers. The personality is viewed as a conflict within the unconscious mind. However, it is the way in which the client perceives and interprets events which is important. Some theories within this approach are termed humanistic while others are theories of the self. An important part of Rogers' self theory is how people evaluate their self-image as this may have a bearing on how they perceive the world and events happening around them. This is often called perceived self. People are also made to think of how they would like to be, compared with what they are. This is known as the ideal self. Self-actualisation occurs when a person chooses what they want to become and progresses to this goal rather than regresses from it. A peak experience occurs when people go through periods of self-actualisation. It is usually characterised by feelings of fulfilment and happiness because clients have reached their goal. In general terms, this approach is subjective in that individuals must examine their own experiences of the world and their reaction to them. *See* Smith et al (2003).

phenothiazines the type of drugs used in treating SCHIZOPHRENIA. The parent drug is chlorpromazine (Largactil). It can be given orally, intramuscularly or intravenously. It has some side effects which include drowsiness, hypotension, hypothermia, rare cholestatic jaundice (reversible when drug stopped), Parkinsonian symptoms and dyskinesias. Thioridazine (Melleril) is from the same family of drugs but, if given a high dosage, it can produce rare retinal damage. Trifluoperazine (Stelazine) tends to produce Parkinsonian symptoms rather than problems with blood pressure and jaundice. It produces alertness rather than drowsiness. *See* Stafford-Clark and Bridges (1990); Smith et al (2003).

phenylketonuria described by Mabry and colleagues in 1963, it is an autosomal recessive (*see* CHROMOSOMES) condition. It involves an error in the metabolism of phenylalanine as the gene lacks a certain chemical. An entirely preventable condition if detected by the GUTHRIE TEST. Children are put on a special diet low in phenylalanine for the rest of their lives. If it is untreated, LEARNING DISABILITY, MICRO-CEPHALY and seizures can result. The face is rounded with prominent glabella and epicanthal folds. Strabismus is frequent. *See* Hosking (1982); Jones (1997); Smith et al (2003); Tortora and Grabowski (2000); Davison et al (2004); http://web.ukonline.co.uk/nspku/.

phenytoin see EPILEPSY.

phobias a neurosis and a possible cause of anxiety. A phobia is an irrational fear which will not be dissipated by any amount of logical discussion. Such an irrational fear may happen only in particular situations. For example, someone who has a phobia of dogs will only show this irrational fear in the presence of dogs and will produce quite normal, rational reactions to other aspects of daily life. As the person approaches a feared situation, the irrational fear may produce an acute anxiety state. Some phobias, like the one just cited, may not affect the person's life significantly, while other social phobias such as agoraphobia, i.e. fear of crowds, enclosed spaces, etc., can cause isolation and loneliness to such a degree that the person's lifestyle can be altered significantly. Sixty per cent of all phobias are agoraphobic by nature with an incidence of 2:1 in favour of males; 8 per cent of phobias are social by nature with a similar incidence in favour of males; animal phobias account for 20 per cent of phobias with an equal sex incidence. Behaviour therapy is often used for the treatment of phobias. *See* Stafford-Clark and Bridges (1990); Davison et al (2004).

phonation the sound that results from the setting of the vocal and ventricular folds in motion. The three main types of phonation are voice, breathy and creaky voice. Those who have DYSARTHRIA or DYSPHONIA can have problems with phonation. *See* Catford (1989).

phonemic jargon *see* JARGON APHASIA (2).

phonetics the study of the articulatory mechanism which produces sounds and the characteristics of speech sound waves and the way sounds are interpreted by the cochlea (*see* EAR) and CORTEX. Starting from the LUNGS, a pulmonic egressive airstream (*see* AIRSTREAMS) is produced and forces the air through the VOCAL TRACT into the mouth where the articulators (*see* ARTICULATION) move in particular sequences to produce the desired sound. The phonetician, who makes this study, describes consonants in terms of place and manner of articulation (*see* ARTICULA-TION) and voicing (*see* ARTICULATION) and vowels (*see* CARDINAL VOWEL SYSTEM) in terms of openness and rounding of lips. Such descriptions of sounds can be used in describing all the languages of the world. There are three different types of phonetics which are studied: ARTICULA-TORY PHONETICS, ACOUSTIC PHONETICS and psycho phonetics (*see* AUDITORY PHONET-ICS). *See* Ladefoged (2001).

Phonological Abilities Test (PAT) devised by Muter and her colleagues, PAT attempts to identify early reading difficulties which have been related to children's phonological skills. It comprises rhyme detection, rhyme production, word completion-syllables and phonemes, phoneme deletion – beginning sounds and end sounds. There is also a speech rate subtest and a letter knowledge subtest. It is suitable for children in the age range of 5;0–7;00. *See* Muter et al (1997) in Appendix I.

Phonological Assessment Battery: Standardised Edition – PhAB devised by Frederickson and colleagues, PhAB is designed to profile children's phonological skills, identify areas of difficulty and assess the impact of intervention programmes. It is based on the steps of phonological awareness taken through-out childhood comprising single sounds, onset and rhyme, phrases, single syllables, whole words and sentences. PhAB has six tests of phonological processing:

Alliteration Test – assessing children's ability to isolate the initial sounds in single syllable words.

Naming Speed Tests – picture and digit naming, assessing how fast children can produce the sounds of words.

Rhyme Test – assessing the ability to identify the rhyme in single syllable words.

Spoonerisms Test – assessing if children can segment single syllable words and synthesise the segments to provide new words or word combinations.

Fluency Tests – assessing the retrieval of phonological information from long-term memory using three different types of word retrieval relying on semantics, alliteration and rhyme.

Non-Word Reading Test – assessing the child's ability to apply the sounds of words to non-words without using other strategies to decode the non-words.

If PhAB is used together with the Test of Word and Grammatical Awareness (TOWGA), the assessor can gain an idea of the child's all-round metalinguistic ability. *See* Frederickson et al (1997) in Appendix I.

Phonological Assessment of Child Speech (PACS) devised by Grunwell in 1985, it is a framework within which the therapist can assess and analyse the child's sound system (*see* PHONOLOGY). Two types of analysis are possible:

1. Contrastive analysis: comparisons are made between the child's phonetic inventory and the adult's sound system as well as with a developmental profile which shows which sounds the child should have learnt at a particular CHRONOLOGICAL AGE. This is the usual type of contrastive analysis. However, Grunwell goes further in PACS and has produced an assessment and analysis

for CONSONANT CLUSTERS. Another addition to the contrastive analysis and assessment used in PACS is a comprehensive analysis and assessment of phonotactic possibilities in the child's pronunciation patterns. Again, the information found is compared with the adult's syllabic and word formation in a matrix format. In describing this part of the PACS assessment and analysis, Grunwell writes: '... PACS attempts to provide a comprehensive framework for analysis and assessment based, in the instances of the Contrastive Analysis and Assessment procedures, on the principles of phonological analysis...' (Grunwell 1987, p. 121).

2. Phonological process analysis: an analysis is made of spontaneous speech samples. The processes used to analyse these samples are described under PHONOLOGICAL PROCESSES. The number of times a particular process occurs is entered on a table as well as examples of the type of process. When the analysis is completed, the child's pronunciation patterns are compared with a developmental profile.

The characteristics of children's phonological disorders are discussed in the PACS manual, namely, persisting normal processes, chronological mismatch, unusual/idiosyncratic processes, variable use of processes and systematic sound preference. Thus, PACS provides a comprehensive assessment and analysis of the child's sound system taking account of developmental processes and how it may compare with the adult's sound system. *See* Grunwell (1985a, b) in Appendix I; Grunwell (1987); Beech et al (1993).

phonological delay this should not be confused with an ARTICULATION DELAY which is phonetically based. It is a delay in producing appropriate adult contrasts between phonemes, e.g. voice/voiceless, fronting/backing, etc. It is a delay because a child may produce /ɡɔɡi/ for [dɔɡi] at the age of 3;6–4;0 years when this substitution should have stopped between 2;0–3;0 years. *See* Grunwell (1987).

phonological disorder the severe form of phonological delay in which the child's sound system (*see* PHONOLOGY) is completely disordered. For example, the child may have no fricatives (*see* ARTICULATION) in their sound system or they may just have fricatives which do not belong in the spoken English sound system e.g. [ɸ,β]. Such a system for children of 4;0–5;0 years would be described as a significant phonological disorder. *See* Grunwell (1987).

phonological dyslexia *see* ACQUIRED DYSLEXIA (1).

Phonological Process Analysis (PPA) devised by Weiner in 1979 for use with children between 2;0 and 5;0 to discover the PHONOLOGICAL PROCESSES used in their speech. Each process is tested in a set of four to eight words illustrated by line drawings. The test contains 136 pictures. The responses are recorded on sheets for each process. The processes are tested in a set of words in sequence. There are also control items to check if the child is producing assimilative or substitution processes. The developmental stages of process acquisition are not used. A phonetic inventory can be produced as well as the processes on the Process Profile Form. *See* Grunwell (1987).

phonological processes rules which are used in natural phonology to describe the simplifications made by a child. These processes include:

1. Weak syllable deletion: children omit one or more unstressed syllables.
'banana'   ['nɑnə]
'pyjamas'   ['dɑməd]
2. Final consonant deletion: children produce open syllables by omitting the final consonant of the word.
'pen'   [pɛ]
'cold'   [ko]

'bib'   [bɪ]
'zip'   [zɪ]
'bath'   [bɑ]
'cat'   [kɑ]

3. Reduplication: children repeat the first syllable in the position of the second syllable.
'mummy'   [mʌmʌ]
'kitten' [kɪkɪ]
4. Consonant harmony: children make consonants in the word phonetically similar. The place of articulation (*see* ARTICULATION) changes but the voicing (*see* ARTICULATION) distinction is maintained between the realisation and the target sound.
'cup'   [pʌp]
'table'   [pebʌ]
'duck'   [kʌk]
'kettle' [kɛk]
'goat'   [gok]
'cat'   [kæk]
5. Cluster reduction: children reduce a group of consonants which begin words.
'smoke'   [mok]
'string'   [srɪŋ]
'skid'   [kɪd]
'splash'   [plæʃ]
'christmas' [kɪsməs]
'scratch'   [skæt]
6. Stopping: children substitute a stop for a fricative or affricate (*see* ARTICULATION) and at the same place of articulation (*see* ARTICULATION).
'fine'   [bain]
'church' [tʌt]
'size'   [taid]
'jump'   [dʌmp]
7. Fronting: children produce all velar sounds at the front of the mouth, usually, as alveolar sounds.
'cat'   [tæt]
'cake'   [tek]/[tet]
'cow'   [taʌ]
'key'   [ti]
8. Gliding: children produce the target liquid sounds /l,r/ as [w,j]
'lunch'   [wʌn]
'red'   [wɛd]

9. Context-sensitive voicing: children change the voicing of obstruents. Voiced obstruents become voiceless word-initially and word-medially while voiceless obstruents become voiced word-finally.

'fat'	[væd]
'cat'	[gæd]
'sad'	[zæt]
'bid'	[pɪt]

See Grunwell (1987).

phonology the study of the sound systems in any given language. A sound system reveals contrasts in sounds and how such contrasts account for different meanings in a language. A phonologist undertakes such a study. These systems are based on phonemes. The phoneme is represented in speech production by the phone. Variations of the phoneme are known as allophones, e.g. the phoneme /p/ can have the allophones /pʰ/ (*see* ASPIRATION), /p'/ (*see* EJECTIVE), etc. When all the allophones are put together, they form a phoneme and the phonemes together within an accent form a phonemic system. In English, there are about 44 phonemes, depending on the accent. *See* Hyman (1975); Grunwell (1987); Carr (1993); Fromkin and Rodman (2003); Ladefoged (2001).

phonotactics rules that describe the possible combinations of sounds in any language. The most basic syllable in English is the vowel (V) with consonants (c) added to each side. In English, a maximum number of three consonants can be added before the vowel while a maximum of four consonants can be added after the vowel as in the word 'strength'. Rules exist for the production of two place consonant clusters:

1. Where C1 is /s/, C2 must be one of the following: /p,t,k,m,n,l,j,f/.
2. Where C2 is one of /w,r,l,j/, C2 may be one of a large number of consonants, predominately obstruents including /p,t,k,b,d,g,f/ etc. (Grunwell 1987, p. 14).

Phonotactics are useful in speech therapy as the therapist can show the sounds which are not contrasting and in which position of the word or cluster the errors occur:

C1 [p,b,t,d,f]		C2 [ɹ]	
'pram'	[pɹam]	'queen'	[tɹin]
'bread'	[bɹ ɛd]	'glove'	[dɹ əv]
'swing'	[fɹ ŋg]	'straw'	[dɹɔ]

(from Grunwell 1987, p. 18)

In her *Phonological Assessment of Child Speech* (1985a) in Appendix I, Grunwell has incorporated an assessment and analysis of phonotactics. *See* Grunwell (1987); Fromkin and Rodman (2003).

phrase structure grammar a grammatical model discussed by Chomsky in *Syntactic Structures* in 1957. The basis of the model is a CONSTITUENT ANALYSIS using rewrite rules. However, Chomsky did not believe it was powerful enough to explain the structure of all sentences in the language. *See* Chomsky (1957); Huddleston (1976); Fromkin and Rodman (2003).

physiology the study of how the body functions. While an anatomist studies structures of the body, a physiologist studies how these structures function. Thus, some of the subjects which interest a physiologist are the workings of the heart, the breathing system, the autonomic and central nervous systems and the digestive tract. *See* J.H. Green (1982); Tortora and Grabowski (2000).

physiotherapy the physiotherapist assesses and treats people who have varying degrees of physical disability. The disability may be congenital, e.g. CEREBRAL PALSY, or acquired, e.g. HEMIPLEGIA, due to a CEREBROVASCULAR ACCIDENT, HEAD INJURY, etc. People will also be shown how to transfer, e.g. moving from a chair into a wheelchair, or from wheelchair to a commode or toilet. If someone is admitted to hospital in a coma, the physiotherapist will make sure their airways are kept clear by suction, and will also use suction if the person is dysphagic (see DYSPHAGIA) and aspirates when taking food if it goes down into the TRACHEA and, in such situations, will work closely with a speech and language therapist.

Piaget Jean Piaget (1896–1980), a Swiss psychologist, who observed children's cognitive behaviour from birth to about 11 years of age. He included his own child, and as a result evolved a theory of cognitive development which proceeded through several distinct stages as the child grew: (1) SENSORIMOTOR STAGE; (2) PREOPERATIONAL STAGE; (3) CONCRETE OPERATIONS; (4) FORMAL OPERATIONS. Piaget's theory of language development is based on the empiricist view according to which a child is believed to be born with a 'tabula rasa' or an empty mind and develops language only by his own experience and experimenting with what he hears in the environment around him. This is opposed to Chomsky's theory of INNATENESS in language development and to the existence of a LANGUAGE ACQUISITION DEVICE. *See* Smith et al (2003); Boden (1994).

PICA *see* PORCH INDEX OF COMMUNICATIVE ABILITIES.

PICAC *see* PORCH INDEX OF COMMUNICATIVE ABILITIES IN CHILDREN.

Pick's disease a rare type of DEMENTIA caused by neuron degeneration in the frontal and temporal lobes of the BRAIN (*see* CEREBRAL HEMISPHERES). The neurons which survive have special characteristics and are known as Pick's cells. It is thought to be a familial disorder. A major characteristic is the change of personality in later life particularly in the person's moral standards. APHASIA can also appear. Treatment is similar to other forms of dementia such as ALZHEIMER'S DISEASE. The prognosis is not good as death can occur within 6–12 months, caused by chest problems. *See* Gilroy and Holliday (1982); Stafford-Clark and Bridges (1990); Kolb and Whishaw (1996); http://www.pdsg.org.uk/

Picsyms a symbol system based on a consistent set of principles. The core system, consisting of 880 line drawings accompanied by written labels, was developed by Carlson (1985). New symbols can be made by following the generative rules that are included with the dictionary of symbols. Information about their transparency with other symbol systems can be found under PICTURE COMMUNICATION SYMBOLS and REBUS. *See* Beukelman and Mirenda (1998).

Pictograms a symbol system with almost 1000 white on black symbols designed to reduce figure–ground discrimination difficulties (Maharaj 1980). *See* Glennen and DeCoste (1997); Beukelman and Mirenda (1998).

Picture Communication Symbols (PCS) a system of more than 3000 simple line drawings with English or no labels. It is used with Boardmaker software so that communication boards, pages for communication books or overlays for some communication aids can be made easily. Research studies have shown that PCS symbols and PICSYMS are found to be more transparent than BLISSYMBOLS by preschool children who have no disabilities and children at school as well as adults with LEARNING DISABILITIES. In a study which compared Blissymbols, Pictogram Ideogram Symbols (now Pictogram symbols), Picsyms and REBUS symbols, PCS symbols and Rebuses were learned more easily across NOUNS, verbs and modifiers. PCS symbols have been used successfully including in people with learning disabilities (Heller et al, 1996; Mirenda and Santogrossi 1985), cerebral palsy (Goossens 1989), deafblindness (Heller et al 1996) and autism (Hamilton and Snell 1993; Rotholz et al 1989). *See* Glennen and DeCoste (1997); Beukelman and Mirenda (1998).

Picture Exchange Communication System (PECS) developed by Bondy and Frost in the mid-1990s in the USA, PECS is an AAC system which starts to teach initiation by teaching the child to exchange a picture of a desired item with a teacher who immediately fulfils the request. The system teaches discrimination of symbols and how to construct simple sentences. Although originally designed for use with children who have AUTISM, it has been used with children and adolescents with various communication disorders. *See* Bondy and Frost (1993, 1995a, b); Frost and Bondy (1994); Glennen and DeCoste (1997); Beukelman and Mirenda (1998); http://www.pecs.org.uk/html/pecs.asp

Pierre Robin syndrome a syndrome caused by hypoplasia of the mandibular area during the seventh week of in utero growth, allowing the TONGUE to be positioned at the posterior of the mouth preventing the palatal shelves meeting in the midline. As the tongue is obstructing the airway, it may have to be sutured to the lower lip or the head placed forward on the chest. Thus the four main characteristics of this syndrome are cleft palate but not cleft lip, respiration problems, small mandible and glossoptosis (drooping of the tongue backwards). *See* Watson et al (2001); Jones (1997); http://www.widesmiles.org/cleftlinks/pierre.html

pill rolling the manifestation of the tremor (*see* PARKINSON'S DISEASE) affecting those who have Parkinson's disease. It appears at the fingers which, with the thumb, produce a rolling motion similar to that of the old apothecaries when they were making pills. *See* Gilroy and Holliday (1982).

pitch *see* AUDITORY PHONETICS.

pivot grammar a grammatical system proposed by Braine in the 1960s. He found that, as children acquired language, they produced sentences containing repeated words in one position while other words were used less often. The former process was called a pivot while the latter was an open class word. The system was used to explain the two-word stage in language acquisition. *See* Cruttenden (1979).

place of articulation *see* ARTICULATION.

placenta part of the chorion which attaches the fetus to the wall of the uterus. Its highly specialised functions allow transfer of nutrients and oxygen from mother to baby and excretion of metabolic products from the fetus. *See* Tortora and Grabowski (2000).

plain a DISTINCTIVE FEATURE proposed by Jakobson and Halle to distinguish sounds which are produced with the mouth open and a high frequency [+PLAIN] from those produced with the mouth more closed and a low frequency [−PLAIN]. It is opposed to flat. *See* Hyman (1975).

plantar response a response obtained by stimulating the sole of the foot with an object. If the response exists, the hallux will flex. If there is extension, this is an abnormal response and is recorded as an extensor plantar response. This indicates an upper motor neuron lesion. *See* Gilroy and Holliday (1982).

play a vital component in the child's development as it allows him to develop manipulative and social skills so that he can learn to cope with his total environment. It functions also as a bridge between the child's internal world of fantasy and the external world of his environment, thus the child plays out his anxieties and fears, his jealousies and feelings of aggression. Play is often used in psychotherapy for treating the child's emotional disorders and conduct disorders. It can also be used in speech therapy to produce a natural setting for children to develop their communication skills, especially with those who suffer from language delay. Garvey has described play happening 'in a period of dramatically expanding knowledge of self, the physical and social world, and systems of communication' (Garvey 1990). Over the years, there has been a considerable body of research which has investigated the relationship of play to language development of both children without a disability (McCune-Nicolich 1981; Corrigan 1982; Shore et al 1984; McCune 1995) and of children who have a variety of disabilities (Mundy et al 1987; Beeghly et al 1990). In 1995

McCune observed children between the ages of 0;08–2;00 playing with a selection of toys and categorised their play into five levels of pretend which she defined as the child's understanding of the play act and what it represented. The sequence moved from pre-symbolic (level 1) to single pretend acts involving self (level 2) to single pretend acts involving self and another (level 3) to combinations of pretend acts (level 4) and finally to hierarchical pretend or planned pretend (level 5). McCune also found a relationship between the developing language and these levels in that there was a relationship between vocabulary size and level 2, word combinations and level 4 and a predominance of word combinations over single words at level 5. In their study of children with disabilities Mundy et al (1987) found significant correlations between symbolic play and both expressive and receptive language measures in a group of children aged 3;00–6;00 who had AUTISM. Beeghly et al (1990) compared the play of young children who had DOWN SYNDROME with that of children with no disability but a similar MENTAL AGE. They produced a summary of findings and found a relationship between MEAN LENGTH OF UTTERANCE (MLU) and symbolic play in both groups but the relationship was strongest in children with Down syndrome aged under 5 years. Beyond this age the relationship was stronger in the children with no disability with whom they had been compared. Lewis et al (2000) set out to assess the relationship between language and conceptual ability as well as the relationship between language and symbolising ability. By letting children play with realistic objects, including miniature representations of real objects, in ways appropriate to their conventional function involves conceptual ability but not symbolising ability. This type of pretend play has been called 'functional pretend play' (Baron-Cohen 1987). Since symbolic pretend play requires both conceptual understanding and symbolising ability, in a similar way to language itself, symbolic play should be more strongly related to language than functional play. Their findings suggested that relationships between solitary pretend play and language development result at least partly from the fact that both pretend play and language involve conceptual knowledge and, in the case of symbolic play, symbolising ability. *See* Garvey (1990); McCune-Nicolich (1981); Wood (1981); Corrigan (1982); Shore et al (1984); Baron-Cohen (1987); Mundy et al (1987); Beeghly et al (1990); McCune (1995); Lewis et al (2000).

play audiometry *see* CONDITIONING TESTS.

play therapy the use of play in treating a child's emotional disorders, conduct disorders and also communication disorders. *See* Wood (1981); Davison et al (2004).

plosive *see* ARTICULATION.

Point and Scan Intro Talker a high-tech communication aid with digitised speech output. It uses MINSPEAK to organise vocabulary to store into the device. There are three modes in which the scanning system can be used with a single switch:

1. A 32-location row/column scanning in which the device first scans through the rows and then, once a row is selected, scans across the chosen row until the desired location is selected.
2. An 8-location circular scan, i.e. the device scans each location in a clockwise direction, and once the selection has been made the scan automatically continues.
3. An eight count in which each activation selects the next location in the scan. Once the desired location has been reached, it is automatically selected after an adjustable period of time.

An optical headpointer can also be used with the Point and Scan Intro Talker in either 8- or 32-locations. All other features are explained in the description of

183

the ordinary INTRO TALKER. *See* Appendix IV (Prentke Romich Company).

polyps organic growths which can appear in nasal cavities and VOCAL FOLDS. They occur on the latter unilaterally, they may be round, vascular, oedematous or inflammatory. A polyp may produce hoarse voice, coughing and perhaps even choking, interfering with the person's PHONATION. Therapy for DYSPHONIA includes voice rest and a complete ban on smoking. *See* Freeman and Fawcus (2001).

pons a structure within the BRAIN. It is part of the HINDBRAIN, measures about 3.5 cm wide and 3 cm long, and is situated above the MEDULLA OBLONGATA. It comprises fibres which make up the middle cerebellar peduncles, while further into its centre, it is essentially a continuation of the medulla oblongata. It is associated with cranial nerves V, VI, VII and VIII (*see* CRANIAL NERVES). The CEREBELLUM is found above the pons. *See* Barr (1988); Kolb and Whishaw (1996); Tortora and Grabowski (2000).

population a grouping of people, objects or abstract material which is to be analysed statistically. On occasion, the population will be so large that it would be impossible to test every member of the population. In such cases, the tester has to pick a random sample and then project the scores of this sample onto the population. For example, the organisations such as Gallup, MORI, Marplan, etc. which test the public's opinion, usually on their political views, take a random sample of the population around the country, ask them questions and work out the results. By statistical analysis, they can work out the voting intentions of the population with varying accuracy. *See* Miller (1984).

Porch Index of Communicative Abilities (PICA) devised by Porch in 1967 (revised 1971) (Porch 1971, in Appendix I), it is a formal assessment, which has been standardised, to test the language function of those with APHASIA. Porch changed the aim of aphasia test-

ing. He wanted to find out which of the person's responses could be reliably and objectively quantified. The 16-point scoring system, unique to Porch, is based on four principles: (1) responsiveness of the patient; (2) accuracy of the patient; (3) promptness of the response; and (4) efficiency of response, i.e. evidence of motor delay. Such a test provides the therapist with an extremely detailed performance record for each person. There are at least 18 test tasks in the form of four verbal tasks, eight gestural tasks and six picture tests. Ten objects are also used and have to be presented in the required order. The therapist must attend a 40-hour workshop to become a registered user. Porch does not follow any particular theory of aphasia. *See* Eisenson (1984); Rosenbek et al (1989); Beech et al (1993).

Porch Index of Communicative Abilities in Children (PICAC) devised by Porch in 1971, it is a formal standardised assessment, for use with children with learning difficulties, either requiring special education or having a SPECIFIC DEVELOPMENTAL LANGUAGE DISORDER. It has two scales, one for children in the 2;0–6;0 age range while the other is for children in the 3;0–12;0 age range. As with PICA, Porch was concerned only with the child's communication, not necessarily with the linguistic or phonological aspects of the child's language. The principles for the 16-point scoring system are the same as for the PICA. *See* Porch (1971) in Appendix I; Beech et al (1993).

Portacom a small, light-tech communication aid with DIGITISED SPEECH which can be used by direct manual selection or by linear or row/column scanning with one or two switches. It has a keyboard of 40 keys. The keys can be grouped together to make larger keys. The Portacom allows for 4, 8 or 16 minutes of recorded messages and the memory will not be erased should the batteries be removed or lose charge. *See* Rumble and Larcher (1998); Appendix IV (Active).

Portage Early Education Programme devised in America in the late 1960s, it has been used in the UK since 1976. The Portage Early Education Programme is a major revision of the earlier Portage Checklist designed specifically for use in the UK. All Americanisms have been removed making the new materials more appropriate for users in the UK. It is a means of finding out the different abilities of children with the mental ages of 0–6 years. It is used mainly with those children who will require special education, severely physically handicapped children and those with a severe delay in acquiring various skills. It is designed for use in the home by parents under the supervision of a speech and language therapist, psychologist or district nurse. After analysing the results, the therapist can give the parents a programme to work on with the child. It assesses motor, cognitive, language and self-help skills and, for very young children, infant stimulation. The subtest on language skills was not appropriate for British children, so a new language subtest was devised – the Wessex Revised Portage Language Checklist. These changes have been incorporated into the revised programme. *See* Cameron and White (1985); Shearer and Shearer (1974).

positron emission tomography (PET) radio-isotopes of oxygen or carbon dioxide are prepared in a cyclotron and injected into the body. The radio-isotope emits positively charged electron-like particles called positrons. These destroy the negative electrons which they find in the body and produce gamma rays. It is the gamma rays which are recorded. All the information is fed into a computer which produces a colour PET scan, showing the localisation of the radio-isotopes in the body. PET scans provide evidence of function in various parts of the body rather than of structures. Such scans provide information concerning blood flow in the BRAIN and HEART, the effects of CEREBROVASCULAR ACCIDENTS or

heart attacks, cancerous growths, the chemical changes in SCHIZOPHRENIA, EPILEPSY, OBSESSIVE–COMPULSIVE DISORDERS and ALZHEIMER'S DISEASE. *See* Kolb and Whishaw (1996); Tortora and Grabowski (2000).

posterior pharyngeal wall the area at the back of the pharynx into which the superior, middle and inferior constrictor muscles (*see* PHARYNX) insert themselves. *See* Tortora and Grabowski (2000).

postlingual hearing loss a HEARING LOSS which occurs after language has been acquired.

postnatal the period of the baby's life following delivery.

postvocalic a description of a consonant following a vowel.

PPA *see* PHONOLOGICAL PROCESS ANALYSIS.

PPVT *see* PEABODY PICTURE VOCABULARY TEST.

Prader-Willi syndrome diagnosed by Prader and his colleagues in 1956, children who have this syndrome are obese and flaccid. They have almond-shaped facial appearance with strabismus. There are varying degrees of LEARNING DISABILITY, an enormous appetite and breathing problems which could result in death. Parents should be advised of a suitable diet. The children have also hypo-gonadism and, in some cases, diabetes mellitus. There is no specific treatment. The prevalence is about 1: 10000 and 1:25000–30000 births. The cause is uncertain but in the 1960s and 1970s researchers hypothesised about a localised effect in the hypothalamic region (*see* HYPOTHALAMUS). More recently, studies have tended to focus on an abnormality in chromosome 15 which affects about 50 per cent of those affected. Many researchers have reported a delay in the child's speech and language with the major problems including multiple articulation errors, reduced intelligibility, language problems and voice problems (primarily hypernasality). DYSFLUENCY and flaccid dysarthria (*see* DYSARTHRIA) have also been found. Apraxia of speech has not

185

been found. Therapy is aimed at improving the child's vocabulary, syntax and morphology. PRAGMATICS may also be a problem. It has been suggested that therapeutic programmes should be personalised for the child as the communicative profiles lack common features. There are differences in severity of articulation and language problems as well as in intelligibility, voice problems and fluency. *See* Hosking (1982); Jones (1997); Kleppe et al (1990); http://www.pwsa-uk.demon.co.uk/

pragmatics the use of particular types of language in different contexts, e.g. by studying SPEECH ACTS such as PERFORMATIVES, FELICITY CONDITIONS, etc. *See* Van Dijk (1980); McTear (1985); Fromkin and Rodman (2003).

Pragmatics Profile of Everyday Communication Skills in Children devised by Dewart and Summers in 1988 for children between 9 months and 10 years. Its aim is to provide a descriptive and qualitative assessment of the pragmatic aspects of language or the way in which children use language. It is based on a structured interview in which the parent describes the child's typical behaviour in a wide range of communication settings. The profile gives qualitative information as a basis for treatment as well as for monitoring progress and efficacy of treatment. The profile takes into account three aspects of pragmatics plus the effect of different contexts on the child's communication:

1. The way the child uses messages to communicate.
2. The child's response to communication.
3. The child's participation in conversational activity.
4. The way the child modifies communication in relation to various contexts.

The questions in the profile are based on concrete and everyday events; thus the parents can use their own unique experiences and knowledge of the child's communication. *See* Dewart and Summers (1988, 1995) in Appendix I; Miller (1990); Beech et al (1993).

Pre-Verbal Communication Schedule devised by Kiernan and Reid in 1987 for children and adults with severe LEARNING DISABILITY who are either non-verbal or who have few words or symbols. It can provide comprehensive diagnostic information which can be used as the basis of a treatment programme. There is a 195-item checklist. It provides detailed diagnostic information about the person's pre-communicative, informal and formal communicative skills, and receptive skills. Scores can be transferred to a special summary sheet which highlights strengths and weaknesses. It can be used with those who have a severe learning disability, with non-speaking deaf children and with those with a severe physical handicap. It can also be used with non-handicapped infants. *See* Kiernan and Reid (1987) in Appendix I; Beech et al (1993).

Predictive Adaptive Lexicon (PAL) software designed by the team led by Professor Alan Newell at the Micro-computer Centre, Dundee University. It was designed for people who have a communication disorder and has been extended for use with children and older people with learning difficulties. PAL has a large dictionary of 5000 words. When the user types a letter, the five most frequently used words starting with that letter appear in a window on the screen. To access the word, the user actuates any of the first five function keys. In this way, the number of key actuations can be significantly reduced. The user continues typing in letters until the desired word is found. The team also developed a word processor called Palstar for use with PAL, although PAL can operate using any word processor. PAL can be operated on an IBM-compatible computer. *See* Swiffin et al (1987); Newell et al (1992).

prelingual hearing loss HEARING LOSS which occurs before the acquisition of language, i.e. up to 18 months of age.

prenatal a stage occurring during pregnancy. At this time, the fetus can be affected by infections from the mother, e.g. TORCH, radiation, nutritional deficiency or abnormalities of the placenta. *See* Illingworth (1987).

preoperational stage the second stage of Piaget's theory of cognitive development. It lasts from about 2;0–7;0 and assumes the child can think independently about what he perceives using his developed sense of symbolisation. However, the child may still have difficulties within his cognitive skills. When posed with a problem, children can only see it from their own perspective, not from anyone else's. This is egocentricity, e.g. Three Mountains Test in Donaldson (1987). Piaget introduced this theory of egocentricity into his theory of language development. He claimed a child could not understand the position of a listener in a two-way conversation and so children used collective monologues with which to communicate, not conversations. He called this egocentric speech. During this stage, the child fails to make inferences about various problems he is set. If the child is told, 'A is greater than B, B is greater than C', and asked what the relationship is between A and C, he fails to respond correctly. However, Donaldson has found that children can make inferences in real situations. Failure to conserve volume, weight, number, etc. also occurs during this stage according to Piaget. However, Donaldson (1987) has shown it depends on how the conservation task is presented to the child for that child to succeed. *See* Beard (1969); Donaldson (1987); Smith et al (2003); Boden (1994).

preparatory blocks *see* BLOCK MODIFICATION.

preposition a constituent (*see* CONSTITUENT ANALYSIS) which is used to precede a NOUN PHRASE, noun or pronouns. It can function as a marker for possession, destination, direction, etc., while syntactically it has a particular place in a sentence. *See* Lyons (1968); Fromkin and Rodman (2003).

prepositional phrase a phrase found in CONSTITUENT ANALYSIS which can be expanded into a preposition plus a noun phrase, e.g. the man went into the shops. *See* Huddleston (1976).

presbycusis a HEARING LOSS which results from the normal ageing process. PURE-TONE AUDIOMETRY shows a high-frequency SENSORINEURAL HEARING LOSS which may also have a conductive component due to changes in the middle ear. People lose speech discrimination although they can have a good understanding of speech if the speaker speaks slower rather than louder. There may also be a general slowing down of processing ability. *See* Katz (1985).

Preschool and Primary Inventory of Phonological Awareness devised by Dodd and her colleagues, this phonological inventory is designed to assess the nature and extent of a child's phonological awareness development. Six subtests, including syllable segmentation, rhyme awareness, alliteration awareness, phoneme segmentation, letter knowledge and phoneme isolation, assess the ability to detect, isolate, manipulate and convert sound units at the syllable, onset-rhyme and phoneme levels. It uses UK norms and has standard scores and percentile ranks. It is suitable for children in the age range of 3;00–6;11. *See* Dodds et al (2000) in Appendix I.

Preschool Language Assessment Instrument (PLAI) devised by Blank and her colleagues, PLAI is based on a model of classroom discourse. Its results show how the child integrates knowledge of vocabulary, concepts, and language structure to follow directions, reflect on information and solve problems. Teaching can be planned better to fit the child's level of functioning. It is suitable to be used with children from the age of 2;09–5;08. *See* Blank et al (1988) in Appendix I.

Preschool Language Scale-3 (UK) (PLS-3^{UK}) devised by Zimmerman et al and adapted by Boucher and Lewis for the UK, PLS-3 is an assessment which uses two broad subscales – AUDITORY COMPRE-HENSION and expressive communication – to assess a variety of language-based skills in children from birth to six years. There are tasks which target: social or interactive communication skills and integrative thinking skills, and tasks which provide opportunities for observing spontaneous interactions with very young children. PLS-3 has been co-normed with the Test of Pretend Play to enable direct comparison between the two assessments. The UK version has been based on a national sample of 339 children and takes into account linguistic and socio-cultural differences between the US and the UK. See Zimmerman et al (1997) in Appendix I; Boucher and Lewis (1997) in Appendix I.

Pre-School Screening Test (PREST) devised by Fawcett and her colleagues, PREST is an individual standardised screening test for children with special educational needs from 3;06–4;05. It consists of two parts: Complete PREST 1 used for routine screening and its subtests include rapid naming, bead threading/paper cutting, digits/letters, repetition, shape copying and corsi frog (visual memory). PREST 2 for children 'at risk' on PREST 1 has subtests which include balance, phonological discrimination, digit span, rhyming, sound order, teddy and form matching. The package includes a training video and a case study while for scoring there is an 'at risk' quotient and a profile graph. See Fawcett et al (2001) in Appendix I.

preterm the description of a baby born before the normal duration of the pregnancy, usually before 37–38 weeks into the pregnancy. Premature labour can be caused by a trauma, e.g. car accident, a multiple pregnancy, or cervical incompetence. As the baby's lungs are immature, breathing problems can occur. The child is kept in an incubator. Liver problems occur producing a high level of bilirubin in the brain which in turn produces kernicterus (a condition involving CEREBRAL PALSY and HEARING

LOSS). The child also has immature bone marrow producing anaemia and a lack of protection from infections. See Illingworth (1987).

prime mover see AGONIST MUSCLE, ANTAGO-NIST.

PRISM see PROFILE IN SEMANTICS.

Profile in Semantics (PRISM) devised by Crystal in 1982 to analyse the child's use of semantics. It was the most experimental of the profiles as very little research has gone into the acquisition of semantics. The profile is based on the acquisition of semantics/grammar and semantics/lexicon. PRISM-G is a three-page chart which analyses the relationship between meaning and grammatical elements of a sentence. PRISM-L is a 16-page analysis because of the amount of vocabulary it has to cover. It is possible for one chart to be used without the other but if the two are used together, an in-depth analysis of the child's semantic system can be discovered. See Crystal (1992).

Profile of Phonology (PROPH) devised by Crystal in 1982, it is a means of analysing the child's sound system (see PHONOLO-GY). There is a transcription page plus a separate three-page section on ways of summarising the data. The therapist takes a language sample of about 100 words but need only transcribe as much of the sample as is necessary to work out the child's phonological problem. This sample is transcribed and then analysed into the segments used by the child. Error realisations are detailed in terms of single consonants, single vowels and consonant clusters. The three types of segments are divided into errors of place and manner of articulation (see ARTICULA-TION). Limited information is given about PHONOLOGICAL PROCESSES. Altogether this profile gives an in-depth analysis of the child's sound system. See Crystal (1992).

Profile of Prosody (PROP) devised by Crystal in 1982 to analyse the suprasegmental (see SUPRASEGMENTAL PHONOLOGY) patterns in the child's speech. It comprises a one-page chart on which is put the pitch, loudness, rate and rhythm patterns of the patient's speech. It is supposed to complement PROPH. A large part of the profile is devoted to the child's use of intonation since most linguistic errors come from this variable. The intonation section is divided into tones and tone units. A summary section is also provided. *See* Crystal (1992).

profound and multiple learning difficulties (PMLD) people who are diagnosed as having PMLD are functioning typically at a developmental level of 2 years or less and may even be below a 1-year level with associated sensory and physical impairments including spasticity, uncoordinated movements, tactile defensiveness and epilepsy. Those who have PMLD have OBJECT PERMANENCE and are beginning to produce intentional behaviour. However, they are not communicating intentionally yet because they have not developed the use of signals consistently to affect the behaviours of other people (Wetherby et al 1988). It has been found that communication can take place if the actions of those with PMLD are interpreted as having significant meanings. McLean and Snyder-McLean (1987) divide this pre-intentional period into reactive and proactive phases. During the reactive phase, responses act as signals that may be interpreted by others while during the proactive phase intentional acts on objects and people have a similar purpose. See McLean and Snyder-McLean (1987); Wetherby et al (1988); Ware (1996); Jones et al (2002).

prolabium the middle part of the top lip which tends to protrude down further than the rest of the lip.

prolonged speech a treatment technique for use with people who stammer. It has five parts:

1. Prolongation: a slowing down of the rate of articulation. This process simplifies the movement from one sound to another which is usually difficult for someone who stammers.

2. Flow: running the words together, thus reducing the stopping and starting in a stammerer's speech.

3. Light/soft contacts are encouraged between the articulators to reduce the tension in the mouth when producing such sounds as /p,b,t,d,k,g/.

4. Pausing: a stammerer believes pausing exhibits DYSFLUENCY and so finds it difficult to understand it is a normal process in daily conversation. People have to be shown how they can use normal pausing.

5. Slowing down is encouraged to help the stammerer produce what is required in (1)–(4).

All these are intended to encourage the feeling of using fluent speech which some stammerers have never experienced. *See* Dalton (1983).

Promoting Aphasics' Communicative Effectiveness (PACE) devised by Davis in 1980, this is a treatment technique used with aphasic patients (*see* APHASIA). It has been designed to produce meaningful interaction between the therapist and the patient. Treatment sessions should resemble everyday face-to-face conversation. PACE is based on four principles: (1) equal participation between therapist and patient; (2) new information being conveyed between the therapist and patient; (3) a free choice of communication between modalities; and (4) feedback from the therapist sounding more natural. When PACE is used effectively, patients enjoy therapy because it is they who are communicating some new information to the therapist or another member of the group. *See* Eisenson (1984); Rosenbek et al (1989); Pulvermüller and Roth (1991).

pronoun a set of words which can be used to replace nouns or noun phrases. There are several types of pronoun:

1. Personal pronoun, e.g. I, you, he, etc.
2. Reflexive pronoun, e.g. myself, yourself, himself, etc.
3. Possessive pronoun, e.g. mine, yours, his, etc.

4. Demonstrative pronoun, e.g. this, that.
5. Indefinite pronoun, e.g. anyone, anybody, etc.
6. Relative pronouns, e.g. who, which, whom, etc.

These pronouns are usually discussed in other areas of linguistics and are discussed under other terms such as DEIXIS (demonstrative pronouns), EMBEDDING (relative pronouns), ANAPHORA (reflexive pronouns). *See* Lyons (1968); Fromkin and Rodman (2003).

PROP *see* PROFILE OF PROSODY.

PROPH *see* PROFILE OF PHONOLOGY.

proprioception an awareness of the exact position of body parts and direction of movement, e.g. to touch one's nose with eyes closed. Such skills are used in a person's daily life, e.g. eating, walking, speaking, etc. If speech is dysarthric (*see* DYSARTHRIA), it may be caused by loss of proprioception, e.g. difficulty in moving the mouth to make the correct sounds. This results in a treatment programme including neuromuscular facilitation. *See* Tortora and Grabowski (2000).

proprioceptive neuromuscular facilitation (PNF) a therapeutic technique used to stimulate and facilitate movement in paralysed muscles. It is most commonly used in conjunction with PHYSIOTHERAPY. The aim is to bombard the affected neurons with a variety of different stimuli. Icing (wiping ice over particular muscle groups) is used extensively. *See* Langley (1987).

prosody a general description of the phonological features of tempo (*see* RATE), rhythm, loudness and pitch. *See* Fromkin and Rodman (2003); Cruttenden (1994).

prosthesis the technical term for a 'brace' used to correct positioning, e.g. teeth in the dental arches. For those with cleft palate, there are devices to put in the mouth to help the baby to feed, and for older children a palatal lift raises the soft palate (*see* MOUTH) and reduces nasalisation in the child's speech. It is also used to describe any aid for the patient. Communication aids are often described as being 'prostheses'.

ProtoType is a smart programme aimed at providing faster typing and spelling support. It allows the person using ProtoType to check their typing before the text is sent to the main application. It can autocorrect spelling as the person types and has autocorrection of common spelling errors as well as having graphic symbols to identify the correct word. Text can be edited in a separate window. *See* Appendix IV (Sensory Software International).

pseudobulbar palsy *see* BULBAR PALSY.

PSI *see* PERCEPTIONS OF STUTTERING INVENTORY.

psychiatry a branch of medicine which provides treatment for those who have a mental illness such as AFFECTIVE DISORDERS, neuroses (*see* NEUROSIS), PSYCHOSES and SCHIZOPHRENIA. The psychiatrist can give treatment in the form PSYCHOTHERAPY and/or drug therapy. *See* Stafford-Clark and Bridges (1990).

psychoanalysis a psychological theory evolved by Sigmund Freud in 1900. The basis of the approach hinges on the two basic motivators in life – sex and aggression. Freud also believed people had certain instincts which guided them through life – the life instinct and the death instinct. The former, he believed, was concerned with the libido and sexual drives, while the latter was concerned with people's destructive feelings leading either to suicide or aggression against others. Both drives are found in young children but are often suppressed by their parents. Thus, the drives become unconscious motives and produce anxiety in the child as he knows he will incur his parents' disapproval if he tries to express them. Within the framework of psychoanalysis, Freud produced a theory for the development of one's personality using the unconscious motives of the id, the conscious ego and the social and moral superego (*see* PERSONALITY). The child's emotional development was described in terms of PSYCHOSEXUAL STAGES OF DEVELOPMENT. In

PSYCHOTHERAPY, psychoanalysis also plays a role. It is based on the Freudian concepts of free association, abreaction, insight, interpretation, transference and working through. During abreaction, the patient can release emotions in a safe environment. Following this, there is a period of insight when the patient is encouraged to discover the root cause of the conflict and how to interpret these emotions. Having discovered the cause, the patient transfers his emotional feelings to the therapist. Thus, patients begin to see the therapist in the role of person(s) with whom they have or have had difficulty in forming a relationship. It may be parents or friends with whom they are having such problems. By discussing such a transference, the patient is often helped to work through his or her feelings. See Smith et al (2003); Davison et al (2004).

psychodrama a therapeutic technique used in social skills training devised by Moreno in 1946. It can be used to produce insight, MODELLING, SYSTEMATIC DESENSITISATION, SOCIAL SKILLS and ASSERTIVE TRAINING. It helps people to share their problems and to make clear their emotions in certain situations, i.e. those in which the people have difficulty in expressing themselves. It can also improve empathy within the group. See Trower et al (1978).

Psycholinguistic Assessments of Language Processing in Aphasia (PALPA) produced by Kay and her colleagues in 1992, PALPA is a comprehensive psycholinguistic assessment of language processing in adult acquired APHASIA. The areas of language processing assessed are orthography and PHONOLOGY, word and picture SEMANTICS, MORPHOLOGY and SYNTAX. Responses are obtained from the client such as lexical decision, repetition and picture naming. Thus, the various tests assess spoken and written input and output. See Kay et al (1992) in Appendix I; Beech et al (1993).

psycholinguistics a subdivision of linguistics in which THEORETICAL LINGUISTICS come together with psychological theories to show the behaviour of children during the acquisition of language, how people are going to decide on what they are going to say, how they will produce it and how the listener understands it. See Clark and Clark (1977); Garnham (1985); Stackhouse and Wells (1993) (psycholinguistic assessment of developmental speech disorders).

psychology a science which studies behaviour and mental functioning in animals and man. The psychologist uses PSYCHOTHERAPY to treat people who produce abnormal behaviour, EMOTIONAL DISORDERS and CONDUCT DISORDERS, LEARNING DISABILITY and a lack of SOCIAL SKILLS. There are different branches of psychology to deal with such problems. The two main branches are clinical and educational psychology. However, psychologists also take part in industry, with firms and companies having their own psychologist, sometimes dealing with time and motion studies and with industrial disputes and personal problems affecting inter-staff relationships. See Smith et al (2003); Davison et al (2004).

psychoses psychotic disorders are those which cause the person to lose contact with reality. Such disorders include major AFFECTIVE DISORDERS, e.g. psychotic DEPRESSION, paranoia and SCHIZOPHRENIA. Such people may also have hallucinations and delusions. See Davison et al (2004).

psychosexual stages of development Freud proposed five distinct stages in the development of the child's personality. He believed children were more aware of different parts of their body at different ages and their manipulation satisfied the id (see PERSONALITY):

1. Oral stage: children are most conscious of their mouths. The pleasures which are satisfied by such manipulation are those of feeding and sucking.
2. Anal stage: satisfaction comes from the act of defecation. Toilet-training usually occurs at this time.

191

psychosomatic

3. Phallic stage: satisfaction comes from manipulation of the genitalia. The Oedipus complex begins to affect the child at this time.
4. Latency stage: not strictly a psychosexual stage of development as the child does not show sexual behaviour. The child turns away from the Oedipal conflict and begins to have an interest in outside friends, school, etc.
5. Genital stage: heterosexual relationships begin to develop.

Many critics believe these stages to be too simple to explain the development of personality. Erikson describes this development in terms of ATTACHMENT. *See* Smith et al (2003).

psychosomatic a description of physical disorders in which emotions play a central role. *See* Stafford-Clark and Bridges (1990); Smith et al (2003).

psychosurgery a treatment technique in which certain parts of the BRAIN are removed by cutting nerve fibres, usually between the frontal lobe and the limbic system or particular areas in the HYPOTHALAMUS. It is a controversial therapy, as although the person is often happier and more relaxed, the brain has been so damaged that the person cannot function normally. New techniques have improved the situation, significantly reducing the amount of intellectual impairment. The procedure helps those with depression or who have suicidal feelings. *See* Kolb and Whishaw (1996); Smith et al (2003); Davison et al (2004).

psychotherapy different types of therapy used by psychologists and psychiatrists with the aim of modifying the person's behaviour, thoughts and emotions. Thus, it is hoped to improve their coping with stress and other behavioural problems. It includes BEHAVIOUR THERAPY, PSYCHOANALYSIS, PSYCHODRAMA, humanistic therapy and GROUP THERAPY. *See* Smith et al (2003); Davison et al (2004).

psychotic depression *see* DEPRESSION.

PTA *see* PURE-TONE AUDIOMETRY.

pterygoid plate *see* MUSCLES OF MASTICATION.

pull-out *see* BLOCK MODIFICATION.

punch-drunk syndrome a medical condition which can lead to DEMENTIA. It is caused by a subdural haematoma which can develop to affect the rest of the brain and produce dementia, tremor and seizures. *See* Stafford-Clark and Bridges (1990); http://www.surfablebooks.com/wbmedical/32447/32805/1.htm.

pure agraphia a type of PURE APHASIA identified by the BOSTON SCHOOL. Patients present with problems of writing and spelling. *See* Goodglass and Kaplan (2000).

pure alexia a type of PURE APHASIA identified by the BOSTON SCHOOL. Patients present with problems of reading, although objects presented to the patient may still be recognised without difficulty. *See* Goodglass and Kaplan (2000).

pure aphasia a type of APHASIA identified by the BOSTON SCHOOL. Only one language modality is affected while all other allied modalities remain intact. *See* Goodglass and Kaplan (2000).

pure-tone audiometry (PTA) behavioural assessment to determine hearing sensitivity in which pure-tone tests determine the type and degree of hearing loss. Pure-tone testing involves the presentation of up to 11 frequencies (125, 250, 500, 750, 1000, 1500, 2000, 3000, 4000, 6000, 8000 Hz) at decreasing and increasing intensities in the range of −10 to 120 dB HL until the person identifies the tone as being present 50 per cent of the time or two-thirds of the time. The tones are presented to both ears at different times and the person whose hearing is being tested presses a button to indicate he/she can hear the sound. Two pathways of hearing are used:

1. Air conduction (AC): the sound waves enter the external auditory canal and are transmitted via the tympanic membrane to the ossicles in the middle ear, to the oval window from where they enter the inner ear. This action stimulates the hair cells on the basilar

membrane. AC involves the whole hearing system, so any damage to any part of it will result in depressed thresholds for air conduction.

2. Bone conduction (BC): a vibrating unit is placed on the mastoid process although it has been suggested that more reliable results are obtained if the vibrator is placed on the frontal bone. Some researchers have proposed greater test–retest reliability and less inter-subject variability because of the kind of bone tissue making up the frontal bone and, by placing the vibrator on the frontal bone, it bypasses the outer and middle ear and directly assesses the functioning of the cochlea. Depressed thresholds will only occur in bone conduction if there is a lesion or damage to the inner ear.

Masking is a technique to produce a constant noise used to prevent the non-test ear from detecting the sound so only the test ear can respond. Thresholds obtained when using masking are known as masked thresholds and should give the true threshold of the test ear. A CONDUCTIVE HEARING LOSS will have depressed AC thresholds (poorer by about 10 dB from normal) but normal BC thresholds while a SENSORINEURAL HEARING LOSS has air and bone conduction thresholds within 10 dB of each other and thresholds higher than 25 dB. The machine which is used to carry out these tests is an audiometer. It produces the frequencies by means of an electronic oscillator. Pure tones are not used in everyday speech but their use in testing gives a good idea of how the person will cope with complex speech signals as they are made of pure tones. The results of pure-tone audiometry are displayed graphi-

cally on an audiogram. This gives frequencies along the horizontal axis and intensities down the vertical axis. The audiologist uses symbols to show which pathway has been tested and in which ear (see box below). When analysing the results on the audiogram, the tester should look for the presence of the air–bone gap, i.e. the difference between the AC and BC curves. This will reveal a conductive hearing loss. The degree of hearing loss is determined by the pure-tone average. The AC thresholds most often used are 500, 1000 and 2000 Hz. They are added and divided by three. The average should match close (within 5 dB) to the SPEECH RECEPTION THRESHOLD (SRT) (the softest intensity bisyllabic word produced emphasising both syllables equally which the person repeats at least 50% of the time) and within 6–8 dB of the speech detection threshold (lowest intensity speech stimulus that a person can detect at least 50% of the time). This gives only a reasonable prediction of the degree of hearing loss. The slope of the curves on the audiogram is also important:

1. Low frequency loss – usually conductive.
2. Flat loss across all frequencies – usually conductive or sensorineural.
3. Ski slope/high-frequency/sloping loss – usually sensorineural.

Audiograms can also show particular features of a person's hearing such as CARHART'S NOTCH, acoustic trauma, NOISE-INDUCED HEARING LOSS and PRESBYCUSIS. There are several classifications to show the degree of hearing loss such as that of D.S. Green (1978). See Katz (1985); Ballantyne and Martin (2001).

pure-tone average see PURE-TONE AUDIOMETRY.

		Unmasked AC	BC		Masked AC	BC
Right ear (red)	R	O	<		Δ	[
Left ear (blue)	L	X	>		□	]

pure vowels vowels that are not diph-thongs. Most of the vowels in Scottish-English are pure vowels, e.g. /put/, /mek/, etc. The Scottish-English vowels system is:

i	ɪ	u
e	ʌ	o
ɛ	a	ɔ

ai	ʌu
ʌi	
ɔi	

See Cruttenden (1994).

pure word deafness a type of PURE APHASIA identified by the BOSTON SCHOOL. The patient's auditory comprehension fails although his expressive language remains unimpaired, as do his reading and writing. *See* Goodglass and Kaplan (2000).

pyramidal system/tract the fibres of the upper neuron (*see* NEURONS) make up this system. As they come out of the BRAIN into the SPINAL CORD, they become known as the corticospinal tracts. They are responsible for voluntary movements. *See* Barr (1988); Kolb and Whishaw (1996); Tortora and Grabowski (2000).

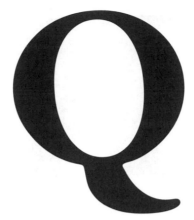

quadriparesis *see* QUADRIPLEGIA.

quadriplegia a physical paralysis which affects all four limbs. Often found in types of CEREBRAL PALSY. If paralysis is not complete and some movements persist, it is called quadriparesis. *See* Hosking (1982).

quality when used in AUDITORY PHONETICS, quality refers to the timbre or resonance of a sound constituted by its different frequencies. Quality can also be used to describe vowels and consonants, e.g. the difference between [i] and [e] can be said to be qualitative. When used in this way, quality is opposed to quantity (*see* LENGTH) or LENGTH. *See* Ladefoged (1993).

quantity *see* LENGTH.

Quick Glance Eye Tracking System developed by Eye Tracking Systems, the Quick Glance Eye Tracking System allows for a person to use a Windows-based computer to use their eyes to operate the computer. The person using the system will be able to open applications on the desktop, open and close pull-down menus as well as any other operation which would have been carried out using the mouse. It works by infra-red light being reflected off the retina of the eye into a camera attached to the base of the monitor. After calibrating the system for someone's eyes, the cursor will follow the person's eye movements. *See* Appendix IV (Eye Tracking Systems).

Quinkey keyboard an input device for the BBC microcomputer for those who cannot use a conventional QWERTY KEYBOARD. It is a one-handed keyboard which bypasses the QWERTY KEYBOARD. The operator produces combinations of keys to produce different characters. The Quinkey keyboard plugs into the analog port at the back of the computer. When the software which comes with Quinkey is loaded, the keyboard becomes operational. There is a Quinkey unit which can have four keyboards all interfaced into the computers for multi-users.

QWERTY keyboard the usual keyboard layout found on typewriters, computer keyboards and other high-tech communication aids manufactured in the UK. The name comes from the first six letters of the top alphabetic row of the keyboard. Similarly, on the Continent some keyboards are known as Azerty keyboards. The positioning of letters on such keyboards depends on the frequency with which letters are used. It is opposed to keyboards which are set out alphabetically from A to Z.

radical behaviourism *see* OPERANT CONDI-
TIONING.

radiogram *see* RADIOGRAPHY.

radiography the process of observing
structures within the body by X-rays.
The film plates on which the images are
printed are known as radiograms while
those who carry out the X-rays are radi-
ologists. A variety of specialised X-ray
examinations are available, e.g. swallowing barium allows the examination
of the act of swallowing. The barium
may then be followed around the
bowel. *See* Pracy et al (1974); Tortora
and Grabowski (2000).

radiologist *see* RADIOGRAPHY.

radiotherapy a therapeutic technique used
to treat malignant tumours without the
person undergoing surgery. Radiotherapy sometimes follows surgery as it
is this combination which can be most
effective for removing a tumour completely. *See* Pracy et al (1974).

raised intracranial pressure *see* INTRACRA-
NIAL PRESSURE.

Ramsay Hunt syndrome a syndrome
which results from infection with
herpes zoster (chickenpox virus). There
may be facial paresis, hyperacusis, loss
of taste which is unilateral, decreased
salivation, pain in the ear and vesicles
in the external canal and/or the eardrum.
See Gilroy and Holliday (1982); http:
//www.umm.edu/ency/article/001647.
htm

ramus of mandible *see* ZYGOMATIC ARCH.

randomisation *see* INDEPENDENT GROUP
DESIGN.

range a measure of dispersion or spread of
some measure. Range is calculated by
subtracting the highest score from the
lowest. However, this is not always useful since the calculation of the range
uses only the two extreme scores. So, if
one or both differs by a large amount
from the other scores, the resulting
range will be affected greatly. The statis-
tician would use the interquartile range
in such circumstances where the range
is divided into quarters. The interquartile range is the difference between the
third and first quartiles. *See* Miller
(1984).

Rapid Screening Test (RST) this test
forms part of the assessment used in the
DERBYSHIRE LANGUAGE SCHEME. It is a
quick way to find out the child's level of
comprehension. After analysing the
results, if it is found that the child
requires further assessment for comprehension, the therapist will administer the DETAILED TEST OF COMPREHENSION.
See Masidlover and Knowles (1987) in
Appendix I.

rate the speed at which people speak. It
may also be described as tempo. An
analysis of rate is made under SUPRASEG-
MENTAL PHONOLOGY. Rate is often tested
in DYSARTHRIA assessments such as the
ROBERTSON DYSARTHRIA PROFILE. It is often
found that those who use a particularly
fast rate have a DYSFLUENCY or DYSPHONIA.

Thus, if they are made to slow down their rate of speech using techniques such as PROLONGED or slowed speech, their dysfluency or dysphonia reduces significantly. *See* Robertson and Thomson (1986); Cruttenden (1994).

rational-emotive therapy (RET) a COGNITIVE BEHAVIOUR THERAPY developed by Ellis in the early 1960s. It is aimed at analysing the individual's distorted perception of life events, not the events themselves. Ellis listed 12 assumptions of distorted cognition which include such beliefs as: 'It is easier to avoid than to face life's difficulties and self-responsibilities', and 'One has no control over one's emotions and one cannot help feeling certain things' (Ellis 1970, quoted in Rachman and Wilson 1980, p. 196). The therapy is aimed mainly at the neurotic population who do not always rehearse their distorted cognitions deliberately but the cognitions appear suddenly and are pervasive in their influence. The onus is put on the individual to identify irrational thoughts and replace them with positive thoughts. The treatment procedure includes discussing the philosophical aims of RET; identifying the irrational thoughts by the client through discussion with the therapist; the therapist points out the irrational thoughts and models a rational method of dealing with them; repetition of the rational thoughts aims at replacing the irrational thoughts; and, finally, the client is given behavioural tasks to reinforce the new rational thought processes. *See* Rachman and Wilson (1980); Davison et al (2004).

Raven's progressive matrices devised by Raven between 1938 and 1977 to assess a person's non-verbal comprehension. The black and white version was published in 1938 for use with adults. The coloured version was published in 1949 for use with young children and adults with varying degrees of LEARNING DISABILITY or other impairments. The advanced version was published in 1962 for use with those of above-average ability between the age of 11;0 and adulthood.

The person is presented with a progression of abstract patterns from which a piece has been removed and hidden in an array of distracting pieces. The person has then to choose the correct piece to fit the pattern. Although designed for use by psychologists, it can be used with those who have APHASIA with associated comprehension deficits as a result of trauma to the brain, e.g. CEREBROVASCULAR ACCIDENT, HEAD INJURY, TUMOURS OF THE CENTRAL NERVOUS SYSTEM, etc. It may be used as an alternative to the Token Test. *See* Aiken (1988).

raw score the score which a child or adult receives after an assessment has been carried out. This score can be turned into a STANDARD SCORE, AGE-EQUIVALENT SCORE or a PERCENTILE SCORE. *See* Smith et al (2003).

RDLS *see* REYNELL DEVELOPMENTAL LANGUAGE SCALES.

REACH Interface Author developed by Applied Human Factors, REACH Interface Author provides over 100 different on-screen keyboards, including the means of creating on-screen keyboards for whoever uses keys, of any size and allows graphics and sounds to be imported into the keyboard. It is suitable for children, adolescents and adults who find it difficult to operate an ordinary computer keyboard. The on-screen keyboards can be operated by switch access or any mouse emulator. Some of the keyboards included on disk include alphabetic and QWERTY KEYBOARDS, keyboards showing both upper and lower case letters, keyboards depicting stories such as 'The Three Pigs', keyboards for games, keyboards for exploring which help develop cause and effect, and keyboards to develop motor skills. *See* Appendix IV (Applied Human Factors).

REACH Smart Key Technology developed by Applied Human Factors, REACH Smart Key Technology is designed to speed up typing with on-screen keyboards used for spelling. When a letter is typed, only the letters which will follow logically the typed

197

letter are left on the screen and a word prediction system gives six words starting with that letter. When the next letter is typed the selection changes to only those letters which follow logically and so on until the word is either typed out in full or predicted in the word bar. When used with a switch or switches for scanning, when there are only a few letters remaining on the screen, the scanning prompt will only scan to those letters and so speed up using an on-screen keyboard with scanning. *See* Appendix IV (Applied Human Factors).

Reading Comprehension Battery for Aphasia devised by LaPointe and Horner, this battery of tests is designed to provide the systematic evaluation of the type and severity of reading impairment in those with APHASIA. The intention was to produce a test, the results of which would lead the therapist to decide on appropriate therapy. The battery comprises 10 subtests:

I	Single word comprehension (visual)
II	Single word comprehension (auditory)
III	Single word comprehension (semantic)
IV	Functional reading
V	Synonyms
VI	Sentence comprehension (picture)
VII	Short paragraph comprehension
VIII&IX	Paragraphs: factual and inferential
X	Morphosyntactic

See LaPointe and Horner (1979) in Appendix I; Rosenbek et al (1989).

realisation in speech pathology, the realisation of a sound usually refers to the wrong sound or PHONOLOGICAL PROCESS produced by a child. In articulation delay/disorder or phonological delay/disorder, it describes the difference between the sound the child uses when producing certain words and the target sound, i.e. the correct sound. It is this difference which is analysed by the speech and language therapist. The aim of treatment is to match the realisation to the target so that the differences disappear. *See* Grunwell (1987).

reality orientation therapy a therapeutic technique used with the confused elderly patient. The confusion is usually caused by trauma to the brain such as CVA, trauma, excess medication, etc. A regular daily routine is maintained while in the hospital with the patient's name, dates, schedule for meals and the patient's timetable. There is usually a reality orientation board in the ward to remind patients of essential information. *See* Wertz (1981).

Rebus devised by Woodcock in 1968 in the form of *The Rebus Reading Series* for use with children with a mild LEARNING DISABILITY. A Rebus is any pictorial representation which acts as a symbol to represent either individual words, phrases or sentences. It has been developed to help those children with language delay or language disorder who may or may not have learning disability. It has been developed into a communication system in the US (Clarke et al 1974) and in the UK (Van Oosterum and Devereux 1985). By 1998 there were more than 3500 rebuses in the British Rebus collection. A study of children and young adults who had no physical disabilities in four age groups found Rebus symbols to be equivalent to PICSYMS in transparency while both were more transparent than BLISSYMBOLS (Musselwhite and Ruscello ,1984). The results of another study found that Rebus and PCS symbols were easier to learn than Picsyms, PIC symbols and Blissymbols (Bloomberg et al 1990) while Rebus symbols were found to be superior to Blissymbols in learning and short-term recall tasks with both typical preschoolers (Ecklund and Reichle 1987) and preschoolers who had language delays (Burroughs et al 1990). All Rebus dictionaries and software products are available from Widgit Software Ltd. *See* Woodcock et al (1968); Clark et al (1974); Kiernan et al (1982); Musselwhite and Ruscello (1984); Van Oosterum and Devereux (1985); Ecklund and Reichle (1987); Bloomberg et al (1990); Burroughs et al (1990); Glennen and DeCoste (1997); Beukelman and Mirenda (1998); Whittle and Detheridge (2001).

received pronunciation (RP) a non-regional accent of British English. It is an accent used to refer to other accents.

receptive aphasia the description of a comprehension (how language is 'received') deficit which someone with APHASIA might have. Its characteristics are similar to Wernicke's aphasia (*see* APHASIA (2)) and is opposed to EXPRESSIVE APHASIA. The degree of receptive aphasia can be determined by administering the TOKEN TEST, the TEST FOR RECEPTION OF GRAMMAR as well as comprehension subtests of formal aphasia assessments such as the BOSTON DIAGNOSTIC APHASIA EXAMINATION, the WESTERN APHASIA BATTERY or the MINNESOTA TEST FOR THE DIFFERENTIAL DIAGNOSIS OF APHASIA. *See* Eisenson (1984); Rosenbek et al (1989).

Receptive-Expressive Emergent Language Scales: Second Edition (REELS) devised by Bzoch and League originally in 1970 and now in its third edition (2003), it is an observational checklist of language development undertaken jointly by the therapist and caregiver. It is suitable for use with children from birth to 3;00 years. Detailed questions about receptive and expressive ability can be asked corresponding to 1 month old, 2 months old and 3 months old; first year of life, second year and third year in normal child development. *See* Bzoch and League (2003) in Appendix I; Beech et al (1993).

recessive condition *see* CHROMOSOMES.

reciprocal assimilation *see* ASSIMILATION (2).

recruitment an abnormal growth in loudness. It occurs when the intensity level of the sound is given a small increase but to the person it can become almost unbearable. For example, an increase of 20dB may sound like an increase of 60 dB. It often occurs with nerve loss or in Ménière's disease. The hearing loss caused by recruitment can mean sufferers cannot hear normal conversation or other environmental sounds. Tests used to detect recruitment include direct tests for recruitment such as the ALTERNATE BINAURAL LOUDNESS BALANCE TEST and the stapedius reflex threshold (*see* IMPEDANCE AUDIOMETRY), and indirect tests for recruitment such as finding out the DIFFERENCE LIMEN, the short increment sensitivity index and BÉKÉSY AUDIOMETRY. *See* Katz (1985); http://www.lowedown.net/recruitment.html

recurrent laryngeal nerve palsy *see* LARYNGEAL NERVE PALSIES (5, 6); TRACHEA.

recurrent utterances also known as speech automatisms, these are stereotyped and repetitive productions made by those with a severe form of APHASIA. *See* Blanken (1991).

reduplication *see* PHONOLOGICAL PROCESSES (3).

REELS *see* RECEPTIVE-EXPRESSIVE EMERGENT LANGUAGE SCALES.

referent a process found in philosophical linguistics. A referent describes what a linguistic unit refers to in the outside world. For example, the word 'book' refers to the object 'book'. However, not all linguistic units have such obvious referents, e.g. the, a, and, is, etc. *See* Lyons (1981); Fromkin and Rodman (2003).

register the way in which people use their VOCAL FOLDS to change the type of voice they can produce. In speaking, there are different types of register such as breathy, creaky and hoarse voice while in singing there are the different voices such as tenor, soprano, falsetto, etc. These voice changes are caused by changes in the thickness, length and tightness in the vocal folds. *See* Catford (1977); Fromkin and Rodman (2003).

regressive assimilation *see* ASSIMILATION (2).

reliability if an assessment is to be worthwhile, it must be reliable, have validity and be discriminating. For an assessment to be reliable, each of the subtests must measure the same variable. For example, in assessments of language, all the subtests must be a measure of various aspects of language, e.g. word finding, reading aloud, comprehension, etc. Thus, there would not be subtests concerning social skills or other non-language functions. It must also be consistent over time, so that if children are tested with a particular test, they should have the same score when tested six months later if no improvement has taken place. This is known as test–retest reliability. *See* Purser (1982); Smith et al (2003).

Remote-Switch Intro Talker a high-tech communication aid which operates like the ordinary INTRO TALKER. Its main difference is the eight single switch sockets on the side of the device. When the device is used in 8-locations each of the individual locations can be operated by a switch. For example, if the device is used with children for group work, each child can have a switch and access a line of a song, poem or story. It is not a scanning device for which a POINT AND SCAN INTRO TALKER is required. *See* Appendix IV (Prentke Romich Company).

Renfrew Language Attainment Scales devised by Renfrew in the late 1960s, revised in the 1970s, 1980s and 1990s, to assess various modalities of the child's communication. There are five tests:

1. Bus Story: assesses continuous language.
2. Action Picture Test: assesses expressive language.
3. Word-finding Vocabulary Scale: assesses the use of words.
4. Auditory Discrimination Screening Test: assesses auditory comprehension.
5. Articulation Attainment Test: assesses use of English consonants.

See Clarke and Clarke (1974); Berry (1976).

Repeatable Battery for the Assessment of

Neuropsychological Status (RBANS™) devised by Randolph, RBANS is a brief, individually administered test that helps measure cognitive decline in adults with neurological problems as a result of CEREBROVASCULAR ACCIDENT (CVA), HEAD INJURY or DEMENTIA. There are 12 subtests which provide samples of five cognitive areas: immediate memory, visuospatial/constructional, attention, language and delayed memory. It is suitable for people in the age range of 20;00–89;00. *See* Randolph (1998) in Appendix I.

repeated measures design an experimental design in which a single subject takes part under both of the experimental conditions. There can be problems using this design and so COUNTERBALANCING may have to be used to be certain the results are not confounded. *See* Miller (1984).

repertory grids an assessment technique used in PERSONAL CONSTRUCT THEORY. If this theory is to be used effectively, the therapist has to find out how the person views the world and so the person's constructs have to be elicited. The person is provided with role constructs, e.g. someone you look up to, someone you dislike, someone who is successful, someone who is not successful, etc., and gives the names or initials of the people they think about. The person, however, should include himself/herself in the role constructs, e.g. me as I am now, me as I would like to be. Once the people have been identified, three are chosen and the person is asked the following question: 'Can you tell me in what important way two of these people are alike and thereby different from the third?' Thus, the person produces constructs. These can be divided into subordinate constructs, e.g. helpful/unhelpful, and superordinate constructs which the therapist finds out using the technique of laddering. In laddering, the therapist takes one of the bipolar constructs, e.g. helpful/unhelpful, and asks the person questions to obtain a more in-depth analysis of the person's personality. The therapist would stop the interview when it was thought a superordinate level had been reached. Both types of constructs (both subordinate and superordinate) are placed on a grid by the person using a rating system of 1–9. Correlations between the ratings of the constructs are worked out by a computer program. *See* Dalton (1983, 1994).

Reporter's Test devised by De Renzi and Ferrari in 1978, it is a formal assessment derived from the TOKEN TEST. Its full name is 'The Reporter's Test: A Sensitive Test to Detect Expressive Disturbances in Aphasics'. The same stimuli are used to test the person's expressive abilities as in the Token Test. So that the person becomes accustomed to the material, the 36-item Short Token Test (*see* TOKEN TEST) is given first. Following this, the 20 tokens are laid out in the prescribed manner. The person is told to pretend there is someone else next to him with a board placed between them. The therapist points to a token, which the person has to tell the 'other' person to point to. The scoring is based on whether the report would or would not allow a correct reproduction by the 'other' person. One point is scored if the response is correct after the first presentation and half a point after the second presentation. The correct names and adjectives must be used. If the score is 18–35 or less, there could be evidence of an EXPRESSIVE APHASIA. The weighting score scale measures the person's verbal output. If the score is 54 or less, there may be evidence for the person having APHASIA. *See* Eisenson (1984).

reserve volume in breathing, the full capacity of the lungs is not used all the time. Most people keep within the level of the TIDAL VOLUME. The rest of the air which could be used is the reserve volume of which there are two types:

1. Inspiratory reserve volume: the volume of air which can be used during varying degrees of deep inspiration.
2. Expiratory reserve volume: the volume of air which can be used for varying degrees of breath expiration.

See J.H. Green (1982); Tortora and Grabowski (2000).

residual air air remaining in the lungs as residual volume.

residual volume air which is always left in the lungs after total expiration. This amounts to about 1200 ml. *See* J.H. Green (1982); Tortora and Grabowski (2000).

resonance a phenomenon which describes the setting in vibration of one structure at its frequency by another structure vibrating at that frequency. In ACOUSTIC PHONETICS it refers to vibrations of air movement in the VOCAL TRACT which are set off by phonation. It occurs, in particular, when the air particles begin to vibrate in the nasal cavities. These cavities can change shape, and increase loudness and frequency at the source of the sound. In disorders of nasality, the degrees of resonance will either be increased (hypernasality) or decreased (hyponasality). *See* Catford (1989); Denes and Pinson (1993).

respiration the process of breathing. There are two elements to respiration: inspiration (breathing in) and expiration (breathing out). The normal type of breathing in the male is ABDOMINAL–DIAPHRAGMATIC RESPIRATION while thoracic respiration (*see* CLAVICULAR) is more common in the female. *See* J.H. Green (1982); Tortora and Grabowski (2000).

respiratory capacity another name for VITAL CAPACITY.

reticular system this system in the BRAIN receives almost all sensory input from the whole CENTRAL NERVOUS SYSTEM. It has a role in such functions of the brain as the sleep-arousal cycle. Its neurons are connected to the motor areas of the brain and SPINAL CORD. *See* Barr (1988); Kolb and Whishaw (1996).

retract the action of the tongue to produce sounds in particular parts of the mouth, e.g. at the back by bunching the tongue at the back to produce velar sounds [k,g] and at the front of the mouth by raising the tongue to the post-alveolar area to produce sounds. *See* Catford (1977).

retrocochlear hearing loss a hearing loss which is caused by damage or a lesion behind the cochlea (*see* EAR), just below the BRAINSTEM. It produces a neural hearing loss. *See* Katz (1985).

Rett's syndrome discovered by Andreas Rett in 1966, it is a very rare syndrome which is found primarily in females. Its prevalence is 1 in 10000 births. Children who have Rett's syndrome will have been developing normally over the first 6–18 months at which time they begin to lose their gross motor control, start producing repetitive movements of their hands (e.g. hand wringing or rubbing) and head growth stops. Their walking is poor and they exhibit over-breathing, air-swallowing and teeth-grinding. Since all these changes make them anxious, they become cut off socially and have severe learning disability, little or no language development and no pretend play. Unlike those children with AUTISM the lack of sociability lessens and they can become quite sociable although all the other features of the syndrome remain. *See* http://www.nichcy.org/pubs/factshe/fs20txt.htm; http://www.autism.org/rett.html; Wing (1996).

reversal a phenomenon used in PSYCHOLIN-GUISTICS. Traditionally, such problems are referred to as spoonerisms or metathesis. A very famous example is one of the many by William Spooner himself: 'You have hissed all my mystery lessons' for 'You have missed all my history lessons.' The phonemes [m] and [h] have been reversed in the mistaken utterance. *See* Clark and Clark (1977).

Revised Token Test *see* TOKEN TEST.

rewrite rules *see* CONSTITUENT ANALYSIS.

Reynell Developmental Language Scales (RDLS) devised by Reynell in 1969 (revised 1977, 2nd revision 1985), it is a formal, standardised assessment to assess the child's development of EXPRESSIVE LANGUAGE and COMPREHENSION. Although it can be used with children between 1;0 and 7;0, it is most sensitive for assessing children between 1;0 and 5;0. It can also be used with physically and visually handicapped children as well as those who have a HEARING LOSS. The RAW SCORE on the comprehension and expressive language tests can be converted to a STANDARD SCORE from which an AGE-EQUIVALENT SCORE can be derived. It was standardised originally on over 1300 UK children between the ages of 1;6 and 7;0. *See* Berry (1976); Reynell (1985) in Appendix I; Beech et al (1993).

Reynell Developmental Language Scales III: The University of Reading Edition (RDLS III) devised by Edwards and her colleagues, RDLS III are new scales based on the previous versions of the Scales but take into account up-to-date knowledge about language impairment as well as research into structural and lexical development in child language. The Expressive Scale from the previous versions, which was not used much previously, has been completely revamped and significant changes have been made to the Comprehension Scale. The pictures and toys used during the administration of the Scales have been chosen to reflect the social and cultural changes which have occurred in the UK since the original Scales were first devised in the later 1960s and early 1970s. Both the Comprehension and Expressive Scales are designed to be administered together so that the person testing the child obtains a complete picture of the child's language development. The Comprehension Scale has 62 items in 10 sections which cover a range of skills including the comprehension of single words, clausal constituents (e.g., 'give me the apple and the teddy'; 'make teddy sit'; 'show me the blue box', etc.), complex grammar where the child has to select one picture out of a choice of four, and inferencing which uses the picture of a 'burger bar' because it crosses cultural boundaries and is known by most children. The child has to point to a person in the picture following a request such as 'whose daughter is having a birthday party?' where the child has to understand what is meant by 'whose' and point to the birthday party and the parent sitting at the table. The Expressive Scale contains 62 items across six main sections which follow broadly those used in the Comprehension Scale. The first section concerns single word naming of objects followed by sections concerning clausal, phrasal and morpho- logical development. The final two sections concern assessing complex structures and the use of auxiliaries in negation and question forming. The Scales are still for children in the age range of 1;06–7;00 and were trialed on 400 children while the Scales were standardised on a further 1074 children aged between 1;03–7;06 in the UK and the Republic of Ireland. *See* Edwards et al (1997) in Appendix I; Edwards et al (1999a, b); Ball (1999); Lees (1999); Law (1999);

rhinitis a disorder found in the nose, affecting its mucous membrane which produces an excess of runny mucus. *See* Pracy et al (1974).

rhythm suprasegmental feature (*see* SUPRASEGMENTAL PHONOLOGY) of speech production in which the listener picks up a regular pattern of units in speech. Commonly, this pattern refers to the use of stressed and unstressed syllables, the use of short and long syllables or using high or low pitch in producing the sentence. In relation to a communication disorder, impaired rhythm is a characteristic of verbal dyspraxia (*see* DEVELOPMENTAL VERBAL DYSPRAXIA). In relation to movement, lack of rhythm is observed in the CLUMSY CHILD SYNDROME. *See* Gordon and McKinley (1980); Ladefoged (2001).

Robertson Dysarthria Profile devised by Robertson in 1982, it is a FORMAL ASSESSMENT to assess the severity of DYSARTHRIA. It concentrates on testing ARTICULATION,

RATE, PROSODY and other suprasegmental phenomena (*see* SUPRASEGMENTAL PHONOLOGY). There are seven subtests:

1. Voice.
2. Respiration.
3. Facial musculature.
4. DIADOCHOKINESIS.
5. Reflexes (e.g. swallow, cough).
6. Articulation.
7. Rate, prosody, intelligibility.

Unlike the FRENCHAY DYSARTHRIA ASSESSMENT, the profile does not produce an aetiology but, instead, will give an in-depth analysis of the dysarthric characteristics of the person's speech. *See* Robertson et al (1986) in Appendix I.

Rochester Method *see* EDUCATION OF HEARING-IMPAIRED CHILDREN.

Rogers *see* PHENOMENOLOGICAL APPROACH.

role reversal a therapeutic technique used commonly in training SOCIAL SKILLS. The person adopts the role of the assertive person and the supervisor takes the non-assertive role. If there is a role conflict, this type of therapy is often difficult to implement. It is part of ASSERTIVE TRAINING. *See* Trower et al (1978).

Royal College of Speech and Language Therapists the professional body concerned with the education of speech and language therapists and with standards of service throughout the UK. The College sets out a code of ethics which every therapist has to follow. It organises working parties to study all forms of communication disorders for which therapists provide treatment. The working parties can be approached at any time for advice on treatment programmes for a specific disorder. Membership of the College is open to all qualified speech and language therapists as well as to students studying speech therapy. The College is financed by a yearly membership subscription for which therapists receive the *International Journal of Language and Communication Disorders* quarterly, the *Bulletin* (a magazine for therapists produced by therapists), a Directory of

College members and a twice-monthly list of vacancies in Health Boards/Trusts in the UK and abroad. Information leaflets about different communication disorders are also available. The College produces position papers concerning various aspects of speech and language therapy, e.g. dysphagia, dysphasia, use of AAC, etc. *See* Jennings (1984); Morris (1994); http://www.rcslt.org

RP *see* RECEIVED PRONUNCIATION.

RST *see* RAPID SCREENING TEST.

rubella also known as German measles. It forms part of the TORCH classification of infectious diseases which can adversely affect a fetus. If the fetus becomes infected, it may die or be miscarried. If the fetus survives, there may be congenital heart disease, the brain may be underdeveloped producing CEREBRAL PALSY, AUTISM and LEARNING DISABILITY. The eyes may have cataracts and there may be a HEARING LOSS. The disease can be prevented by the mother undergoing immunisation before child-bearing years. This is usually carried out in the UK in the early senior school. *See* Hosking (1982); http://www.sense.org. uk/sensory_impairment/rubella2.html

S-24 a shortened form of Erikson's (1969) S-scale, it is an assessment designed to find out the attitudes of a person to various communication situations. It is used commonly with stammerers. The individual is asked to give a true/false response to 24 statements, e.g. 'I often ask questions in groups'. The statements cover how stammerers view their speaking ability, how they cope with anxiety-provoking situations, e.g. speaking in groups or to someone in authority, and what situations they try to avoid. *See* Dalton (1983).

salient letter encoding an encoding system in which the initial letter of some or all the words of a phrase are stored into the memory of the system being used so that when they are accessed, the device or software will speak out that phrase. For example, 'Can I have a cup of coffee?' could be stored using the three letter 'C's (i.e. CCC) so that when they are accessed the given phrase will be spoken. This requires some degree of literacy and can result in clashes with other phrases such as 'Can I have a can of coke?' and so the person using the system would have to learn that CCC1 meant 'Can I have a cup of coffee?' while CCC2 meant 'Can I have a can of coke?'. *See* Beukelman and Mirenda (1998).

salivary glands there are three pairs of large salivary glands. The ducts from these glands open into the mouth. The glands are:

1. Parotid gland: wedge-shaped structure lying behind the MANDIBLE and below the EAR and in front of the mastoid process. It grows at the same rate as the person. Cranial nerve VII (*see* CRANIAL NERVES) runs through the gland. The duct runs over the buccinator and masseter muscle (*see* MUSCLES OF FACIAL EXPRESSION) and exits at the second molar. The purpose of the secretion of the gland is to keep the mouth moist, lubricate the passage of food and initiate digestion by the presence of ptyalin which breaks down starch.
2. Submandibular gland: it opens through a duct in the floor of the mouth and runs posteriorly under the mandible. The gland measures 2–3 cm deep, wide and high. The duct opening is at the side of the lingual frenulum (*see* MOUTH). It is a mixed serous/mucus producing gland.
3. Sublingual salivary gland: it is situated under the floor of the mouth and is both the shape and size of an almond. It opens into the mouth by several ducts. It is a mixed serous/mucus producing gland.

These glands are controlled by secretory motor nerves. The parotid gland is supplied by the parasympathetic fibres from the glossopharyngeal nerve (*see* CRANIAL NERVES) while the other two salivary glands are supplied by the facial nerve (*see* CRANIAL NERVES). The salivary glands are compound racemose glands because they branch into several parts: lobes–lobules–branching ducts–dilated alveoli. These three glands together produce 1–1.5 litres of saliva per day. *See* Tortora and Grabowski (2000).

salpingopharyngeus muscle *see* PHARYNX.

sample

1. A sample of language is often taken by a speech therapist for analysis as the person's language in a free situation is often more natural than in an assessment situation. It is an INFORMAL ASSESSMENT and can be analysed by any of the linguistic profiles devised by Crystal or just by the therapist's intuition and experience. *See* Crystal and Varley (1998).
2. *See* POPULATION.

Sandwell Bilingual Screening Assessment (SBSA) devised by Duncan et al for children of 6;0–9;0 years whose first language is Panjabi. It is a picture-based screening test for children who have problems acquiring English as a second language. By analysing the results of the SBSA, the therapist can decide if the problems are in the child's poor language skills or as a result of some pathological cause which will require therapeutic intervention from a speech therapist. The child is presented with 44 line drawings with questions being asked both in Panjabi and English. Two grammatical profiles are produced for each language. The scores in either language are compared with the norm tables in the manual to establish if problems exist in one or both languages. The norms have been obtained from 300 Panjabi and English children. *See* Duncan et al (1987) in Appendix I.

sarcoma a malignant tumour which arises from CONNECTIVE TISSUE. Thus, a fibrosarcoma arises from fibrous tissue, an osteosarcoma arises from BONE while a chondrosarcoma arises from CARTILAGE. *See* Tortora and Grabowski (2000).

Saussure Ferdinand de Saussure (1857–1913) is the founding father of modern linguistics. The linguistic theories he proposed were set out in the *Cours de Linguistique Générale* in 1913. Saussure did not write this book himself. It was published posthumously from the notes of his students who had attended three series of lectures he gave before his death. When all the notes were collected, it was found there were repetition and some inconsistencies. However, all the information was gathered by Bally and Sechehaye and, to overcome the problems already mentioned, they concentrated their work on the third series of lectures as well as taking information from the other two series of lectures and Saussure's personal notes. Later, Rudolf Engler published Saussure's students' notes in 1967. There was much linguistic discussion before Saussure that was confined to the historical study of language. He proposed that it should be possible to stop at a particular time either past or present and describe the language processes which occur. This is the study of synchronic linguistics and is an important part of the historical description of linguistics. However, one of the main standpoints for his linguistics theory is 'language is a system of signs'. These signs are arbitrary by nature in that the 'signifier' for 'television' is a sequence of sounds which could be equally well represented by other sound sequences such as 'bimp', 'gapo' or 'glick', etc. However, this arbitrariness is lessened with some processes such as onomatopoeia, e.g. 'splash', 'miaow', etc. These words are not arbitrary as they are imitative of the action described. There are also sound sequences which are combined to produce new signs, e.g. typewriter, as this sign is associated with the object it names. Saussure proposed a more complex explanation for the arbitrariness of the signifier and the signified. He tried to show they were arbitrary over time. For example, the word 'gay' in the nineteenth century and early part of the twentieth century meant 'happy', 'lively', etc. while in the last 20–30 years it has come to refer to someone's sexuality. Thus, the signifier and the signified are themselves arbitrary. 'La langue' describes the groups of forms which are used to make up a particular language while 'la parole' is the actual physical manifestation of language, i.e. the speech acts and how meaning is communicated. *See* Saussure (1916); Lepschy (1982); Culler (1986).

SCAN-A: A Screening Test for Auditory Processing Disorders in Adolescents and Adults devised by Keith, SCAN-A is designed to find out if there is a problem with auditory processing. It has the same subtests as SCAN-C (filtered words, auditory figure–ground, competing words and competing sentences) but can be used with just an audio cassette. It is also suitable for those in the age range of 12;00–50;00. *See* Keith (1994) in Appendix I.

SCAN-C: Test for Auditory Processing Disorders in Children – Revised devised by Keith, SCAN-C examines the child repeating stimulus words or sentences heard on a CD using four subtests: filtered words, auditory figure–ground, competing words and competing sentences. It is suitable for children in the age range of 5;00–11;00. *See* Keith (1999) in Appendix I.

ScanBuddy developed by Applied Human Factors, ScanBuddy allows a person who cannot access a computer by hand to access it using a single switch or two switches so that the Windows desktop is scanned and applications can be opened and closed as well as being able to pull down menus and make selections. It can be used in conjunction with REACH INTERFACE AUTHOR and SOOTHSAYER. *See* Appendix IV (Applied Human Factors).

scanning most of the communication aids which are used presently can be accessed directly with either the person using a hand(s) or using a headpointer system in the form of a headstick or an optical/infra-red headpointer system, or, alternatively, the devices can be accessed by the use of one or two switches which can be mounted so that the person has the most reliable means of accessing the communication aid. In these communication aids, different parameters can be set up such as: the scan rate; a timed delay between hitting the switch and it accessing the symbol or the words so that there is time to correct an erroneous hit; the way in which the scanning occurs and whether it is row/column or column/row, linear or circular. If the person using the switch also has visual problems auditory prompts can be turned on so that he or she can hear, usually through an earphone, the names of the symbol or letter as the device scans the overlay or keyboard, and the person hits the switch when he or she hears the required auditory prompts. Switches can also be used to operate many on-screen keyboards with similar parameters to set up. *See* Glennen and DeCoste (1997); Beukelman and Mirenda (1998).

schema, schemata *see* ASSIMILATION (2).

schizophrenia a syndrome or group of mental illnesses characterised by specific psychological symptoms which interfere with an individual's thinking, emoting and behaviour and with each of these in a characteristic way. The person can have THOUGHT DISORDERS, FLATTENING OF AFFECT and disorders of speech and language. There are three main types of schizophrenia:

1. Hebephrenic schizophrenia: disorganised features of movements, ideas and moods.
2. Catatonic schizophrenia: odd movements caused by motor disturbances.
3. Paranoic schizophrenia: characterised by delusions which are often grandiose in nature.

As already mentioned, some people who have schizophrenia have associated problems in communication. These include: (1) PERSEVERATION in syntax; (2) repetition of words and syllables; (3) disruption of semantic memory; (4)

clang associations; (5) ECHOLALIA and palilalia; (6) echopraxia; (7) mutism; (8) poverty of thought and speech; (9) concreteness; (10) PHONATION problems; and (11) FLATTENING OF AFFECT. A therapist will have to take a language sample for analysis and plan a treatment programme accordingly. Medical treatment can be treated by the PHENOTHIAZINE family of drugs. *See* Davison et al (2004); Goren et al (1996); http://www.schizophrenia.com/

Schuell in 1964, Schuell and her colleagues put forward a classification of aphasia comprising five major categories and two minor syndromes:

1. Simple aphasia: a breakdown in the symbolic use of language, resulting in a reduction in language, WORD-FINDING DIFFICULTIES with syntactic problems plus phonemic or jargon errors depending on the severity of the aphasia, and comprehension errors depending on the length and complexity of what is said.
2. Aphasia with visual involvement.
3. Aphasia with persistent dysfluency.
4. Aphasia with scattered findings: the individual has some functional language, is not severely disabled but may have dysarthria.
5. Aphasia with sensory motor involvement: mild aphasia with persistent dysarthria.

The two minor syndromes are:

1. Aphasia with intermittent auditory imperception.
2. Irreversible aphasia syndrome: a sudden loss in all modalities and loss of all functional language.

Schuell believed that aphasia was not modality-specific but affected all language modalities. Following this theory, she devised the MINNESOTA TEST FOR THE DIFFERENTIAL DIAGNOSIS OF APHASIA (MTDDA). *See* Eisenson (1984); Rosenbek et al (1989).

schwa perhaps the most common vowel found in English. It is used to transcribe the last sound in 'after' [æftə], and when a stressed vowel becomes unstressed and is the pronounced sound in words such as 'a', 'an', 'the', etc. *See* Ladefoged (2001).

Schwann cell a cell which covers the myelin sheath covering the nerve's axon. It is divided into the sections of the nerve between the nodes of Ranvier. The myelin is formed by the membrane of the Schwann cell. When Wallerian degeneration takes place, it is the Schwann cells which are affected. *See* Barr (1988); Kolb and Whishaw (1996).

ScreenDoors an on-screen keyboard for PCs using Windows, Screen-Doors produces a movable and resizeable window. It has good graphics and fonts on the keyboard. It offers word prediction and context specific dictionaries that can be created for different subjects. Selections are made through a puff switch. ScreenDoors runs in the Multi-Finder environment on System 6.3 or higher. It requires a hard drive and at least two megabytes of RAM memory. *See* Appendix IV (Madentec).

screening audiometry audiometric tests which are carried out quickly with individuals (usually children or in a pre-school clinic). The frequencies are tested at a constant intensity level. This is also known as sweep testing. *See* Katz (1985).

screening tests tests which can be carried out quickly to discover the severity of any disorder, e.g. APHASIA, DYSARTHRIA, etc. Such tests include the Whurr APHASIA SCREENING TEST and the FRENCHAY APHASIA SCREENING TEST (FAST). They are designed to provide an indication as to the type of in-depth assessment which should follow. *See* Byers Brown (1981); Stott et al (2002, Introduction).

SDLD *see* SPECIFIC DEVELOPMENTAL LANGUAGE DISORDER.

secondary articulation an articulation which occurs with little or no narrowing of the articulators while producing the secondary articulation. For example, a palatalised fricative (*see* ARTICULA-

TION) where the friction is the primary articulation and the palatalisation is the secondary articulation. *See* Ladefoged (2001).

secretory motor nerves *see* SALIVARY GLANDS.

segmental phonology a study of the phonemes (*see* PHONOLOGY) in any given language. Phonemes are regarded as the segments under study. It is opposed to SUPRASEGMENTAL PHONOLOGY. *See* Hyman (1975).

seizure a descriptive term for fits or convulsions (compare EPILEPSY). *See* Kolb and Whishaw (1996).

self-actualisation *see* PHENOMENOLOGICAL APPROACH.

self-characterisation an assessment used in PERSONAL CONSTRUCT THEORY. It is part of the 'credulous' approach. People are asked to describe themselves in a non-threatening way as if their best friend were making the description. The request is presented thus: 'I want you to write a character sketch of (person's name), just as if he were the principal character in a play. Write it as it might be written by a friend who knew him very intimately and very sympathetically, perhaps better than anyone ever really could know him. Be sure to write it in the third person. For example, start out by writing, '(person's name) is a...' *See* Dalton (1983, 1994).

self-instructional training (SIT) developed by Meichenbaum in 1977, SIT is a COGNITIVE BEHAVIOUR THERAPY. It is based in part on Ellis's RATIONAL-EMOTIVE THERAPY as well as on the developmental sequence which children use to develop internal speech and verbal-symbolic control over their behaviour. The therapist using SIT takes the client through the following stages:

1. The client is trained to identify maladaptive behaviour or thoughts (self-statements).
2. The therapist models appropriate behaviour while talking the client through effective action strategies using self-statements which are positive, which stress the client's adequacy, and reduce feelings of failure.
3. The client performs the target behaviour and rehearses the appropriate self-instructions aloud followed by rehearsing them internally. The therapist provides positive feedback to ensure constructive problem-solving self-talk which replaces anxiety-produced cognitions associated with the behaviour. *See* Rachman and Wilson (1980); Davison et al (2004).

self-theory *see* PHENOMENOLOGICAL APPROACH.

semantic field a conceptually identified group of lexical items, e.g. kinship relations, colour terms, constitutes a semantic field. The meanings of the lexical items that make up the field are in part determined by the sense relations they contract with one another within the field.

semantic-pragmatic language disorder a rare disorder in which there is gross impairment of semantics and severely restricted pragmatic use of language. Comprehension is also limited. Children can demonstrate deficits in abstract comprehension and formulation of discourse as well as making atypical choices of words, inordinate use of scripts and seem not to need a conversational partner because of their verbose output as well as having poor turn-taking skills. They also have difficulty staying on topic. Some children with SPLD may be over-literal, and their ability to infer may also be restricted. Phonology may be normal or near normal. There has also been discussion concerning the classification of semantic-pragmatic disorder and how it relates to AUTISM and SPECIFIC LANGUAGE IMPAIRMENT. Bishop et al (2000) showed children diagnosed as having SPLD do not necessarily have additional grammatical or semantic problems. This led Bishop (2000) to propose a new label of 'pragmatic language impairment'. *See* Allen (1988, 1989); Adams and Bishop (1989); Bishop and Adams (1989); Rapin and Allen (1992); Boucher (1998a, b); Rapin and Allen (1998); Botting (1998); Bowler and Lister Brook (1998); Bishop et al (2000); Bishop (2000); Adams (2001).

semantic relations one approach to the early utterance of children has tried to account for them in terms of the semantic relations they express, rather than in terms of grammatical patterns. Such relations were proposed by Brown (1973):

agent + action	man put
action + object	kick ball
agent + object	mummy shoe
action + locative	go home
entity + locative	book table
possessor + possessed	daddy car
entity + attributive	cup blue
demonstrative + entity	that book

See Lyons (1981).

semantics the study of meaning. Within modern linguistics, the most important areas have been lexical (structural) semantics – which has concerned itself with structural relations in the vocabulary, e.g. autonomy, synonymy, hyponymy – and truth-conditional semantics. This is an approach to sentence meaning which holds that (at least part of) sentence meaning is characterised in terms of the conditions (in the real or possible world) under which a sentence can be held to express a statement that is true. *See* Lyons (1981); Fromkin and Rodman (2003).

semi-vowels the sounds subsumed under this term are sometimes known as approximants (*see* ARTICULATION). They are classified as consonants but have a vowel-like quality in that they are produced without closure or friction. The sounds which follow this pattern in English are [j, w]. *See* Fromkin and Rodman (2003); Ladefoged (2001).

senile dementia *see* ALZHEIMER'S DISEASE.

sensation level (SL) a measure of the level of a sound above the person's hearing threshold. It is measured in decibels (dB). For example, if the hearing threshold is 60 dB HL and a sound is presented at 90 dB HL, the sensation level is 30 dB SL (sensation level). *See* Katz (1985).

sensitivity training a therapeutic technique used commonly in SOCIAL SKILLS training. It takes the form of the participants learning from their own immediate and direct experiences within the group. It is not so much a procedure for learning social skills but a way of learning sensitivity to others, improving interpersonal relationships and improving the person's self-confidence. There are two types of techniques used for this end – ENCOUNTER GROUPS and T-GROUPS. *See* Trower et al (1978); Davison et al (2004).

sensorimotor stage the first of Piaget's four stages of cognitive development in children. The stage lasts from birth to 2 years of age and concerns the child's ability to perceive objects but not to think about them. In other words, the child can only act upon an object when it is within his vision but not if it is hidden. This is Piaget's theory of OBJECT PERMANENCE where he showed object permanence did not exist in young children. The development of imitation and play are important in the child's ability to symbolise objects. Towards the end of this stage, the child may use deferred imitation, i.e. the ability to act out events which the child has stored in memory, and play with objects using them to symbolise other objects. This idea of symbolisation is the mainstay of Piaget's theory of language development. He believed a child could not develop language until he or she had acquired symbolisation. More concisely, Piaget believed language did not appear until the cognitive events underlying symbolisation have been achieved and thus language develops out of cognition. *See* Beard (1969); Smith et al (2003); Boden (1994).

sensorineural hearing loss this is caused by a lesion or damage to the inner ear, to the auditory nerve, to the BRAINSTEM or to the auditory cortex. It can be improved by wearing a HEARING AID, using an assistive hearing device which amplifies sound or changing behaviour, e.g. making sure the speaker is in the same room as the listener. Those with this type of hearing loss often talk too loudly because they cannot hear their own voice and sometimes they have vertigo and often TINNITUS. They have difficulty picking up speech especially if they are in a noisy environment or having a conversation in a group. There is no air–bone gap (*see* PURE-TONE AUDIOMETRY) whilst the loss varies from mild to severe. *See* Katz (1985); Smith et al (2003).

sensory aphasia acoustic agnostic APHASIA identified by Luria in 1966. The main difficulty lies in discriminating speech sounds and this leads to impaired understanding of word meaning. Because of the inability to analyse words into their sound components cueing-in through the initial sound of the word does not help. *See* Lesser (1988); Kolb and Whishaw (1996).

sentence the largest unit in grammar within which distributional patterns can be recognised. Lyons has referred to it as 'the largest unit of grammatical description' (Lyons 1968, p. 172). Note, however, that it can be defined, either in traditional terms as a list of patterns defined in terms of some set of elements, e.g. SVO, SVA, SVC, etc., or more recently as the product of a set of defining rules. 'Sentence' is a theoretical term of linguistic description. *See* Lyons (1968); Fromkin and Rodman (2003).

Sentence Comprehension Test devised by Wheldall, Hobsbaum and Mittler in 1977 (revised 1987), it is a FORMAL ASSESSMENT to test the child's understanding of grammatical constructions. It can only be used with children of 3;0–5;6 years. It comprises 15 subtests, each of which have a different grammatical structure. Each subtest has four items from which the child has to choose the correct one. A subtest is passed if the child scores three or more

in each subtest which produces a profile score out of 60 items from which the therapist decides whether or not therapy is required. In the 1986 edition, five subtests were left out as well as several items (there are only 10 subtests) and the pictures have been redrawn. There is also a Panjabi version. *See* Wheldall (1987) in Appendix I; Beech et al (1993).

separation anxiety a possible cause of EMOTIONAL DISORDER which children may have. Feelings of fear and anxiety are quite common and are normal reactions in children to certain circumstances but when these feelings begin to interfere with everyday life, they become abnormal. During children's early life, they are very sensitive and vulnerable to traumatic events and separation is one such event. The mother, often regarded by the child as being someone special (since she is usually the parent with whom bonding first takes place), may have to leave home suddenly, for example, to have another child or for other medical reasons. If the child has been adequately prepared for this separation, there will be less of a problem accepting the situation than if the mother disappears suddenly and no preparation has taken place. In the latter case, the child becomes 'lost' and has severe anxiety. PSYCHOTHERAPY of all kinds has been used successfully with such children. FAMILY THERAPY and/or parental counselling is also useful. *See* Rutter (1975); Davison et al (2004).

serial speech the type of language which is automatic to most people, e.g. days of the week, months of the year, alphabet, counting, etc. For some of those with APHASIA, it may be the only language which is intact. Thus, in many aphasia assessments, subtests for serial speech are included. *See* Eisenson (1984).

serous cells these produce a water-like substance. *See* SALIVARY GLANDS.

serous otitis media *see* OTITIS MEDIA (3).

servo system in speech, a cybernetic theory proposed by Fairbanks in 1954 to explain speech production. He describes an effector unit, a feedback loop and a comparator device whereby output may be compared with intention, error detected and necessary corrections made.

sex chromosomes *see* CHROMOSOMES.

Sheffield Screening Test for Acquired Language Disorders devised by Syder and colleagues in 1994, this screening test can be used to assess the presence of high level language disorders as a result of trauma to the brain. It is in three sections; the first allows some assessment of the person's functional communication while the second and third allow an assessment of receptive and expressive language problems. It takes 10 minutes to administer. The test has been standardised on 112 people aged 30–91 years. *See* Syder et al (1994) in Appendix I.

Short Token Test *see* TOKEN TEST.

shunt a device fitted into the BRAIN to drain the fluid causing pressure in the FOURTH VENTRICLE in people with hydrocephalus. There are two types of shunt treatment – the Spitz-Holter shunt and the Pudenz shunt. *See* Hosking (1982).

shwa *see* SCHWA.

sibilant a subtype of fricative (*see* ARTICULATION). The fricatives in English are [f, v, θ, ð, s, z, ʃ, ʒ]. Some fricatives are produced with greater acoustic energy and hence a higher pitch. This produces a loud hissing noise. These fricatives, i.e. [s, z, ʃ, ʒ] are sibilants and thus opposed to the non-sibilants, i.e., [f, v, θ, ð]. *See* Ladefoged (2001).

sibling rivalry it is common knowledge that there is almost always some degree of rivalry between or among siblings. This may take the form of play-fighting or trying to do better at school, etc. It is usually caused by just wanting to do better than the other sibling to obtain more praise from parents. However, if parents go out of their way overtly to show preference to one sibling rather than to another, the one to whom preference is not given may produce feelings of aggression either to the other

sibling or to parents or both. These feelings can produce either CONDUCT DISORDERS or EMOTIONAL DISORDERS such as ELECTIVE MUTISM. For example, if children wish to be vindictive towards the parents, they may decide not to speak at school and so make life as difficult as possible. *See* Rutter (1975).

sigh/yawn technique *see* YAWN/SIGH.

sign *see* SAUSSURE.

sign languages a type of ALTERNATIVE AUGMENTATIVE COMMUNICATION system taught to those who have difficulty in using EXPRESSIVE LANGUAGE. A sign language has its own grammar and has similar characteristics to any oral language, i.e. historical change, puns, humour, arbitrariness, etc. Such languages include BRITISH SIGN LANGUAGE (BSL) and American Sign Language (ASL) for use with those who have a hearing loss. *See* Kiernan et al (1982); Glennen and DeCoste (1997); Beukelman and Mirenda (1998).

sign systems a type of AUGMENTATIVE AND ALTERNATIVE COMMUNICATION system taught to those who have difficulty in using expressive language or whose speech is significantly unintelligible. A sign system is not a language in itself although it has signs which represent words and, in some cases, morphological endings. It does not have its own grammar but follows the order in spoken English as it has a sign for each keyword in the sentence. Such examples are the PAGET-GORMAN SIGN SYSTEM and MAKATON vocabulary. *See* Kiernan et al (1982); Beukelman and Mirenda (1998).

Signalong devised by Kennard and Grove in 1991, Signalong is a sign supporting system based loosely around the word levels of the DERBYSHIRE LANGUAGE SCHEME. It was a response to what was seen as a prescriptive set of vocabulary as used in MAKATON. Therefore the Signalong Group's aim is to seek to offer a wide-ranging selection of signs to facilitate communication which will enable people with LEARNING DISABILITIES to take more control of their own lives and to make more of their own decisions. Phase 1 of the signs was published in 1992 and there are a total of four basic vocabulary manuals. It is based on BRITISH SIGN LANGUAGE with nearly all the signs being unaltered and the most iconic (see ICONICITY) ones being chosen where there is a choice. There are CD-ROMs available with 'Annie', an animation of a girl performing the signs with a recorded voice speaking the words. *See* http://www.sign-along.org.uk

signed English a SIGN SYSTEM designed in the early 1970s to represent oral English. The hand signs can be used with speech which makes the message to be communicated very clear. It can be used with children who have a HEARING LOSS and/or LEARNING DISABILITY. Each sign has a semantic relationship with each English word. There are more than 3100 signs and 14 sign markers for morphological endings. It was the first sign system to be used with children who had AUTISTIC SPECTRUM DISORDER. *See* Creedon (1973); Bornstein and Hamilton (1978); Beukelman and Mirenda (1998).

signifier, signified *see* SAUSSURE.

simple aphasia proposed by Schuell in the 1960s, it refers to a reduction in the ability to use all language modalities without accompanying DYSPRAXIA or DYSARTHRIA. *See* Eisenson (1984).

simple depression *see* DEPRESSION.

singer's nodes/nodules *see* VOCAL NODULES.

single case study in studies of the efficacy of certain treatment techniques, it has been found difficult to use test designs such as the INDEPENDENT GROUP, MATCHED GROUP and REPEATED MEASURES. Thus, statisticians proposed the single case study. In this type of study, the subjects have to act as their own controls. The aim is to test the subject during periods of treatment and non-treatment. The best design for such studies is the ABA design. This means that during 'A' (no treatment) the person is tested, during 'B' treatment is given followed by 'A' when the person is retested using similar stimuli as were used during the treatment sessions. For example, if the person has naming problems and therapy is given to improve his naming skills, the therapist might take 50 pictures, test the person, take half the cards and give treatment to help him to name these pictures and then retest using all 50 pictures. *See* Coltheart (1983).

SIT *see* SELF-INSTRUCTIONAL TRAINING.

skew *see* CENTRAL TENDENCY.

ski slope hearing loss *see* PURE-TONE AUDIOMETRY.

Skinner's boxes *see* OPERANT CONDITIONING.

skull a structure formed by the bones of the cranium and MANDIBLE. The bones all fit together strongly except for the mandible which swings quite freely so that the mouth can open and close. The function of the skull is to protect the BRAIN. Other areas of the skull are the orbits which are filled by the eyes and their respective nerves and muscles, the nasal cavities (*see* NOSE) and the MOUTH. *See* Tortora and Grabowski (2000).

SL *see* SENSATION LEVEL.

slit a particular configuration of the TONGUE for producing fricatives (*see* ARTICULATION). The tongue is flat for the fricatives [f, v, ʃ, ʒ] while it is grooved for the fricatives [s, z]. *See* Catford (1977).

sloping hearing loss *see* PURE-TONE AUDIOMETRY.

smooth muscle produces slow contraction over long distances. It is supplied by the AUTONOMIC NERVOUS SYSTEM (ANS). Its fibres are spindle-like and have thin ends while the central part is thicker and contains the nucleus of the muscle. Smooth muscle is involuntary muscle tissue supplied by involuntary nerves and certain hormones. It is found in the gut, respiratory passages, urinogenital system, iris of eye and blood vessel walls. *See* Leeson et al (1985); Tortora and Grabowski (2000).

social skills a person produces socially acceptable behaviour and the behaviour produces the desired effect on others. Any child or adult who does not possess such skills has to be given a treatment programme to teach him/her how to cope in various situations through experience. Such treatment takes the form of ASSERTIVE TRAINING, SENSITIVITY TRAINING and PSYCHODRAMA. *See* Trower et al (1978); Davison et al (2004).

Social Use of Language Programme devised by Rinaldi in 1992, this programme is designed to improve the social communication skills of children and adolescents with mild to moderate learning disabilities, speech impairment or hearing difficulties. It is possible to assess a person's different social communication skills, both verbal and non-verbal, as well as to implement an effective educational therapy programme. It uses group activities such as games, role-playing exercises and problem solving for assessment and remediation. *See* Rinaldi (1992) in Appendix I.

socialised conduct disorder *see* CONDUCT DISORDER.

sociolinguistics the study of accents and dialects used in different regions of a country. It discusses also the different varieties of language used in social contexts and the role of linguistic minorities in a multi-racial society. *See* Trudgill (1995); Woll and Barnett (1998) (sociolinguistics and AAC).

sodium valproate a drug treatment for EPILEPSY.

soft palate *see* MOUTH.

sonorant a MAJOR CLASS FEATURE proposed by Chomsky and Halle to distinguish sounds produced without any blocking of the VOCAL TRACT [+SONORANT], i.e. liquids, nasals and laterals, from those which are produced with an obstruction [−SONORANT]. *See* Fromkin and Rodman (2003); Ladefoged (2001).

sonority a phenomenon in auditory phonetics which examines loudness relative to pitch, stress and duration. *See* Ladefoged (2001).

SoothSayer developed by Applied Human Factors, SoothSayer is a word prediction system designed to make a saving on keystrokes. When the first few letters of a word are typed the word beginning with the typed letter appears in the word bar. By selecting the required word, it is sent to the open application. It speaks out letters, words or sentences as typed and learns words which are not in the Dictionary. SoothSayer takes account of word frequency and recency as well as finishing a word automatically when it is the only possible word. *See* Appendix IV (Applied Human Factors).

sound pressure level measured at a given point along the propagation of the sound wave. It decreases as distance from source increases. It is measured in dynes/cm^2 or pascals (Pa). *See* Denes and Pinson (1993).

sound system *see* PHONOLOGY.

source features a classification in Chomsky and Halle's DISTINCTIVE FEATURES. The others are MAJOR CLASS FEATURES, cavity features, manner of articulation features and prosodic features. The features describe the modification which happens to the airstream producing voice and strident sounds. *See* Hyman (1975).

South Tyneside Assessment of Phonology (STAP) devised by Armstrong and Ainley in 1988, STAP is an assessment of the child's phonological development. The 27 pictures give 74 items to be named providing consonant phonemes and clusters in all positions appearing in more than one context. *See* Armstrong and Ainley (1988) in Appendix I.

South Tyneside Assessment of Syntactic Structures (STASS) devised by Armstrong and Ainley in 1988, STASS is an assessment of children's expressive speech. The 32 coloured illustrations are designed to elicit grammatical structures at clause, phrase and word levels in stages I–IV of the LARSP chart as well as auxiliary verbs, pronouns and prepositions. It is suitable for children in the age range of 3;00–7;00. *See* Armstrong and Ainley (1988) in Appendix I.

spastic cerebral palsy *see* CEREBRAL PALSY.

spastic dysarthria *see* DYSARTHRIA.

spastic dysphonia a type of DYSPHONIA in which the voice becomes strained and staccato owing to intermittent spasm of the vocal folds. It occurs equally frequently in men and women. The cause is not understood as there appears to be no obvious pathology. *See* Greene and Mathieson (1989).

spasticity a condition produced by a lesion to the upper motor neurons (*see* NEURONS) causing hypertonia, i.e. excessive tone of the muscles. The person's speech is characterised by spastic DYSARTHRIA. *See* Tortora and Grabowski (2000).

speak more fluently a technique of remediation for those who stammer. Little attention is paid to any underlying psychological causes. It concentrates on removing the stammer completely and making the person totally fluent. Therapists using this theory aim for total fluency – an ACCEPTABLE STAMMER is regarded as failure. The MONTEREY FLUENCY PROGRAMME is based on this theory, as is PROLONGED SPEECH. *See* Dalton (1983).

SpeakEasy a basic message system which can hold 12 single messages totalling 4 minutes and 20 seconds while six keys allow for 10-second messages, four keys allow for 20-second messages and two keys allow 60-second messages. Each of these can be accessed by a switch although there is no scanning. The device can be attached by a cable to toys which can be operated with auditory reinforcement. It can be carried by a shoulder strap. *See* Glennen and DeCoste (1997); Rumble and Larcher (1998); Appendix IV (AbleNet).

speaker's nodes/nodules *see* VOCAL NODULES.

special education a description of the education received by children who have varying degrees of LEARNING DISABILITY. The classes are often small, and outside agencies such as SPEECH AND LANGUAGE THERAPY, PHYSIOTHERAPY and PSYCHOLOGY are involved in the education of such children. However, it is becoming more usual for these children to be integrated into mainstream education with their own support teacher who works with them on a one-to-one basis, although there are subjects in which they participate with the rest of the class.

Special Needs Assessment Software devised by Douglas in 1990, it aims to establish the educational needs of young children with severe physical difficulties and/or LEARNING DISABILITY. There are two separate tests:

1. Cognitive development test: assesses the child's cognitive skills in such tests as visual discrimination matching, observational memory, visual sequencing, etc. Results can be interpreted using a criterion-referenced scoring system, or by comparison with norms for able bodied children aged 2;6–6;0 years.
2. Verbal comprehension test: a test of the child's language comprehension in such areas as the use of prepositions, verb tenses, adjective comprehension and use of number concepts. Interpretation of results is similar to that of the cognitive development test.

Responses for both tests can be made using any input device suitable for the child. The software can run on a BBC B or Master microcomputer with a single 40-track disk drive. A hard copy of the results can be obtained from a printer although the results also appear on the screen. *See* Douglas (1990) in Appendix I.

specific developmental language disorder (SDLD) a communication disorder affecting children. The causes are not the same as those which produce LANGUAGE DELAY. The child will have one of the following:

1. A phonological delay during the child's early years.
2. A grammatical problem with expressive language.
3. A high non-verbal IQ and a low verbal IQ.
4. Disorder of prosody.
5. Limited symbolic play.
6. Visual sequential memory superior to auditory sequential memory.

215

7. Degree of frustration from producing a language performance below the child's intellectual level.

If a child is to be diagnosed as suffering from SLI, he or she may or may not present with some of the following causes:

1. Developmental articulatory, verbal or constructional apraxia.
2. Minor neurological problems.
3. Comprehension problems.
4. LANDAU-KLEFFNER SYNDROME.
5. DYSLEXIA or DYSGRAPHIA.

This DIFFERENTIAL DIAGNOSIS from language delay, which has a different set of causes, can only be carried out by a speech and language therapist. SDLD must be differentiated from language delay if treatment is to be successful. There has been discussion about the educational provision for children who have SDLD in language units in the UK. *See* Wyke (1978); Stott et al (2002).

specific language impairment (SLI) a developmental deficit in language in the absence of a number of other diagnostic features such as hearing loss, autism, cerebral palsy, emotional disorder or environmental deprivation which accounts for approximately half a million children between the ages of 3;00–16;00 (AFASIC 1989 quoted in van der Lely 1993). Lely (op cit) described subgroups of SLI: those which include semantic pragmatic SLI, those with primarily phonological SLI and those with primarily grammatical SLI, which Haynes (1992) has called 'classic SLI'. Lely investigated a subgroup who had persistent grammatical deficits in both expression and comprehension of language. Her investigation aimed to find out the children's grammatical knowledge of sentence comprehension and, more precisely, their ability to learn the semantic and syntactic properties of verbs. She also carried out an investigation into verbal short-term memory and analysed the expressive morpho-grammatical characteristics of the children. Her results showed that the short-term memory abilities of children with SLI and those who had no SLI showed no difference. Her conclusion was that their problem with comprehension and expression may be caused by a specific linguistic deficit in one of the 'mechanisms' or modules in universal grammar and that this subgroup of SLI children may be unable to use syntactic cues to help learn semantic properties of verbs, but semantic cues may facilitate learning the syntactic properties of verbs. O'Hara (1997) showed that children with SLI were less adept at 'syntactic bootstrapping' (where children were asked to infer a meaning from a sentence with a novel verb in it, depending on its grammatical relation with the rest of the sentence) than those children developing language normally. One possible reason was processing errors. Sturn and Johnston (1999) made one of the first investigations into the cognitive functions of speech in children who have SLI. By giving their groups a bridge building exercise, they came up with results which, they stated themselves, need to be taken with caution. Their main conclusion seemed to be that whatever differences exist, in the reduction of use of modals or utterances relating to the bridge building task, they are due to a general reduction in the amount of speech rather than to any specific failure, or inability, to use speech in the service of thought. SLI is specific to language but during the last few years, there has been evidence to show non-linguistic cognitive difficulties including deficits in attention (Tallal et al 1989) and perceptual deficits (Tallal et al 1993) in children who have SLI. For example, Hill (2001), following a review of the literature relating language impairment to motor disorders, concludes that SLI is not *just* a specific disorder of language, but rather that children with SLI generally experience a broader range of difficulties, of which motor incoordination is one. Hammer et al (2001) investigated the difference in parenting and the interaction of parents between children of preschool and kindergarten age and that of parents whose children had SLI. They found that while ordinary conversational topics took place with equal frequencies between parents with normally developing language and those whose language was not following such developmental progress, differences existed where parents with the children developing language normally would read stories, discuss daily events, activities and feelings, parents with children who had SLI taught them the alphabet and interacted differently. However, the authors stress that this does not mean there is a causal link for SLI but the children's style may have had an effect on the parents' behaviours. Throughout the 1990s, there has been discussion about verb learning and verb use in preschool children with SLI which suggested that there are deficits in a number of areas including semantic, syntactic and morphological aspects supporting the claim that inordinate difficulties with verbs are a characteristic of SLI. However, in a study of 100 school-age children, Thordardottir and Weisman (2001) found that no differences were apparent between groups of children with SLI and those developing language normally in general lexical diversity or verb diversity in samples of a set number of tokens. They concluded that the results of their study did not suggest that verb diversity constitutes an area of specific deficit in spontaneous production for children with SLI and both groups could not be distinguished in their use of high-frequency verbs. It has been proposed that children with SLI have a problem developing their phonology system. In a study by Orsolini et al (2001), the authors showed that normal phonological development by children aged between 4–6 years is characterised by some difficulties with articulatory planning while the impaired phonological development of children with SLI is characterised by a coming together of different factors but not in a uniform way such

as an extremely slow articulatory development shown by a limited number of vocal actions, a deficit in building sequentially structured representations where an auditory-phonetic content has to be linked to articulatory patterns in a precise way and a difficulty in monitoring auditory stimuli. Anderson (2001) carried out a study into how children with SLI learn a morphologically rich language such as Spanish as there have been studies looking not just at learning morphology in English but also Italian and Hebrew. He found significant differences across the group of children who had SLI and the group of children developing language normally for both comprehension and production of the inflectional morpheme regardless of how it was taught to them. In a study investigating the use of lexical fields by children with SLI, Johnston et al (2001) carried out two studies where Study 1 analysed longitudinal language samples collected from 26 children with SLI and 25 children with normal language development aged 4;04 and 2;11 respectively while Study 2 analysed samples from children with SLI with more severe delays at an earlier language stage where there were 10 children with SLI and 10 children developing language normally. They found in the first study that SLI children used cognitive state predicates (those which refer directly or by implication to the knowledge state of the speaker, listener or a third party. The set consists of 30 entries including 'know', 'pretend', 'sure', 'think' and 'understand' less frequently than their mean age peers and with no greater frequency or variety than their younger, language peers while in the second study children with SLI used more predicates referring to communication events only. Their conclusion was that children with SLI provided no convincing evidence of advanced lexical usage throughout the domain of cognitive state predicates. Evans (2002) looked at strategies used by children with SLI to comprehend language. *See van der Lely*

(1993); O'Hara and Johnston (1997); Botting et al (1998a, b); Lindsay and Dockrell (1998); Nelson (1998); Greenhalgh and Mason (1998); Donlan (1998); Sturn and Johnston (1999); Anderson (2001); Botting and Conti-Ramsden (2001); Hammer et al (2001); Hill (2001); Johnston et al (2001); Orsolini, et al (2001); Thordardottir and Weismer (2001); Evans (2002).

spectrography an acoustic approach to representing all speech sounds in a way which shows the basic acoustic components which reflect the articulatory features of speech sounds. The spectrograph was invented in the late 1940s. Every sound consists of frequencies with each of these frequencies shown on the spectrograph. The spectrogram has a time scale along the horizontal axis while the frequency is measured down the vertical axis. The frequencies show up as light or dark marks depending on their intensity. In a typical spectrogram, there are dark bands known as formants, i.e. groups of harmonics whose intensity is greater than those of the surrounding harmonics. Each formant is numbered from the bottom of the spectrogram. The lowest formant is F1, while the next formant is F2, etc. It is the different frequencies of each formant which account for the different vowel sounds which are heard. See Ladefoged (2001).

speech acts speech acts describe the presumed intention of the speaker when expressing an utterance in relation to the hearer. Speakers may, for instance, be directive, commanding or requesting a hearer to do something. Or they may be expressive, in using utterances to convey their own feelings or attitudes, e.g. apologising, welcoming. Various other categories have been proposed. Searle has stated, 'speech acts are the basic or minimal units of linguistic communication' (Searle 1969, p. 16) *See* Searle (1969); Clark and Clark (1977); Fromkin and Rodman (2003).

speech and language therapist a term used in the UK to describe the person who assesses, diagnoses and treats people with communication disorders.

speech and language therapy the assessment, diagnosis and treatment of all types of communication disorders as well as DYSPHAGIA, DYSPHONIA and LARYNGECTOMY affecting both children and adults. In 1990, it was decided by a ballot of all members of the ROYAL COLLEGE OF SPEECH AND LANGUAGE THERAPISTS to change the name of the profession in the UK from speech therapy to speech and language therapy. *See* Crystal (1984).

speech audiometry audiometric tests used to find out the degree to which a person has speech recognition problems which cannot be discovered by using PURE-TONE AUDIOMETRY alone as well as identifying the benefits from having a hearing aid. The test comprises lists of single words, sentences, meaningless speech sounds known as logotoms or nonsense syllables. However, the vocabulary used needs to be within the cognitive and linguistic abilities of the person so that he/she can understand it. Although speech audiometers are not made specifically for carrying out these tests, a pure tone audiometer is used with a speech channel. The speech audiogram shows on the x-axis the level of the speech signal while on the y-axis there is the percentage of words or sounds recognised correctly. For each point on the audiogram one complete list of the test material must be used. Speech audiometry is particularly important in assessing the ability of a child to recognise speech and may have important implications for their education. Toy tests may be used with very young children. When assessing an adult's suitability for a COCHLEAR IMPLANT, sentence recognition tests using hearing aids play a vital part in deciding if an implant is going to be of greater benefit than the use of a hearing aid. *See* Hood (1981); Martin (1997); Ballantyne and Martin (2001).

speech chain the means by which a speaker transmits information to a listener. The speaker forms an utterance by selecting the words and making up the correct order in the BRAIN. This is the performance part of the speech chain. These words are sent by nerve impulses along the VOCAL TRACT, uttered by the articulators, whereupon they are transferred into sound waves. These waves are acoustic energy which are sent across the gap between speaker and listener. The latter receives them through the EAR where they undergo a physiological change in the form of nerve impulses to the brain where they are decoded so that the listener can understand the utterance. Thus, one human can communicate through the medium of speech to another human – a feature of man's existence which raises him above other animal life. In speech and language therapy, the therapist has often to find out which part of this chain is broken, e.g. the route taken by the nerve impulses to activate the facial nerve (*see* CRANIAL NERVE VII) and muscles of the tongue is interrupted as in DYSARTHRIA. It could also be that the person has difficulty in formulating an utterance either by not finding the required word to use or not being able to put the words in the correct order, as in APHASIA, or it may be the feedback system which does not function, as with a HEARING LOSS. When this broken link is found by ASSESSMENT, a TREATMENT PROGRAMME can begin to repair it. *See* Denes and Pinson (1993).

speech discrimination test a test used in SPEECH AUDIOMETRY for assessing the person's ability to understand speech at levels above the threshold of hearing. Usually lists of 10 words are presented to the person. The words have been phonetically balanced. One list is presented at ±30 dB above the SPEECH RECEPTION THRESHOLD. Correct repetitions are scored as percentages. The next list is presented at 10 dB higher followed by another list at 10 dB higher than the previous list. The curve of discrimination scores is shown on a graph. *See* Hood (1981).

speech pathology

1. The title used for speech and language therapy in the US and Canada.
2. The study of disordered communication.

speech pattern audiometry an audiological test to find out the person's ability to perceive speech, making use of the acoustic speech pattern information fundamental to speech perception by decoding the complex waveform into a set of speech patterns. Particular speech patterns are very important in signalling certain features of the sound and constitute acoustic cues. MINIMAL PAIRS are used, e.g., 'pea' and 'key', manipulating elements of the speech pattern but keeping a degree of speech naturalness since speech synthesis is used from the computer. The person undergoing the test is asked to press the picture of the word on a touch-sensitive response box. Speech pattern audiometry goes a stage further than discrimination tests which only assess the ability to hear a difference between two sounds whereas in speech pattern audiometry the person is assigning the sound to a specific phonemic category which is central to the process of speech perception. *See* Hazan et al (1995).

speech perception the way in which sound segments are interpreted by an individual depending on acoustic features of phonemes or longer phrases. *See* Denes and Pinson (1993).

speech production *see* ARTICULATION; CARDINAL VOWEL SYSTEM; SPECTROGRAPHY; VOCAL FOLDS.

speech reception threshold (SRT) the level in dB, at which 50 per cent of bisyllabic words are repeated accurately. Three words are presented at a level of ±25 dB above PTA. The person repeats the words and then the test level descends in 5 dB steps until the person fails to repeat one or more words. This is followed by six words at each level. The SRT is the level at which three or four words out of six are repeated correctly. *See* Hood (1981).

219

speech synthesis the production of speech by use of a microprocessor to simulate the human voice. It is also called voice synthesis. The quality of the speech output depends on the cost of the synthesiser used. During 1989 and 1990, researchers at the Microcomputer Centre at Dundee University were trying to develop a speech synthesiser to produce emotion in speech. Thus, if the operator produces the statement on the computer 'I am happy', the speech output will sound happy and a similar outcome will happen for other emotions such as 'sadness', 'doubting', etc. At the present time, DECTALK is regarded as being the best speech synthesiser available and is being used with many voice output communication aids. *See* Bishop (1985); Mirenda and Beukelman (1987); Keller (1994); Mirenda and Beukelman (1990); Crabtree et al (1990); Venkatagari (1991); Raghavendra (1993); Higgenbotham et al (1994); McNaughton (1994); Fucci et al (1995); Higgenbotham and Baird (1995); Scherz and Beer (1995); Sutton et al (1995); Venkatagari and Ramabadran (1995) (digital speech synthesis); Reynolds and Jefferson (1996); Glennen and DeCoste (1997); Govenflo and Govenflo (1997); Koul and Hanners (1997); Reynolds and Jefferson (1999); Reynolds et al (2000); Drager and Reichie (2001); Ratcliff et al (2002) (speech naturalness in AAC).

spina bifida a congenital abnormality of the SPINAL CORD. The most common condition is spina bifida occulta. It occurs between the lumbar vertebrae and the sacral vertebrae. There is a failure in the fusion of the vertebral arch and an abnormality in the overlying skin. Twenty per cent of children with a closed lesion have normal intelligence and no physical handicaps. HYDROCEPHALUS commonly develops in children with spina bifida. According to recent research, children with spina bifida form the largest subgroup of the hydrocephalic population. In the USA, research was undertaken to find out if there were language problems in this group. It had been thought that these children had an inability to produce utterances that met basic semantic-pragmatic requirements. This problem takes several forms:

1. Production of numerous utterances of the topic or task in hand.
2. Utterances are often over-personalised.
3. Production of automatic social phrases such as 'thank you' and 'how are you' at an abnormally high rate and inappropriately.
4. Frequent imitation of words and phrases of others rather than answering questions or otherwise contributing to the discussion.
5. Utterances are often semantically anomalous or bizarre. There were also thought to be problems in comprehension as well as expressive language.

Syntax was at the age-appropriate level although there were semantic-pragmatic problems. The conclusions of the study were that, although children with spina bifida hydrocephalus may have some language difficulties, those who are intellectually normal do not have such problems – at least in the semantic-pragmatic domain. The authors propose it may be the degree of associated LEARNING DISABILITY that accounts for linguistic difficulties. *See* Hosking (1982); Byrne et al (1990); http://www.asbah.org/index.html

spinal cord a cylinder-like structure which is situated in the canal of the vertebral column. It is about 45 cm long and about 1 cm wide. It extends up the magnum foramen to the MEDULLA OBLONGATA. At the end of the spinal cord is the causa equina (a collection of lumbosacral roots); in the middle of these roots is the filum terminale which attaches to the coccyx. There are two enlargements which enervate the limbs:

1. Cervical enlargement supplies the upper limbs.
2. Lumbosacral enlargement supplies the lower limbs.

It is composed of grey and white matter. *See* Barr (1988); Kolb and Whishaw (1996); Tortora and Grabowski (2000).

spontaneous recovery spontaneous recovery occurs without the intervention of professional skills. It can occur during the first 2–6 months following the onset of a disorder such as APHASIA, but some people may not go through spontaneous recovery. *See* Eisenson (1984).

spontaneous speech a description of language which a person produces every day. It is opposed to elicited language (*see* ELICITATION) or speech where the therapist is trying to get the person to say particular words or phrases. A language assessment, whether it is formal or informal, should always include a subtest from which an analysis could be made of the person's spontaneous speech.

spread an aspect of lip movement when producing vowels such as [i, e, ɛ, a] found in the primary CARDINAL VOWEL SYSTEM. It is opposed to lip rounding. *See* Ladefoged (2001).

spreadsheet a means of making calculations using tables of figures, e.g. producing annual accounts, keeping running totals for budgets. It can scroll both horizontally and vertically if there is not enough space on the screen to take the full spreadsheet. The computer carries out calculations when certain formulae are used. These formulae may vary according to the particular spreadsheet being used. *See* Bishop (1985).

Springboard a high-tech communication aid which uses MINSPEAK with a dynamic display and digitised speech. It has up to 50 minutes recording time and can be used in 4, 8, 15 or 32 locations. There is a dynamic activity row for extended vocabulary and it has a battery life of 8–10 hours. It can be used with UNITY or an adapted version of LANGUAGE, LEARNING AND LIVING. *See* Appendix IV (Prentke Romich Company).

SRT *see* SPEECH RECEPTION THRESHOLD.

stammer a disorder of fluency which appears to have a multifactorial aetiology. Consequently there are many theories of intervention. Chief among putative causes are: (1) organic factors such as minimal brain damage; a forced change in cerebral dominance (*see* DOMINANCE; heredity or IQ level; (2) neurotic causes in the form of emotional predisposition; a compulsive neurosis; CONVERSION REACTION or learnt behaviour. This last proposition makes use of CLASSICAL CONDITIONING and OPERANT CONDITIONING. Avoidance reaction is another psychological cause which has been proposed. However, nowadays it is argued that stammering could be caused by a combination of some of these factors. Treatment techniques fall into two main theories – SPEAK MORE FLUENTLY and STAMMER MORE FLUENTLY. *See* Dalton (1983).

stammer more fluently a treatment approach used with those who have a STAMMER. It takes into account the underlying psychological symptoms which may affect the stammerer. One of the major therapeutic techniques used is van Riper's BLOCK MODIFICATION. This approach is also known as stutter more fluently. *See* Dalton (1983).

standard deviation a measure of dispersion of all the values from the MEAN. The greater the dispersion of the values, the bigger the standard deviation. This means that measuring the difference of values from the mean will give us negative and positive deviations. Each deviation is squared to give the variance but to get the deviation back to the same units as the observed values, we take the square root of the variance. *See* Miller (1984).

standard score a score obtained in various assessments from the RAW SCORE. It is based on the STANDARD DEVIATION. *See* Smith et al (2003).

Standard theory an early form of TRANS-FORMATIONAL GRAMMAR (TG) proposed by Chomsky (1965) (*see* CHOMSKYAN LINGUISTICS). In it he proposed a deep structure from which, by a series of transformations, a surface structure would appear. It is the surface structure which is spoken or written. *See* Chomsky (1965); Huddleston (1976).

standardisation *see* STANDARDISED TESTS.

standardised tests to standardise a test it must be given to a large number of the population covering the age range for which it is intended to be used. In this way, the tester can discover the most frequent or normal responses of the different age groups, and thence be enabled to compare the scores obtained from those with a particular disorder with those of the norm for the age groups. In some tests, the mental age and resulting IQ can also be calculated.

Stanford-Binet Intelligence Scales assessments to test children's intelligence levels. Binet published his first test in 1905 with the help of Theodore Simon (1873–1961), a French psychologist. These tests became known throughout the world and translations into English followed. The scale, which became widely used, had been translated and adapted by Lewis Terman of Stanford University. Terman introduced the INTELLIGENCE QUOTIENT to the scales, while Stern, a German psychologist, proposed the IQ scale. There have been three editions subsequently since 1916. The latest edition (4th edition) was published in 1985. Its age range is similar to that of the other editions – 2 years to adulthood. It tests four areas:

1. Cognitive ability.
2. Verbal reasoning.
3. Quantitative reasoning.
4. Abstract/visual reasoning and short-term memory.

The scale comprises 15 subtests: vocabulary, comprehension, verbal relations, pattern analysis, matrices, paper folding and cutting, copying, quantities, number series, equation building, memory for digits, sentences, objects and beads. *See* Aiken (1988).

stapedectomy the removal of the stapes (*see* EAR) by surgery. *See* Pracy et al (1974).

stapedius reflex *see* IMPEDANCE AUDIOMETRY.

stapes *see* EAR.

Starset software which allows the operator to produce or adapt computer programs for use with the concept keyboard.

statementing following the 1981 Education Act, Education Authorities have a statutory obligation to see that SPECIAL EDUCATION is provided for all those children in need. To this end a multidisciplinary assessment is carried out and a written statement of advice is given. This formal statement is reviewed annually. Children with language impairment are included in this process.

static impedance *see* IMPEDANCE AUDIOMETRY.

statistics the discipline which produces ways of measuring random samples allowing inferences to be drawn from the data about the population as a whole from which it came. There are two main types of statistics – INFERENTIAL STATISTICS and DESCRIPTIVE STATISTICS. In the former, measures of CENTRAL TENDENCY and dispersion are used, while in the latter parametric and non-parametric tests (*see* PARAMETRIC TESTS) are used to analyse the data obtained from experiments. *See* Miller (1984); Smith et al (2003).

status epilepticus *see* EPILEPSY.

Step-by-Step communicator a light tech system similar to the ONE STEP COMMUNICATOR but with the capacity to take up to 45 messages recorded in a maximum of 75 seconds. The messages can be accessed by direct manual selection or with a single switch attached to it and can be accessed only in the order in which they were recorded. *See* Rumble and Larcher (1998); Appendix IV (AbleNet).

Step-by-Step with Levels communicator a light tech system similar to the STEP-BY-STEP COMMUNICATOR but it can be used on different levels for different types of information, songs, poems or whatever. There can be as many levels as the person wants within the 75 seconds. *See* Appendix IV (AbleNet).

Stepping Stones devised by Robertson, Stepping Stones is a keyword MINSPEAK APPLICATION PROGRAM using 32 icons, which can be used on an ALPHA TALKER, DELTA TALKER, LIBERATOR COMMUNICATION AID or PATHFINDER. It is a precursor to using the whole 128-location LANGUAGE, LEARNING AND LIVING (LLL) programme teaching similar icon sequences although not having the grammatical element of LLL. In 2002, Robertson also designed a version of Stepping Stones for the SPRINGBOARD communication aid. *See* Robertson (1995, 2002).

sternocleidomastoid muscle a muscle in the neck which runs from behind the EAR to the clavicle. *See* Tortora and Grabowski (2000).

sternohyoid muscle *see* LARYNX.

stirrup *see* EAR.

stoma a hole left in the neck after LARYNGECTOMY or TRACHEOTOMY. It is used for breathing. If a person who has had this operation collapses, mouth-to-mouth resuscitation will not help, he will have to be given mouth-to-stoma resuscitation. People who have undergone this operation can produce OESOPHAGEAL VOICE by occluding the stoma. *See* Edels (1984).

stop a description of a sound which is produced by a complete blocking of the vocal tract. Thus, stops can be used to classify plosives (*see* ARTICULATION). *See* Ladefoged (2001).

stress

1. *See* SUPRASEGMENTAL PHONOLOGY.
2. *See* HYSTERIA.

striated muscle voluntary muscle tissue, striated or skeletal muscle is attached mainly to bones and moves parts of the skeleton. It is known as voluntary muscle because it can contract or relax under conscious control and is called striated because of the alternating dark and light striations which are found under microscopic examination. It is innervated by the somatic nervous system. *See* Leeson et al (1985); Tortora and Grabowski (2000).

strident a DISTINCTIVE FEATURE proposed by Chomsky and Halle to distinguish sounds produced with high frequency and intensity (*see* ACOUSTIC PHONETICS) as in [f, s, ʃ, ʒ] [+STRIDENT] from those produced with low frequency and intensity [−STRIDENT]. It is opposed to non-strident. *See* Hyman (1975).

stroke the layman's term for CEREBROVASCULAR ACCIDENT (CVA).

structural brain disease a possible cause of EPILEPSY. Almost any disease of the BRAIN which produces a focus for discharging neurons will cause epileptic convulsions. The disease could be due to a TUMOUR OF THE CENTRAL NERVOUS SYSTEM, a BRAIN ABSCESS or degenerative disorders causing degeneration of neurons, etc. *See* Ginsbergh (1999).

structured programming a method of designing a program which breaks the task down into functional units or modules and builds the program from these modules. This is also called top-down programming.

Sturge-Weber syndrome its main characteristics are a port-wine naevus on the scalp, and other vascular abnormalities both intracranially and elsewhere in the body. These may produce LEARNING DISABILITY (about 30 per cent), HEMIPLEGIA (about 30–40 per cent) and EPILEPSY (about 90 per cent). *See* Salmon (1978); http://www.sturgeweber.org.uk/

stutter *see* STAMMER.

Stuttering Prediction Instrument for Young Children devised by Riley, the instrument is designed to let clinicians determine the severity and potential chronicity of childhood dysfluency and can be used with children between 3 and 11 years of age. There are five sections including the history of the child; the child's, parents' and others' reactions to the child's stammer; part-word repetitions; prolongations and the frequency of the stammer. *See* Beech et al (1993).

Stuttering Severity Instrument for Children and Adults devised by Riley, the instrument is a STANDARDISED assessment of the quantity and quality of the dysfluency and can be used with either children or adults. It measures three parameters:

1. Frequency of repetition, prolongation of sounds and syllables.
2. Estimated duration of the longest blocks.
3. Observable physical concomitants.

The scores from these categories give a RAW SCORE, and the total is converted into a PERCENTILE SCORE and severity rating. The tape records speech samples for analysis and the therapist notes any EXTRANEOUS MOVEMENTS rating them from 0 (none) to 5 (severe and painful). *See* Beech et al (1993).

stuttering stages a description, proposed by van Riper, of the sequences found in stammerers as their dysfluency progresses:

1. Primary stuttering stage: easy repetitions of words and syllables of a sentence without emotion or stress.
2. Secondary stuttering stage: the person becomes more conscious of his DYSFLUENCY and begins to anticipate the situation in which the person will stammer.
3. Transitional stuttering stage: occurs between the primary and secondary stages in which emotions accompany the easy repetitions of the primary stuttering stage.

See Dalton and Hardcastle (1989).

Stycar Hearing Test devised by Sheridan to be used with children between the ages of 6 months and 7 years. It uses very simple and familiar objects, words and pictures. Its aim is to test the child's ability to hear meaningful speech with different frequency and intensity components. The test contains several different subtests for different age groups. These subtests take the form of toy tests, cube tests, doll vocabulary, picture vocabulary, word lists and sentences. Thus, the tester can identify sounds which are producing difficulties for the child. *See* Sheridan (1973) in Appendix I.

Stycar Language Test devised by Sheridan to assess the normal development of children concerning comprehension, expression and use of language forms such as mime, models, picture and especially spoken-verbal language. It can be used with 'normal' children (1–7 years) and older children with developmental delay. It uses real objects, toys and pictures and the child's performance is recorded descriptively. The clinician makes a detailed observation of the child's ability to use 'language codes' such as verbal, gestural and two-dimensional as well as other symbolic activity such as play and other aspects of development such as physical manipulation. There are three tests: Common Objects Test, Miniature Toy Test and Picture Book Test. *See* Sheridan (1976) in Appendix I; Beech et al (1993).

Stycar Tests devised by Sheridan in 1973, this is a series of assessments plotting normal development from birth to 5;0 years. Four parameters of development are examined: motor, vision, hearing and speech, and social and play development.

styloglossus muscle *see* EXTRINSIC MUSCLES OF THE TONGUE.

stylohyoid muscle *see* MUSCLES FOR SWALLOWING.

styloid process a projection found in the skull which extends down and forward from the temporal bone and measures 2 cm long and 3 mm wide. It is the attachment point for muscles and ligaments which are marked by using stylo- as a prefix to their complete name. *See* Tortora and Grabowski (2000).

stylopharyngeus muscle *see* MUSCLES FOR SWALLOWING.

subarachnoid space this is the space which contains the CEREBROSPINAL FLUID and is enclosed by the arachnoid membrane. Berry aneurysms (*see* CERE-BROVASCULAR ACCIDENT) cause bleeding into the subarachnoid space. *See* Barr (1988).

subglottic a description of the position of all structures or lesions below the GLOTTIS. It is opposed to supraglottic.

sublingual salivary gland *see* SALIVARY GLANDS.

submandibular salivary gland *see* SALIVARY GLANDS.

submucous cleft palate *see* CLEFT PALATE.

suction a DISTINCTIVE FEATURE proposed by Chomsky and Halle to describe sounds made in a specific way by the GLOTTIS and velum such as implosives and clicks (*see* VELARIC AIRSTREAM) [+SUCTION]. *See* Hyman (1975).

suffix MORPHOLOGY identifies separate units which are used in the formation of words. Those that occur at the ends of words are referred to as suffixes, e.g. '-ness' in 'happiness', '-er' in 'robber', '-s' in 'hats', etc. *See* Matthews (1974).

sulcus in the BRAIN, a sulcus appears as a groove surrounded by elevated areas called gyri (*see* GYRUS). *See* Barr (1988); Kolb and Whishaw (1996).

sulcus terminalis *see* TONGUE.

superego *see* PERSONALITY.

Superhawk a high-tech communication aid which allows for 120 messages each of up to 5 seconds in length in 72 levels and using between 1 to 72 locations. Overlays can be set up so that the person using the system can choose vocabulary between the different levels. Adapted toys and appliances can also be operated from it. It can be accessed by direct manual selection or by attaching four separate switches which activate four specific locations. Memory will not be lost if the batteries lose their charge completely. *See* Rumble and Larcher (1998); Appendix IV (AdamLab).

superior constrictor muscle *see* PHARYNX.

supplementary movements a classification for DISTINCTIVE FEATURES proposed by Chomsky and Halle. They are used to distinguish manner of articulation (*see* ARTICULATION). The two distinctive fea-

tures subsumed by this term are SUCTION and pressure which describe such sounds as EJECTIVES, IMPLOSIVES and clicks. *See* Hyman (1975).

suppurative otitis media *see* OTITIS MEDIA.

supraglottic a description of the position of the structures or lesions found above the GLOTTIS. It is opposed to subglottic.

suprasegmental phonology the study of stress and intonation. Stress often marks the difference between verbs and nouns, e.g. re'cord/'record; (') is the diacritic used to mark stress. A speaker's intonation contours are usually described in terms of pitch direction, e.g. fall–rise. The pitch range could be higher or lower than the average range or widened or narrowed until it becomes a monotone. A tone group is the part of the sentence which contains changes in pitch. In the tone group, there is normally one single syllable which receives a major pitch change – the tonic syllable or nuclear syllable. The direction change of the tonic syllable, also known as the nucleus, is most important in understanding speech since it usually gives information concerning attitudes of the speaker:

`yes (falling)	–	the answer is 'yes'
´yes (high-rise)	–	did you say 'yes'
‚yes (low-rise)	–	please go on, I'm listening
ˇyes (fall-rise)	–	I'm doubtful
^yes (rise-fall)	–	I'm certain
		(based on Ladefoged).

Thus, a person can show by changing their way of producing the tonic syllable the meaning of what they say. Some people who have DYSARTHRIA have lost the distinctions used in stress and intonation patterns and so cannot make changes to meaning as exemplified above. *See* Fromkin and Rodman (2003); Ladefoged (2001).

surface structure *see* TRANSFORMATIONAL GRAMMAR.

swallowing the transfer of the food bolus from the MOUTH to the stomach avoiding the airway, i.e. the TRACHEA. It is also known as the process of deglutition. The bolus goes through stages before it reaches the stomach after it is prepared by the saliva from the SALIVARY GLANDS:

1. Oral stage: the food is chewed in the mouth and prepared into a bolus. It is transferred to the back of the mouth by the tip of the tongue being raised towards the alveolar ridge. As the tongue contracts, the bolus is moved near the PHARYNX. This is a wholly voluntary process.
2. Pharyngeal stage: the bolus leaves the mouth and enters the oropharynx (see PHARYNX), the muscles of which are stimulated from the MEDULLA OBLONGATA via the glossopharyngeal nerve (see CRANIAL NERVES). The bolus could leave this area by four potential routes – the mouth, nasopharynx (see PHARYNX), LARYNX/TRACHEA or OESOPHAGUS but muscle contraction closes off all the exits except the one to the oesophagus.
3. Oesophageal stage: the bolus reaches the top of the oesophagus. As it is a flat tube, the bolus has to wait for the muscle at the top to relax and produce a contraction to push the bolus into it. The bolus is propelled down the oesophagus by a series of peristaltic waves. When the bolus reaches the lower end of the oesophagus, there is a sphincter into the stomach which the last peristaltic contraction opens to allow the bolus to enter into the stomach.

See Tortora and Grabowski (2000).

sweep testing see SCREENING AUDIOMETRY.

switches most high-tech communication aids and specially designed computer software can be operated by various kinds of switches for those who cannot operate the communication aid or computer by the keyboard. Particular companies which produce communication aids often produce switches designed for their own aids. However, nearly all the switches produced are similar in their function. The most common

switches used are:

1. Plate switch: by touching a rocking plate the aid can be operated. In some models, it may be a double switch so that the person can operate the device in two ways.
2. Foot switch: for gross foot movement.
3. Joystick: allows for scanning up/down, side to side and diagonally, or any combination of these. There are four-way and eight-way joysticks.
4. Wobblesticks: can be hit in any direction to operate the scanning. Used with those who have gross uncontrollable movements.
5. Head-operated: either microswitches can be placed on a neck halter so that the person can operate them with the chin, or a switch can be attached to the back of the chair and can be operated by head movement.
6. Flexitube switch: operated by the person sucking or blowing down the tube.

It is important that the therapist carries out a good motor assessment, so that the appropriate switch can be chosen to help the person use the communication aid or computer. See Enderby (1987); Glennen and DeCoste (1997); Beukelman and Mirenda (1998).

syllable a unit of speech which is longer than a sound but shorter than a word. Each unit can be pronounced as a single unit as in 'pic-ture'. A syllable has been described in different ways. One way of describing it is as an increase in the pressure in the speaker's lungs and as being more sonorous than other parts of the word. In PHONOLOGY, the syllable is described in terms of PHONOTACTICS. See Fromkin and Rodman (2003); Ladefoged (2001).

Symbolic Play Test devised by Lowe and Costello in 1976 (revised 2nd edition 1988), it is an observational assessment for very young children and provides information about symbolic and conceptual development. It takes the form of a collection of small toys with which the child plays. The level of play is assessed against a checklist. There is practically no verbal requirement on the part of either the assessor or the child. *See* Lowe and Costello (1988) in Appendix I; Lewis et al (1992); Beech et al (1993).

symbolisation *see* SENSORIMOTOR STAGE.

sympathetic nervous system one of the two divisions of the AUTONOMIC NERVOUS SYSTEM becoming highly active when the person becomes very excited. Thus, it is often known as the 'fight, fright, flight' system. The chemical transmitted to the muscle is noradrenaline. As part of the AUTONOMIC NERVOUS SYSTEM (ANS), it innervates SMOOTH MUSCLE. *See* Green (1978); Tortora and Grabowski (2000).

symphysis menti *see* MANDIBLE.

synapse a junction between two nerves where there is a transfer of nerve impulses by the emission of chemicals from one to another. *See* Green (1978); Kolb and Whishaw (1996).

synchronic linguistics *see* SAUSSURE.

syndrome a grouping of several characteristic clinical features common to a particular disease or condition. *See* Tortora and Grabowski (2000).

syntactic-pragmatic syndrome a rare disorder in which there is gross impairment of syntax and severely restricted pragmatic use of language. Comprehension is also limited. Phonology may be normal or near normal.

syntagmatic relations the linear description of sentences. Rules define the order in which elements occur. *See* Lyons (1968).

syntax grammar is sometimes subdivided into MORPHOLOGY, the study of the formation of words, and syntax, the study of the formation of sentences. Within this very general definition, there are a variety of approaches in the modern era to the characterisation of the structure of sentences. *See also* GENERATIVE GRAMMAR and CASE GRAMMAR. *See* Lyons (1968); Stockwell (1977); Fromkin and Rodman (2003).

synthesised speech *see* SPEECH SYNTHESIS.

systematic desensitisation a BEHAVIOUR THERAPY based on CLASSICAL CONDITIONING. It has as its aim the gradual reduction of a learned anxiety. The client tells the therapist what is causing the anxiety. He is relaxed and asked to rate his fear on a fear thermometer. Thus, the therapist can construct an anxiety hierarchy. As the client continues to relax he is asked to imagine the least feared stimulus and after it has been overcome due to the relaxation, the next most feared stimulus is treated similarly and so on. However, it is uncertain for how long fears can be extinguished using this procedure. *See* Smith et al (2003).

t-groups a therapeutic technique used in the sensitivity training approach to social skill training. In these groups, the clients make their own decisions as the therapist takes a back seat. Clients have to make up their minds who is going to be a group leader and what their feelings for each other are, while some may fail to participate completely. If necessary, the therapist will show them how to express such feelings for each other and their reactions to each other, and will encourage openness. The clients themselves may provide a model. *See* Trower et al (1978).

t-**tests** a parametric (*see* PARAMETRIC TESTS) statistical test which measures the two factors of difference in means and the standard error of the difference in means. While values should conform to a NORMAL DISTRIBUTION and have the same variance or homogeneity of variance, the *t*-test is robust sufficiently to take account of any contravention of these two conditions. The independent *t*-test is used when analysing results after using the INDEPENDENT GROUP DESIGN while the *t*-test for related samples is used after using the REPEATED MEASURES DESIGN. *See* Miller 1984).

TACL *see* TEST FOR AUDITORY COMPREHENSION OF LANGUAGE.

tactile a description of the action of touching an object. *See* Kolb and Whishaw (1996); Tortora and Grabowski (2000).

tag question a structure with interrogative form which is placed at the end of an utterance and has a particular discourse function:

1. It's raining, isn't it?
2. She isn't coming, is she?

Generally, the tag question in English (other languages, e.g. French, with an unchanging structure, *n'est-ce pas*, provide a simpler form) is a subject pronoun which matches the number and gender of the subject noun phrase of the sentence to which it is attached. It also generally repeats the auxiliary verb of the main sentence but has reverse polarity to the main sentence (though there are exceptions to both these statements). The tag has a conversational function in seeking or encouraging a response by one's conversational partner. The type of response depends on the intonation of the tag. *See* Brown and Miller (1991).

Talking Lifestyles devised by Whitton and Zloch, a vocabulary package for the ORAC communication aid. It is designed to give users a vocabulary to suit their needs. The overlay is divided into three areas for grammatical parts of speech, the symbols where the majority of the vocabulary is stored and alternate keys which produce opposites etc. There are over 20000 pre-stored words, phrases and messages on a 128-overlay. *See* Whitton and Zloch (1995).

Talking Screen for Windows a dynamic communication system which uses symbols. Pages of symbols are linked together in a vocabulary structure similar to a communication book. The symbols can be used to access messages using SPEECH SYNTHESIS, DIGITISED SPEECH, video clips, and environmental controls. Talking Screen uses PICTURE COMMUNICATION SYMBOLS (PCS) as well as REBUS or BLISSYMBOLS. Pages can have from one symbol up to a total of 128 pictures. *See* Glennen and DeCoste (1997); Appendix 4 (Words+).

TalksBac devised by Waller and her colleagues at the University of Dundee, Scotland, TalksBac is a computerised, word-based system designed for people who have nonfluent aphasia but can recognise familiar words and short sentences. There are two programmes: the 'carer' programme where personal sentences and stories are typed into the TalksBac database while the 'user' programme allows the person using the system to retrieve these conversational items by offering probable items based on previous use of the system since the system adapts itself to usage by individuals. *See* Waller et al (1998); Appendix IV (Don Johnston Development Equipment Inc.).

TalkTrac a small communication aid using DIGITISED SPEECH allowing for four messages to be stored on it with a maximum recording time of 75 seconds. It uses a rechargeable battery. It fits around the wrist of a child or adult. *See* Appendix IV (AbleNet).

tamber *see* TIMBRE.

Tana Talker a small communication aid which allows for 11 different messages to be stored into it by the person's facilitator. Each message can be changed when required. *See* Appendix IV (Hartana Developments Ltd.)

target a description of the correct production of a sound. It is opposed to REALISATION.

taste the tongue is the organ in the body which is responsible for the sense of taste. For this purpose, it is divided into the following parts:

1. The anterior two-thirds of the tongue detects a bitter taste and is innervated by cranial nerve VII (*see* CRANIAL NERVES).
2. The posterior one-third of the tongue detects a salt/sweet taste and is innervated by cranial nerve IX (*see* CRANIAL NERVES).
3. The anterior two-thirds of the tongue (except the taste buds) are supplied by the chorda tympani nerve, a branch of cranial nerve VII (*see* CRANIAL NERVES).

See Green (1978); Smith et al (2003); Tortora and Grabowski (2000).

taste buds these produce the sensation of taste and are found in the papillae which cover the anterior two-thirds of the tongue. There are three types of papillae:

1. Circumvallate papillae: mushroom-shaped and surrounded by a ditch or moat in which are found rows of taste buds (8–12 in a row) in front of the sulcus terminalis.
2. Fungiform papillae: little puff-like balls with a moat around them in which are found more taste buds.
3. Filiform papillae: small, conical-shaped lumps which contain no taste buds.

The taste buds are supplied by cranial nerve IX (*see* CRANIAL NERVES). *See* Tortora and Grabowski (2000).

teacher's nodes/nodules *see* VOCAL NODULES.

Teaching Talking devised by Locke and Beech in 1992, Teaching Talking allows for structured screening and intervention programmes to help teachers in mainstream nursery, infant and junior schools. It is suitable to be used with children between the ages of 3 and 11 years. *See* Locke and Beech (1992) in Appendix I.

teeth bone-like excrescences developing out of the jaw. Their function is to chew food and grind it down into smaller pieces for digestion. Each person has 32 teeth: eight incisors, four canines, eight premolars and 12 molars. *See* Tortora and Grabowski (2000).

Teflon injection a method whereby Teflon is injected in a paralysed vocal fold to provide an increase in mass and thus facilitate approximation with the normally functioning vocal fold. It is used in the treatment of LARYNGEAL NERVE PALSIES. *See* Freeman and Fawcus (2001).

Tellus 2 a computer-based system which can be used as a communication aid when communication software is loaded into it. It uses a touchscreen although it can also be accessed by joystick, mouse or trackball and SCANNING using one or two switches. There is also an option for auditory scanning. The person using the system can also import their own photographs and drawings as well as recording their own sounds and messages or their favourite songs by another person. The Tellus 2 has a built-in word processor and is linked to icons, can be wheelchair mounted and has an infrared transmitter so that the person using it can operate the TV, video, etc. or whatever is operated by an infra-red hand control. *See* Appendix IV (Technology and Integration).

tempo *see* RATE.

temporal lobe *see* CEREBRAL HEMISPHERES.

temporalis muscle *see* MUSCLES OF MASTICATION.

temporary tracheostomy *see* TRACHEOTOMY.

temporomandibular joint the joint between the temporal and mandibular bones. It allows the jaw to open and close.

temporomandibular joint syndrome the failure of the joint to allow the jaw to open and close which leads to difficulty in chewing (*see* MUSCLES OF MASTICATION). There may be other characteristics to the syndrome affecting the person's hearing as well as causing discomfort in the muscles and a clicking of the joint. *See* Tortora and Grabowski (2000).

tensor veli palatini muscle the muscle which operates the soft palate (*see* MOUTH) and is shaped like a triangle as it starts from the skull and runs along the Eustachian tube (*see* EAR). It has its apex at the pterygoid hamulus. Its nerve supply comes from cranial nerve Viii (*see* CRANIAL NERVES). Its functions are to open the auditory tube and, on contraction, to tense the soft palate (*see* MOUTH). *See* Watson et al (2001).

Test for Auditory Comprehension of Language (TACL) devised by Carrow-Woolfolk in 1976 (revised 1985 and 1998), it is an assessment which has been standardised to test the child's auditory verbal understanding of semantic, syntactic and morphological structures. It takes the form of line drawings and involves the selection of one out of four in response to an auditory stimulus. It covers an age range of 3;00–9;00 years. Raw scores can be converted into STANDARD SCORES, AGE-EQUIVALENT SCORES or PERCENTILE SCORES. It is standardised on a North American population. *See* Carrow-Woolfolk (1998) in Appendix I; Beech et al (1993).

Test for Reception of Grammar (TROG) devised by Bishop in 1984, it is a formal, standardised assessment to test children's auditory verbal comprehension. However, it can be used to gain a more in-depth analysis of an aphasic person's auditory verbal comprehension, although it has not been standardised for this population. The material consists of 80 line drawings which are divided into four blocks of 20, each containing four test sentences of increasing syntactic complexity. All four items in each section must be correct before proceeding to the next level. Scoring is either according to AGE-EQUIVALENT SCORES or PERCENTILE SCORES when used with children. *See* Bishop (1984); Beech et al (1993).

Test of Language Competence – Expanded Edition (TLC-Expanded) devised by Wiig and Secord, TLC-Expanded combines the Test of Language Competence with a downward extension for children between the ages of 5;00–9;00. This allows for the assessment of emerging METALINGUISTIC abilities and linguistic strategy acquisition in children and adolescents from 5;00– 18;00. Emphasis is placed on assessing a child's ability to perceive, interpret and respond to the contextual and situational demands of conversation in addition to basic semantic and syntactic abilities. *See* Wiig and Secord (1989) in Appendix I.

Test of Phonological Awareness (TOPA) devised by Torgesen and Bryant, TOPA assesses children's phonological awareness and who may be at risk of having difficulties with reading. It can be used with children in the age range of 5;00–8;00. *See* Torgesen and Bryant (1997) in Appendix I.

Test of Pragmatic Language (TOPL) devised by Phelps-Tarasaki and Phelps-Gunn, TOPL is designed to be used as part of a complete battery to evaluate social language skills and use. It provides information in six core sub-components of pragmatics language: physical setting, audience, topic, purpose (speech acts), visual gestural cues and abstraction. It has been standardised on a sample of 1016 students and can be used with children in the age range of 5;00–13;00. *See* Phelps-Tarasaki and Phelps-Gunn (1992) in Appendix I.

Test of Pretend Play (ToPP) devised by Lewis and Boucher, ToPP is designed to assess three types of symbolic play: substituting one object for another object or person; attributing an imagined property to an object or person; and reference to an absent object, person or substance. It can be used with children in the age range of 1–6 years. There is a non-verbal version for children up to 3 years of age and older children with poorer comprehension to follow the language used in the verbal version as well as a verbal version for children of 3 years and above. ToPP has been co-normed with the PLS-3[UK] to allow for direct comparison between the two assessments. *See* Lewis and Boucher (1997) in Appendix I.

Test of Word and Grammatical Awareness – TOWGA devised by Shaw, TOWGA is designed to give a quick measure of awareness of words and grammar at the same time. It has six subtests:

Subtest A: Segmenting sentences into words – the child points to a square on a counting board to identify each word in the item.

Subtest B: Detecting the first words in a sentence – the child repeats the first word in each test item after the tester has said the item.

Subtest C: Presence/absence judgement – the child has to say whether or not a word is present in each item.

Subtest D: Correct/incorrect judgement – with the use of pictures, the child indicates whether statements are grammatically correct or incorrect.

Subtest E: Detecting the repeated word in a sentence – the child has to say which word occurs twice in each item.

Subtest F: Detecting the first word in a sentence – similar to Subtest B but the words are polysyllabic.

TOWGA is suitable for children in the age range of 4;00–6;08 and can be used to assess children with SPECIFIC LANGUAGE IMPAIRMENT, to plan appropriate therapy for specific difficulties encountered and evaluate progress and outcomes of therapy. TOWGA can also be used in conjunction with PhAB which will give an all-round view of the child's metalinguistic abilities. *See* Shaw (2000) in Appendix 1.

Test of Word Finding devised by German originally in 1986 with its second edition in 2000, it assesses children aged between 4;00–12;11 years who have a lexical retrieval deficit. It comprises four different types of naming task: picture naming, sentence completion naming, picture naming verbs and picture naming categories. Results are based on accuracy and speed of response. Scores are computed as STANDARD SCORES and PERCENTILE SCORES. It is standardised on a North American population. *See* German (2000) in Appendix I; Beech et al (1993).

Test of Word Knowledge (TOWK) devised by Wiig and Secord, TOWK is designed

231

for use as part of a total diagnostic language battery evaluating students' ability to understand and use vocabulary. It has two levels where the first includes the following core subtests: expressive vocabulary, word definitions, receptive vocabulary and word opposites. The supplementary subtest of synonyms is for use with 6;00–8;00-year-old children. The second level includes the following core subtests: word definitions, multiple contexts, synonyms and figurative usage. There are also supplementary subtests of receptive vocabulary, expressive vocabulary and conjunctions and transition words. Level 1 is suitable for children in the age range of 5;00–8;00 while Level 2 is suitable for children and adolescents in the age range of 8;00–17;00. *See* Wiig and Secord (1992) in Appendix I.

text-to-speech synthesis *see* SPEECH SYNTHESIS.

TG *see* TRANSFORMATIONAL GRAMMAR.

thalamus a large part of the DIENCEPHALON which measures about 3 cm in length and comprises four-fifths of the DIENCEPHALON. It comprises two oval-shaped pieces of grey matter and it forms the side of the THIRD VENTRICLE. Each piece can be found deep in the CEREBRAL HEMISPHERES above the MIDBRAIN. Various nuclei can be found within it, e.g. those for hearing, vision and general sensation plus taste. Some of the other nuclei act as synapses controlling voluntary motor actions and arousal. It acts also on information from the senses such as temperature, touch and pressure. *See* Barr (1988); Kolb and Whishaw (1996); Tortora and Grabowski (2000).

theoretical linguistics a term used to contrast particularly with applied linguistics. Some linguists would disavow the possibility of a distinction. *See* Lyons (1968).

thermal paper special paper which can be used with dot-matrix printers. The paper has a special coating which is removed by the electric current from the styluses on the printing head to produce the required characters.

third ventricle it is divided by the THALAMUS and between the lateral ventricles which are linked to the third ventricle by the interventricular foramen. The CEREBROSPINAL FLUID flows into the third ventricle from its initial starting point in the lateral ventricles and before it enters the FOURTH VENTRICLE from where it passes around the rest of the BRAIN. *See* Barr (1988); Tortora and Grabowski (2000).

thoracic respiration *see* CLAVICULAR.

thought disorder a symptom of SCHIZOPHRENIA. There are two different kinds of thought disorder – form and content. Form consists of:

1. Incoherence in conversation.
2. Neologisms.
3. Loose associations: while the person communicates successfully with the listener, he has difficulty sticking to the one topic.
4. Clang associations: the words used are put in a certain order because of their rhyme rather than their syntax.
5. Poverty of speech: either the amount of discourse is increased or it conveys little information.
6. Perseveration.
7. Blocking.

Content consists of:

1. Delusions.
2. Delusional percept: a normal perception which has a special meaning for the person and often a delusional system develops quickly.
3. Somatic passivity: inability to rouse the person by outside forces operating on his body.
4. Thought insertion: thoughts, different from those of the person, are placed in the person's mind from an outside agent.
5. Thought withdrawal: the person believes their thoughts are being removed from their mind without warning.
6. Thought broadcast: the person believes their thoughts are being transmitted to others.

7. 'Made' feelings where people who have schizophrenia believe that others are projecting their feelings and emotions onto them.
8. 'Made' volitional acts where people with schizophrenia believe they have lost control of their body and what they are doing is being caused by an outside agent.
9. 'Made' impulses where people with schizophrenia believe what they do is caused by an outside agent which forces them to do something.

See Davison et al (2004).

thyrohyoid muscle *see* LARYNX.

thyroid cartilage *see* LARYNX.

thyroid gland *see* TRACHEA.

TIAs *see* TRANSIENT ISCHAEMIC ATTACKS.

tic repeated jerky movements usually of the face or neck. GILLES DE LA TOURETTE SYN-DROME is a grouping together of symptoms, one of which is meaningless grunting. *See* Stafford-Clark and Bridges (1990); Kolb and Whishaw (1996); Tortora and Grabowski (2000).

tidal volume the amount of air taken into the LUNGS when breathing normally. *See* RESERVE VOLUME; Tortora and Grabowski (2000).

timbre the ability on the part of the listener to distinguish different characteristics of sound even if the loudness, pitch and length (*see* AUDITORY PHONETICS) are the same. It is often referred to as QUALITY or tamber. *See* Abercrombie (1967).

timing the process of moving the articulators into the correct sequences for producing sounds and making them into words. This can produce important features in rhythm (*see* PROSODY) and other prosodic features. *See* Clark and Clark (1977).

tinnitus the perception of rushing, roaring, ringing noises in the ear. During the last century, it was thought that tinnitus had a similar cause to hearing loss and was associated with the cochlea (*see* EAR). However, when it was found that sound is perceived in the auditory cortex, searches for treatment and research into tinnitus changed direction. In fact Hazell quotes 30 per cent of his patients with long-term tinnitus had normal audiograms and there were no problems with the functioning of their cochleas. The most recent and most effective treatment of tinnitus, which is still being developed, is tinnitus retraining therapy (TRT) which is part of directive counselling. As all the parts of the neuronal networks which comprise the auditory system are active electrically during life, any sound which is generated causes the background electrical activity to lessen. If the auditory system stops receiving information because the environment becomes unnaturally quiet or because of a hearing loss, the background activity increases. This is why tinnitus can be heard by anyone in a quiet environment as long as they listen carefully. Thus, each time the environment is quiet enough and there are no distractions tinnitus will be heard and cause varying degrees of distress. People who come to seek help for tinnitus are those who have a degree of aversive conditioned response which may range from mild changes to their autonomic activity to a powerful phobic reaction with continuous anxiety and panic states. So, TRT uses a combination of teaching, behavioural and sound therapy techniques based on Jastreboff's neurophysiological model of tinnitus with the goal of removing completely any reaction or conditioned response to tinnitus or external sounds. The problems caused by tinnitus only exist when they are producing unpleasant reactions. *See* Katz (1985); Hazell (2001).

Tinnitus Questionnaire (TQ) devised by Hallam, TQ is designed to measure coping strategies or beliefs in relation to TIN-NITUS by measuring three core factors: sleep disturbance, emotional distress and auditory perceptual difficulties. *See* Hallam (1997) in Appendix I.

toggle function key a key which can switch between one of two functions.

token economy a behaviour therapy based on OPERANT CONDITIONING. Basically, people will receive a reward if they overcome the anxiety-provoking situation. The tokens which are given are intended to act as sufficient reinforcers to reduce the aberrant behaviour and promote the behaviour of the norm. *See* Kazdin (1981).

Token Test devised by DeRenzi and Vignolo in 1962, it is a formal assessment to test the auditory comprehension of those with APHASIA. The test material comprises 20 tokens which differ in size, shape and colour. The original Token Test was divided into five parts; the first four used auditory commands of increasing length while the fifth contained commands of increasing grammatical complexity. DeRenzi and Faglioni reported their use of a shortened form of the Token Test where 36 graded commands are presented in six sections. The Revised Token Test devised by McNeil and Prescott in 1978 gives more control over the syntactic variables, and performance can be plotted graphically to reveal variance in performance patterns across subtests. The Short Token Test was devised by Spellacy and Spreen in 1969. *See* DeRenzi and Vignolo (1962) in Appendix I; DeRenzi and Faglioni (1978) in Appendix I; McNeil and Prescott (1978) in Appendix I; Johns (1981); Rosenbek et al (1989); Kolb and Whishaw (1996).

Token Test for Children devised by DiSimoni, it is a test of children's comprehension and is based on the TOKEN TEST. It can be used with children between the ages of 3;0 and 12;6 years of age. Various objects (usually shapes of different colours) are placed in a standardised manner. Spoken commands are given to the child to manipulate the objects. The commands become progressively longer and more complex. It is a rapid screening test which may indicate that further testing of the lexicon and syntax is required. *See* DiSimoni (1978) in Appendix I; Beech et al (1993).

tone *see* SUPRASEGMENTAL PHONOLOGY.

tone group *see* SUPRASEGMENTAL PHONOLOGY.

tongue the floor of the mouth is formed by the tongue, which when lifted is held down by the MUCOUS MEMBRANE – the lingual frenulum. On either side of the frenulum are two papillae or bumps on top of which is the opening of the submandibular SALIVARY GLANDS, while below the tongue there are two swellings which are called sublingual salivary glands (*see* SALIVARY GLANDS). The tongue can be divided into two parts and the line where the division occurs is the sulcus terminalis, i.e. the inverted 'v' shape. The foramen caecum is at the apex of the 'v' or small depression. The surface is covered by stratified squamous epithelium partly keratinised. The anterior two-thirds are covered by papillae while the underside is smooth mucous membrane similar to the rest of the surface. In these papillae, the taste buds can be found. The posterior one-third is covered by the lingual tonsil. Immediately behind the tonsil are two depressions or valleys called vallecula while behind the ridge is the EPIGLOTTIS. The tongue is moved by six muscles – three INTRINSIC MUSCLES OF THE TONGUE and three EXTRINSIC MUSCLES OF THE TONGUE. The tongue is an active articulator used in speech and is also used in the processes of swallowing and chewing. *See* Tortora and Grabowski (2000).

tongue thrust the involuntary forward movement of the tongue, often found in children who have CEREBRAL PALSY. It can produce ARTICULATION DELAY or ARTICULATION DISORDER, and can affect the eating process as the food can be pushed out by the tongue. Treatment for both problems can be given by speech and language therapy.

tongue-tie the layman's term for ANKYLOGLOSSUS.

tonic a stage in which all the muscles contract during a fit in grand-mal EPILEPSY. It can also be a minor fit producing muscle contractions, keeping the muscles tight. *See* Gilroy and Holliday (1982).

tonic syllable *see* SUPRASEGMENTAL PHONOLOGY.

tonicity *see* SUPRASEGMENTAL PHONOLOGY.

tonsil there are three tonsils at the back of the mouth – the pharyngeal, palatine and lingual tonsils. *See* Tortora and Grabowski (2000).

tonsillectomy the operation which removes infected and enlarged tonsils. The palatine tonsil or true tonsil is removed. It may produce hypernasality which can be treated by speech and language therapy. *See* Pracy et al (1974).

TORCH an acronym for the four conditions which can affect a fetus:

1. TOXOPLASMOSIS.
2. RUBELLA.
3. CYTOMEGALOVIRUS.
4. HERPES SIMPLEX.

total communication *see* EDUCATION OF HEARING-IMPAIRED CHILDREN.

touchscreen an input device which allows a computer program to be operated without the use of a keyboard. The operator touches the screen surface to make selections.

TouchSpeak a portable communication aid for adults who have APHASIA. It uses a central vocabulary database and has prestored vocabularies which can be customised. The device uses SPEECH SYNTHESIS and DIGITISED SPEECH. *See* Appendix IV (Richard Hill and Associates).

TouchTalker a high-tech communication aid with synthetic speech output (DECTALK). It uses MINSPEAK to organise vocabulary to store into the device. It has a memory of about 40KB. It can only be accessed by direct manual selection. The device can be set into 8, 32 or 128 locations and if the TouchTalker uses the ENHANCED MINSPEAK OPERATING SYSTEM (EMOS) it can also be set into the 'alternative' overlay. There are various MINSPEAK APPLICATION PROGRAMS (MAPS) which can be transferred into the device. The memory can be backed up on a computer. It can also be used for computer emulation and can be linked to the DIRECTOR, an environmental control. *See* Glennen and DeCoste (1997); Appendix IV (Prentke Romich Company).

toxoplasmosis an infection which can cause brain damage if transferred *in utero* through the placenta to the fetus. It is caused by ingestion of food which has come into contact with protozoal organisms found in cat faeces. It forms part of the TORCH classification of infections which can affect a fetus. Many adults have serological evidence of previous infection which has not been identified by a clinical illness. *See* Gilroy and Holliday (1982); http://co.essortment.com/toxoplasmosis_revu.htm

trace conditioning *see* CLASSICAL CONDITIONING.

trachea the trachea is commonly referred to as the windpipe. It is about 10 cm long and 2 cm wide, extending from the sixth cervical vertebra down to the fifth thoracic vertebra. At this point, it divides into the left and right bronchi. In outline, it is more or less circular but it is actually flattened at the back because running down its whole length is the OESOPHAGUS. It is surrounded by three important structures in the neck – carotid artery, jugular vein, and vagus nerve (*see* CRANIAL NERVES). The nerve behind the trachea is the recurrent laryngeal nerve which supplies nearly all the muscles of the LARYNX. It can be easily picked out on X-ray as it has 20 tracheal rings made of hyaline while the rest of the wall comprises CONNECTIVE TISSUE and SMOOTH MUSCLE. It is lined by ciliated columnar EPITHELIUM with mucous cells. At the front, opposite the third tracheal ring, is the thyroid gland. On inspiration, the trachea lengthens and changes shape as its walls are elastic. Its main function is to provide air during inspiration. *See* Tortora and Grabowski (2000).

tracheostomy *see* TRACHEOTOMY.

tracheotomy an operation to open into the TRACHEA when a person has severe problems in breathing. A tube is inserted into a hole in the neck to aid breathing. *See*

235

Pracy et al (1974); Adamson and Dunbar (1991) (communication development in young children with tracheotomies); Tortora and Grabowski (2000).

trackball an input device which either replaces the mouse and is used along with a QWERTY KEYBOARD or replaces the QWERTY KEYBOARD when using an on-screen keyboard with a word processor. It consists of a ball which can be rolled by the palm of the hand to move the cursor or draw lines to produce graphics.

traditional grammar *see* SYNTAX.

trait approach an approach to psychology which has as its aim finding out the characteristics which make the person act the way he does. Traits are descriptions of behaviour characteristics such as aggressiveness, emotional stability, agreeableness, etc. In fact, a trait is any characteristic which differs significantly from person to person. It does not explain the person's behaviour. A method for measuring traits is factor analysis. The method allows the therapist to reduce a large number of measures to a small number of independent dimensions. Cattell developed a 16 personality factor questionnaire. The client is asked over 100 questions to which he need only reply 'yes/no', and from his replies Cattell could work out the person's personality profile. For the trait approach to be effective, each person's profile should be compared in different situations to find out in which situation the person's traits are most affected. *See* Smith et al (2003).

transcortical motor aphasia a major form of APHASIA described by the BOSTON SCHOOL. It produces non-fluency, but repetition and comprehension remain relatively intact while naming, reading aloud and writing are impaired. The lesion occurs in the perisylvian areas of the BRAIN. *See* Goodglass and Kaplan (2000); Rosenbek et al (1989); Kolb and Whishaw (1996).

transcortical sensory aphasia a major form of APHASIA described by the BOSTON SCHOOL. It produces fluent language full of neologisms (*see* JARGON APHASIA (4)) and PARAPHASIAS, impaired comprehension, naming, reading comprehension and writing, while reading aloud is affected to varying degrees and repetition remains unaffected. *See* Goodglass and Kaplan (2000); Rosenbek et al (1989); Kolb and Whishaw (1996).

transcription systems ways in which a person's speech can be represented usually by the symbols on the IPA chart (*see* Appendix III). When it is used by a speech and language therapist, it shows which sounds have changed and to what they have changed. There are three types of transcription:

1. Phonemic transcription, also known as broad transcription. Each symbol represents all allophonic (*see* PHONOLOGY) variations.
2. Allophonic transcription, also known as narrow transcription. A more technical transcription as it requires the representation of all allophonic variations of each phoneme (*see* PHONOLOGY). DIACRITICS are also used to make the transcription as accurate as possible.
3. Impressionistic transcription is carried out without regard to the phonemic or allophonic interpretation of the sounds.

In speech and language therapy, (1) and (2) are most commonly used to transcribe the speech of children with ARTICULATION DELAY or ARTICULATION DISORDER, or PHONOLOGICAL DELAY or PHONOLOGICAL DISORDER. *See* Abercrombie (1967); Grunwell (1987).

transformational grammar (TG) a theory of SYNTAX proposed by Chomsky (*see* CHOMSKYAN LINGUISTICS) in 1957 after he had set aside the other two theories of finite state grammar and phrase structure grammar. His initial description of such grammar was: 'a grammatical transformation (T) operates on a given string...with a given constituent structure and converts it into a new string with a new derived constituent structure' (Chomsky 1957, p. 44). In 1965, he put forward the STANDARD THEORY of TG. The transformations which he proposed to operate between the deep and surface structures were designed to delete, substitute, insert, move and raise strings so that the person could arrive at the spoken or written utterance. Chomsky believed the most important study for linguists was the syntactic component of language, and to arrive at the correct syntactical structures it was not necessary to deal with the semantic component. Both surface and deep structures represent the phonetic and semantic components interpreted in language. Chomsky went so far as to claim syntax was 'autonomous' and had little to do with semantics. Chomsky found he had to revise the standard theory and so he proposed the Extended Standard Theory (EST). In this theory, Chomsky began to accept the role of semantics in the surface structure. This apparent change was caused by the failure of the Standard Theory to account for the use of stress. In such sentences, the meaning change depends on which word is stressed. Chomsky's problem was: do such sentences all have the same deep structure or different deep structures?

1. Is Bill coming on TUESDAY?
2. Is BILL coming on Tuesday?
3. IS Bill coming on Tuesday?

In the Standard Theory, Chomsky would have had to give all these sentences the same deep structure because transformational rules could not change the meaning of the deep sentence between the deep and surface structures. To overcome this problem, he proposed transformational rules which allowed for markers to be placed in the deep and surface structures so that both structures would affect the semantics of the sentence. This is sometimes called Interpretive Semantics Grammar. In 1973, Chomsky revised EST to the Revised Extended Standard Theory (REST). This theory removed the relationship of the deep structure to the semantic component as in EST, so that all semantic information could be read off from the surface structure. To accomplish this, he introduced the Trace Theory. A trace 't' is an empty node left behind after a NOUN PHRASE has been removed. Thus, the passive transformation becomes as shown in the box below: (1') shows the trace from where the NP 'John' has been removed to the beginning of the sentence. Thus, traces are like chains in that when linked together, the NP can be traced to its original position. The latest development of Chomsky's theory is referred to as 'Government and Binding'. *See* Chomsky (1982); Steinberg (1982); Salkie (1990); Lyons (1991); Fromkin and Rodman (2003).

transient ischaemic attacks (TIAs) episodes of temporary ischaemia of the BRAIN or BRAINSTEM producing a transient loss of cerebral function presumed due to a vascular event which resolves within 24 hours. The attacks begin suddenly and symptoms and signs are present for a few minutes before disappearing. The common symptoms and signs are weakness of a limb or face, loss of sensation or transient blindness in one eye (amaurosis fugax). Some people may have just a single attack while others have several at different time intervals. There are many possible causes for TIAs and it is likely that no cause will be found. It is believed the vast majority of attacks are due to small emboli formed from blood

deep structure	(1)	Mary kissed John
surface structure	(1')	John was kissed t (by Mary)
		i i

platelets with some fibrin thrombus. These emboli originate chiefly in the first centimetre of the internal carotid artery (*see* CAROTID ARTERY) which has become ulcerated due to the formation of atheroma (*see* above). In addition, they may originate on the aortic valves, the damaged wall of the left ventricle (after a heart attack) or in the mitral valve or left atrium (*see* HEART) in people with rheumatic heart disease. Other suggested causes are abnormalities of the blood constituents such as hypercoagulability or reduced cerebral perfusion such as diminished effective cardiac output, steal syndromes, kinking and compression of extracranial vessels. *See* Gilroy and Holliday (1982); Kaye (1991); Tortora and Grabowski (2000); http://www.vssgbi.org/patient-info/tia.html

translucency *see* ICONICITY.

transparency see ICONICITY.

transverse muscle *see* INTRINSIC MUSCLES OF THE TONGUE.

trauma any injury which occurs to parts or structures in the body or severe feelings of stress caused by the external environment. *See* Kaye (1991).

Treacher Collins syndrome a syndrome described by Treacher Collins in 1900, although the first reported case was made by Thomson in 1846. In the 1940s, the condition was also known as mandibulofacial dysostosis. About 40 per cent of those with this condition have a CLEFT PALATE. The characteristic facial appearance is downward slanting eyes with an underdeveloped mandible and maxilla. There are also abnormalities of the EAR such as lack of a pinna causing HEARING LOSS. The hearing loss may produce learning difficulties but the syndrome is not associated with learning disability. *See* Watson et al (2001); Jones (1997); http://www.treachercollins.co.uk/

treatment programme the plan of therapy produced by a therapist for each individual client based on the assessments which have been carried out. This may include some published therapeutic techniques, e.g. PROMOTING APHASICS' COMMUNICATIVE EFFECTIVENESS, MELODIC INTONATION THERAPY, NUFFIELD DYSPRAXIA PROGRAMME, etc., various forms of AUGMENTATIVE AND ALTERNATIVE COMMUNICATION or therapy devised by the therapist based on experience of what has worked best in the past with those with similar disorders. However, there must be flexibility built into a treatment programme if the person does not respond appropriately.

tree diagram a hierarchical structure which is used to analyse constituents (*see* CONSTITUENT ANALYSIS). The constituents are all linked by branches and the points where the branches meet are nodes:

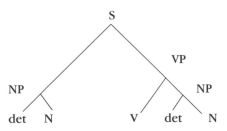

The S (sentence) is said to dominate the NP (noun phrase) which dominates the det (determiner), N (noun) and VP (verb phrase) which are said to dominate V (verb) and the second noun phrase. Tree diagrams are also known as phrase markers. *See* Huddleston (1976); Fromkin and Rodman (2003) (phrase structured trees).

tremor a rhythmic, involuntary and purposeless contraction of muscle groups. There are three main types of tremor:

1. Essential tremor: a benign tremor which is usually bilateral, beginning in the fingers and hands. It may be inherited as an autosomal dominant trait (*see* CHROMOSOMES). It is caused by an imbalance of neurotransmitter substances in the BASAL GANGLIA. It can appear in either young children or the elderly. The tremor worsens if the person is emotionally upset. It is

associated with mild cerebellar signs. The main drug treatment is a ß-receptor blocker such as propranolol and diazepam.

2. Intention tremor: it increases with movement and involves upper extremities, often occurring at the end of the movement. This may be found in those with cerebellar disease. The same drug treatment is used as for essential tremor.

3. Parkinsonian tremor (*see* PARKINSON'S DISEASE).

See Gilroy and Holliday (1982); Tortora and Grabowski (2000).

tricyclics *see* ANTIDEPRESSANT DRUGS.

trigeminal nerve *see* CRANIAL NERVES.

trill *see* ARTICULATION.

Triple C – Checklist of Communication Competencies devised by Bloomberg and West in 1999 in Australia, the Triple C is a screening checklist designed to assess the communication skills of adolescents and adults who have severe or profound intellectual, physical or sensory disabilities. Triple C gives a checklist of abilities which are grouped together to form communication stages and so find out the approximate stage at which the person is communicating. It can be given by the person's primary caregiver or someone familiar with them although the results should be discussed with a speech and language therapist before any intervention is planned. There is a video to help identify the six stages of communication development. *See* http://www.scopevic.org.au/info_publications.html; Bloomberg and West (1999) in Appendix I.

triplegia a physical handicap which affects three limbs – usually both legs and one arm – and is often found in those who have CEREBRAL PALSY.

trisomy-21 *see* DOWN SYNDROME.

TROG *see* TEST FOR RECEPTION OF GRAMMAR.

true tonsil *see* MOUTH.

tuberous sclerosis often thought to have been described first by von Recklinghausen over 100 years ago, Bournville is usually credited for its recognition in 1880. Hamartomatous lesions develop in many tissues, especially the skin and the brain. The condition has three principal features:

1. EPILEPSY.
2. LEARNING DISABILITY.
3. Skin disorder.

However, not every child has all three features. About 40 per cent have a skin disorder while 60 per cent have a degree of learning disability and almost all have a form of epilepsy. *See* Hosking (1982); Jones (1997); http://www.tuberous-sclerosis.org/

tumour the medical term for a cancerous (*see* CANCER) growth found in tissues in the body.

tumours of the central nervous system these are some of the commonest cancerous (*see* CANCER) growths in the glia of the BRAIN:

1. Oligodendrogliomas: these tumours, which may become malignant, produce a greyish-red area in the brain giving a honeycomb effect. They are most often found in the frontal lobe of the CEREBRAL HEMISPHERES. As they grow slowly, they produce a gradual headache and a generalised seizure. They appear in people between the ages of 30 and 40 years. They comprise 5 per cent of all gliomas. Treatment takes the form of surgical removal followed by RADIOTHERAPY with the post-operative life span likely to be about 5–7 years.

2. Meningiomas: these comprise 10 per cent of all intracranial tumours. They usually appear in the later years of life and are more common in women. Treatment takes the form of surgical removal. The prognosis is good as long as complete removal has taken place. Otherwise the tumour may reappear and necessitate a second operation a few years later.

3. Neurofibromas: this type of tumour

can be inherited as an autosomal dominant trait (*see* CHROMOSOMES). These peripheral tumours may be associated with intracerebral gliomas. They may appear on the cranial or peripheral nerves of the brain and SPINAL CORD and produce raised pressure in the head, aphasic symptoms (*see* APHASIA), HEMIPLEGIA, problems in the visual fields as well as seizures. Headaches are not a common symptom. There may also be café-au-lait spots on the skin. The tumours are usually multiple and some may become malignant.

4. Astrocytomas: these tumours are locally invasive. They appear most commonly in the frontal, temporal and parietal lobes (*see* CEREBRAL HEMISPHERES), basal ganglia and occipital lobes (*see* CEREBRAL HEMISPHERES) in decreasing order of frequency. Headaches are often felt on one side of the brain which become more generalised, and raised INTRACRANIAL PRESSURE develops. Treatment takes the form of surgical removal followed by radiotherapy.

5. Medulloblastomas: these grow very quickly and are very invasive from metastatic seeding. These tumours account for about 20 per cent of all intracranial tumours in childhood. They are common in children below the age of 10 years and rarer in older children. The posterior fossa is the site for these lesions. As they grow near the FOURTH VENTRICLE, HYDROCEPHALUS can often develop. Treatment takes the form of surgical removal followed by radiotherapy while the hydrocephalus can be treated with ventricular SHUNTS. The prognosis depends on how much of the tumour has been removed and the efficacy of the radiotherapy.

See Gilroy and Holliday (1982); Kaye (1991); Kolb and Whishaw (1996).

turn a sociolinguistic phenomenon. TURN TAKING in conversation is crucial for a conversation to take place. *See* Clark and Clark (1977).

turn taking the pattern of reciprocal interchange which takes place in normal conversational situations. It is absent or deficient in some types of language disorder.

Turner's syndrome Turner described, in 1938, a condition which involved small stature, sexual infantilism, webbed neck and cubitus valgus in seven females. It is a sex chromosome (*see* CHROMOSOMES) abnormality where 45 chromosomes are present with one X but no Y chromosome. Thus, it is also known as an XO syndrome. It is not particularly associated with LEARNING DISABILITY. However, there can be associated disorders of the neck, kidneys, ovaries and heart. The child is likely to have educational difficulties such as reading problems. *See* Salmon (1978); Jones (1997); Kolb and Whishaw (1996); http://www.tss.org.uk/

turtle either a robotic machine which can be moved by a child giving it commands from the computer or a small triangle which can be moved about the screen. *See* LOGOTRON LOGO.

tympanic membrane *see* EAR.

tympanogram classification *see* IMPEDANCE AUDIOMETRY.

tympanometry *see* IMPEDANCE AUDIOMETRY.

ultrasonography a non-invasive technique

originally devised to assess the growth of the fetus. It can show how the fetus is placed in the placenta, the amount of fetal growth which has taken place and can identify any disorder of the spine, thus showing any possibility of the child having SPINA BIFIDA. It may also show if there are to be multiple births. It is now more widely used as an imaging technique for organ enlargement, tumours, blood flow, presence of gallstones, etc. It is a popular technique because it is totally safe, cheap and easily repeatable. *See* Tortora and Grabowski (2000).

unconditioned response *see* CLASSICAL CONDITIONING.

unconditioned stimulus *see* CLASSICAL CONDITIONING.

unconscious motives *see* PSYCHOANALYSIS.

underextension the opposite of OVER-EXTENSION. During the stage of underextension, the child uses one word for a particular object. So, the child may use the word 'teddy' for his own teddy but not for the teddies belonging to his siblings or friends. However, at a later stage, he could call other teddies by their correct name and overextend its use to an object which may have similar characteristics to a teddy bear, but is another object. *See* Clark and Clark (1977).

understanding *see* COMPREHENSION.

Understanding Ambiguity: An Assessment of Pragmatic Meaning devised by Rinaldi in 1996, Understanding Ambiguity helps to identify children experiencing difficulty with understanding ambiguous communication. It comprises two assessments, each of which is relevant to a different type of ambiguity: Multiple Meaning in Context (only suitable for use with children aged 10+ years) – homonyms, idioms and multiple meaning phrases are used, and Inconsistent Messages of Emotion – here the speaker, on audio tape and video, deliberately creates ambiguity by contradicting the words in the utterance which convey one emotion, by using facial expressions and tone of voice to create a different emotion. The emotions used are sadness, anger and pleasure. It is suitable for children in the age range of 8;00 to 13;00 years. *See* Rinaldi (1996) in Appendix I.

undifferentiated jargon *see* JARGON APHASIA (1).

unilateral a lesion or disease which affects one side of the body or structure in the body. It is opposed to bilateral.

unilateral abductor paralysis *see* LARYNGEAL NERVE PALSIES.

unilateral adductor paralysis *see* LARYNGEAL NERVE PALSIES.

unintelligible speech the speech of a person who has a very severe communication problem. For children, this may be an articulation or phonological delay or disorder. For adults, this may be caused by an ACQUIRED DYSPRAXIA or severe DYSARTHRIA. It is often the case that close relatives can make out what the person

241

is saying but strangers cannot. *See* Grunwell (1987).

unit any item in a syntactic, phonetic, semantic or morphological description. A unit in any of these areas of linguistics describes the focus for discussion. *See* Lyons (1968).

Unity 32 for Pathfinder devised for the Pathfinder using MINSPEAK, Unity 32 has two versions, the first being primarily single-hit words comprising 2100 'root' words while the other version uses sequences of icons for an expanded vocabulary comprising the 2100 root words of version 1 as well as 200 'core' words and phrases.

In the Single Hit vocabulary, one selection causes items to appear in the activity row. In the Sequenced Version this happens on selecting a key, while selecting a second key reveals a new set of vocabulary items allowing easy access to additional vocabulary. *See* Appendix IV (Prentke Romich Company).

Unity 128 devised by Badman et al, it is a MINSPEAK APPLICATION PROGRAM designed using the WORDS STRATEGY paradigm and similar overlay. It is aimed at any age range and from mild learning disability to no learning disability. Unity can start at about 3 years of age and is suitable for childhood, adolescence and adulthood, so there will be no need to learn a new program when the child reaches the cut-off point with a program like IEP+. It uses symbols combined with grammatical labels for nouns, verbs and all their endings, adjectives, prepositions and adverbs as well as using categorisation for a larger set of vocabulary. There are four overlays, the main difference being the gradual increase of grammatical labels until the third and fourth overlays when all the grammatical labels are on the overlay. On the third overlay these labels are represented with icons while on the fourth there is just the written label as with Words Strategy. *See* Badman et al (1995); Glennen and DeCoste (1997).

upper motor neuron *see* NEURONS.

UR (unconditioned response) *see* CLASSICAL CONDITIONING.

US (unconditioned stimulus) *see* CLASSICAL CONDITIONING.

utterance as opposed to sentence, or some other theoretical term referring to an identifiable linguistic unit, i.e. defined within some theoretical approach, utterance is a pre-theoretical term referring to some stretch of speech prior to analysis. *See* Lyons (1968).

uvula a piece of tissue hanging down from the back of the soft palate and between the isthmus of fauces (*see* MOUTH). The uvular muscle runs along the middle of the soft palate (*see* MOUTH) and moves the uvula. Although this may not have been thought to be of much use, research now suggests that the muscle contracts and leads to a VELOPHARYNGEAL closure. *See* Watson et al (2001); Tortora and Grabowski (2000).

uvular *see* ARTICULATION.

uvular muscle *see* UVULA.

vagus nerve *see* CRANIAL NERVES.

vallecula *see* TONGUE.

Vanguard a high-tech communication aid which uses both digitised and synthetic speech. It is the first communication aid using the MINSPEAK method of encoding vocabulary to use a touchscreen. It can use screens of 4, 8, 32 and 45 locations with an activity row being the top row of the 45-location screen. It allows for embellished icons which means that while regular Minspeak ICON sequences can be used, the person using the Vanguard can press an icon for 'drinks' and instead of needing to remember the second icon of the sequence the second icon can show the picture of the real drink. The activity row is for fringe vocabulary which is not used on an everyday basis. Although the activity row has only nine locations, there can be more rows attached to make up an activity. It can be accessed using direct manual selection, single/dual or two-switch scanning, infra-red headpointing and joystick. The Vanguard can be used as an Environmental Controller as it can learn infra-red signals to operate televisions, videos, hi-fis and so on. It can also be used as a computer keyboard emulator as it has its own computer mode which allows the person not only to write into any word processor but also to open applications and pull-down menus. By using serial keys in either Windows or Macintosh, the Vanguard can emulate into either operating system. When using spell mode, the person can also use the Word Prediction feature. *See* Rumble and Larcher (1998); Appendix IV (Prentke Romich Company).

vascular a description of structures or problems in the blood supply to the body.

VDU *see* VISUAL DISPLAY UNIT.

velar *see* ARTICULATION.

velaric airstream an airstream used to produce clicks which are also described as velaric ingressive stops. Clicks which can be produced are bilabial click . , tongue tip [!], lateral click [|||] (as in the 'gee-up' sound for horses) and retroflex click [ǂ]. In English, clicks are only used to express the speaker's feelings and not linguistically as in such languages as Hottentot in which all four types of clicks are used to produce linguistic meaning. *See* Ladefoged (2001).

velopharyngeal a description of structures or disorders between the soft palate (*see* MOUTH) and the back wall of the nasopharynx (see PHARYNX). When the structures in this area close, it is known as velopharyngeal closure. This closure takes place during speech and swallowing so that the oropharynx (*see* PHARYNX) is separated from the nasopharynx by the raising of the soft palate and the moving inward of the walls of the pharynx. A failure of this closure is known as velopharyngeal incompetence. If the soft palate or velum fails to reach the back wall of the pharynx because of damage or because it is too short to reach the wall, it is known as velopharyngeal insufficiency. *See* Watson et al (2001).

velopharyngeal closure *see* VELOPHARYN-GEAL.

velopharyngeal incompetence *see* VELOPHARYNGEAL.

velopharyngeal insufficiency *see* VELOPHARYNGEAL.

ventricles *see* THIRD VENTRICLE; FOURTH VENTRICLE.

Verb and Sentence Test (VAST) devised by Bastiaanse and colleagues, VAST assesses verb and sentence processing for people who have APHASIA with each subtest linked to a remediation programme. VAST has 10 subtests covering the comprehension and production of verbs. *See* VAST in Appendix I.

verb particle a term used in some grammatical approaches to refer to the unit in phrasal verb sequences in English which are preposition-like but do not always function as prepositions, e.g. 'up, 'off, 'away' as in (1)–(3).

(1) We ran a bill up.
(2) She took her hat off.
(3) He threw the rubbish away.

See Crystal et al (1989).

verb phrase *see* CONSTITUENT ANALYSIS; Fromkin and Rodman (2003).

verbal auditory agnosia a very severe form of AGNOSIA. Superficially the child may appear deaf and there may be some HEARING LOSS but this is not sufficient to account for complete lack of AUDITORY COMPREHENSION. Consequently EXPRESSIVE LANGUAGE is also severely affected. Also known as congenital auditory imperception.

verbal dyspraxia *see* DEVELOPMENTAL VERBAL DYSPRAXIA.

Verbal Motor Production Assessment for Children (VMPAC) devised by Hayden and Square, VMPAC evaluates step-by-step children's motor speech system. It can be used with any children who have a problem with their speech and the assessor will find out if it is caused by the presence of a motor disruption. It assesses three areas: global motor control, focal oromotor control and sequencing as well as two supplementary areas in connected speech and language control and speech characteristics. It is suitable for children in the age range of 3;00–12;00. *See* Hayden and Square (1999) in Appendix I.

verbal paraphasia *see* PARAPHASIA.

vertical muscle *see* INTRINSIC MUSCLES OF THE TONGUE.

vestibular schwannoma also known as acoustic neuroma, the commonest tumour of the temporal bone. It arises from the Schwann cells covering the superior or inferior vestibular nerves where the glial cells change to Schwann cells and account for between 6 and 10 per cent of all intracranial tumours and 80 to 90 per cent of all tumours in the cerebellopontine angle, i.e. the angle between the PONS and the CEREBELLUM. They occur in about two people per 100 000 population per year and are slow growing benign tumours that do not spread to other tissues or structures in the body. When they are just in the internal auditory canal (*see* EAR), they cause problems only to the vestibular and cohlear nerves but as they start to grow out of the internal canal they push medially, superiorly and inferiorly, eventually pressing on the BRAINSTEM causing a rise in INTRACRANIAL PRESSURE and possibly death. The most reliable way of making a diagnosis is using MAGNETIC RESONANCE IMAGING (MRI). The commonest clinical sign of a person with vestibular schwannoma is progressive SENSORINEURAL HEARING LOSS caused by slowly increasing compression on the cochlear nerve. In 15 to 25 per cent of people with vestibular schwannoma the hearing loss can be sudden. There may also be unilateral or asymmetric TINNITUS or balance disturbance. If the tumour does become larger, there are associated clinical signs of motor incoordination, pain or paraesthesia in the face since the trigeminal (cranial nerve V) nerve is involved, as well as headaches, diplopia and vomiting due to raised intracranial pressure. The audiogram (*see* PURE-TONE AUDIOMETRY) shows an asymmetrical sensorineural hearing loss which is worse in the higher frequencies. Surgery may be considered and/or radiotherapy. *See* Burton (2001).

vestibular system *see* EAR.

vestibulocochlear nerve also known as acoustic nerve. *See* CRANIAL NERVES III.

videofluoroscopy a radiographic technique to visualise the movement of contrast medium in the body, e.g. the pharyngeal stage of swallowing. The person is given barium mixed with small quantities of food or fluid. The swallowing process is recorded on video film for subsequent analysis which is carried out frame-by-frame so that the therapist can accurately assess the time taken for the person to trigger a swallow and examine closely what happens during different stages of the swallow. Since a lateral view and a head-on view are given of the person swallowing, the therapist can see all the structures in the head and neck which may be defective in the swallowing process. The findings may include aspiration of the bolus, pooling in the vallecula or the pyriform sinuses, the destination of pooled material, spillage of material into the PHARYNX before the swallow is triggered, and delay in the activation of the swallow reflex. *See* Langley (1987).

visible speech *see* FINGERSPELLING.

VisioBoard an alternative INPUT DEVICE to access a PC using Windows. It tracks not only eye movement but also head movement using two cameras housed in the casing which contains the monitor. Selections are made by stare, eye blinks or an external switch. Unlike some other eye-gaze systems, VisioBoard will still work with background light. *See* Appendix IV (Metrovision).

Visispeech a real-time analysis and display system. It can be used with the BBC microcomputer and Apple microcomputer. Visispeech shows many aspects of voice visually. It can help in the assessment of voice quality of people with DYSPHONIA or HEARING LOSS and those with DYSARTHRIA who have pitch problems. There are three displays:

1. Pitch.
2. Energy.
3. Voicing.

Visispeech II has an easy key access as it operates with one actuation of each of the function keys on a BBC computer. There is also a histogram program which provides graphical representations of the frequency distribution. Histograms and the three energy displays can be saved on disk as well as being printed out so that an assessment can be kept and progress monitored accurately.

visual display unit a unit which displays text or graphics produced from the memory of the computer. It forms the display section of a terminal.

vital capacity the greatest TIDAL VOLUME, i.e. the biggest breath a person can take in and let out. *See* Green (1978); Tortora and Grabowski (2000).

Vocab+ a word-based system which can be used on a high-tech communication aid or on a PC running Windows or Windows CE. On the opening screen, as well as the alphabet there are 30 words which account for 30 per cent of what is said, while the next 1000 words, which account for 85 per cent of what is said, can be accessed by pressing the initial letter and finding the word on the page of words which appears starting with that letter, while the words which cannot be found by either of the previous two methods can be found using word prediction. *See* Appendix IV (Vocab Voice Systems Ltd).

vocal abuse *see* VOCAL NODULES.

vocal cords *see* VOCAL FOLDS.

vocal folds found in the LARYNX, they vibrate while a person is speaking. It is the vibration which produces the voice quality in speech. The process of producing voice is known as PHONATION. They may also be called vocal cords. Any growths or struc-

245

tural damage to the folds can produce DYSPHONIA. See Catford (1977); Tortora and Grabowski (2000).

vocal misuse *see* VOCAL NODULES.

vocal nodules growths that appear on the posterior third of the vocal folds. They can occur in both children and adults through vocal abuse or misuse. This takes the form of excessive shouting, abnormal phonation patterns and excessive strain on the vocal folds. The nodules increase in size because of the persistent rubbing together of the strained folds; compare the appearance of corns on the feet after wearing ill-fitting shoes. The nodules prevent the folds from closing normally during phonation and harsh or hoarse voice can occur. Treatment takes the form of relaxation exercises and voice exercises which prevent the vocal folds from coming together harshly, e.g. YAWN/SIGH. Voice rest, where the person has to use the voice as little as possible, may be necessary. This may require the person to take time off work and not live such an active social life for a period of time. Voice rest gives therapy the optimum conditions for improving the voice. See Freeman and Fawcus (2001).

Vocal Profile Analysis devised by Laver in 1980, it is based on a phonetic analysis of voice quality. The interrelationship of different points in the vocal tract is considered together with different types of phonation. Analysis is based on visual and auditory information. Specialised courses are offered for training in the skills necessary to carry out the analysis. *See* Freeman and Fawcus (2001); Beech et al (1993).

vocal tract the whole system through which sounds are produced. It begins with an expulsion of air from the LUNGS which moves up through the TRACHEA and LARYNX in which the VOCAL FOLDS are located. From this point, the air reaches the MOUTH where it is modified by the muscles of the face and tongue to produce the required sound. *See* Catford (1977).

vocalic a MAJOR CLASS FEATURE set up in the DISTINCTIVE FEATURE theory of PHONOLOGY. It distinguishes sounds which are made with a free passage of air through the VOCAL TRACT. In a spectrogram (*see* SPECTROGRAPHY), there is a distinct formant structure [+VOCALIC]. *See* Hyman (1975).

vocalis muscle *see* LARYNX.

voice disorders *see* DYSPHONIA.

voice onset time (VOT) the gap between the release of a closure and the start of voicing, i.e. when the VOCAL FOLDS begin to vibrate. If the sound produced is a voiced plosive /b/, the vocal folds vibrate throughout its production while if the sound is an unaspirated plosive /d/, there is a delay before voicing starts while in a voiceless aspirated plosive /t/ the delay can be much longer depending on the amount of aspiration. *See* Ladefoged (2001).

voice quality *see* REGISTER.

voice rest *see* VOCAL NODULES.

voice synthesis *see* SPEECH SYNTHESIS.

voicing *see* ARTICULATION.

volatile memory computer memory which loses its contents when power is switched off. *See* Brookshear (1991).

VOT *see* VOICE ONSET TIME.

vowel *see* CARDINAL VOWEL SYSTEM.

vowel system different languages have different vowel systems as have different accents of the same language. There are also a number of varieties of English which have different systems such as Scottish English, American English, Australian English, etc. See Fromkin and Rodman (2003); Ladefoged (1993).

VP (verb phrase) *see* CONSTITUENT ANALYSIS.

W

WAIS-R *see* WECHSLER ADULT INTELLIGENCE SCALE – REVISED.

warble tone a tone emitted from a machine which varies in intensity levels. It is part of the DISTRACTION TESTS used to test the hearing of young children. If the child hears the tone, he will turn his head to the side on which the tone has been presented. If he cannot hear the tone, he will continue to look at the person in front of him who is distracting him with toys.

Warnock Report a UK Government report published in 1978 entitled 'Children with Special Needs'. It recommended use of the term 'children with learning difficulties' to replace the former 'educationally subnormal'. They were then to be graded as being mild, moderate or severe with an additional 'specific' category where the difficulty related to one area. *See* Beech et al (1993).

Wechsler Adult Intelligence Scale – Revised (WAIS-R) the first version of WAIS was published in 1939 and revised in 1955. The latest edition was published in 1981. There are 11 subtests, five performance tests and six verbal tests. It can be used with adults in the age range of 16–74 years of age. The subtests have been designed from the easiest to the most difficult and administration is stopped after the person has failed a certain number of items. The RAW SCORE is converted into a STANDARD SCORE with a mean of 10 and a STANDARD DEVIATION of 3. When the six scaled scores of the verbal subtests and the five performance subtests are added together as well as the scaled scores on all the 11 subtests, the three sums are converted to IQ scores – verbal, performance and full-scale.

The IQs have deviations with a mean of 100 and a standard deviation of 15. *See* Aiken (1988); Smith et al (2003); Beech et al (1993); Davison et al (2004).

Wechsler Intelligence Scale for Children – Revised (WISC-R) the original WISC was developed in 1949. The revised version of WISC was published in 1974. It can be administered to children between the ages of 6;0 and 16;0. There are five verbal and five performance subtests with an additional two alternative subtests which are to be used with the child if one of the performance subtests is spoiled or proves difficult to administer. The test usually lasts one hour and the tester receives verbal, performance and full-scale IQ. *See* Aiken (1988); Smith et al (2003); Davison et al (2004).

Wechsler tests tests produced by David Wechsler in the 1930s and 1940s. He produced a test for children: WECHSLER INTELLIGENCE SCALE FOR CHILDREN – REVISED (WISC-R), and for adults: WECHSLER ADULT INTELLIGENCE SCALE – REVISED (WAIS-R). *See* Kolb and Whishaw (1996).

Wernicke-Korsakoff syndrome a SYNDROME which can lead to DEMENTIA. It is produced by a vitamin deficiency of thiamine in the BRAIN. Such deficiency of thiamine occurs in alcoholism, starvation and malnutrition. It has two stages:

1. Wernicke's encephalopathy: the person becomes disoriented in time and place, becomes drowsy, develops abnormalities of the eyes and ataxia. This is caused by the person taking alcohol only, without having anything to eat. Such a condition could be fatal unless the person is given an injection of thiamine. If there is a delay in giving thiamine, the person may recover but will be left with Korsakoff's syndrome.

2. Korsakoff's syndrome: during this part of the syndrome, the person has problems with short-term memory. Proceeding from Wernicke's encephalopathy, the person cannot remember what he has been doing. He cannot find his way to places, and if he does, he cannot get back. People have difficulty forming new memories and they make up stories as they go along. The person should be put on adequate diet with vitamin supplementation and should abstain from alcohol.

See Stafford-Clark and Bridges (1990); Kolb and Whishaw (1996); http://www.healthcentral.com/mhc/top/000771.cfm

Wernicke's aphasia a type of APHASIA first described by Wernicke in 1874 and one of the major types of aphasia identified by the BOSTON SCHOOL. It occurs in Wernicke's area (see CEREBRAL HEMISPHERES) and consequently the predominant feature is impairment in auditory verbal comprehension. See also APHASIA (2). *See* Goodglass and Kaplan (2000); Rosenbek et al (1989); Kolb and Whishaw (1996).

Western Aphasia Battery (WAB) devised by Kertesz, the WAB is an assessment of APHASIA following the LOCATIONIST position whereby the aphasic person is classified into an exclusive category depending on the results, and it uses the modality approach whereby the different modalities of expression, auditory comprehension, reading and writing are tested. The subtests in the Western Aphasia Battery aim to assess content, fluency, auditory comprehension, repetition and naming as well as reading, writing and calculation. RAVEN'S PROGRESSIVE MATRICES are also included in the battery to assess non-verbal visual thinking and there are also subtests for assessing drawing, block design and praxis. After the test is completed, there are two scores – the Aphasia Quotient and a Cortical Quotient. *See* Kertesz (1982) in Appendix I; Rosenbek et al (1989); Beech et al (1993).

wh- questions question words which begin with 'wh-', i.e. why, what, who, when, which, where. 'How' is also included in this classification as it behaves in a similar way to other 'wh-' words. This type of question is opposed to YES/NO QUESTIONS. *See* Fromkin and Rodman (2003).

wh- words *see* WH- QUESTIONS.

Wiig Criterion Referenced Inventory of Language (Wiig CRIL) devised by Wiig, CRIL is a complete inventory of consistent, criterion-referenced language probes that help bridge the gap between diagnosis and intervention. It targets language objectives with language probe sets organised into four modules – SEMANTICS, PRAGMATICS, MORPHOLOGY and SYNTAX. The items are presented in a variety of formats such as picture naming, sentence completion, parallel production and SPEECH ACT elicitation. The child responds orally to each one and is given 10 opportunities with each objective. It can be used with children in the age range of 4;00–13;00. *See* Wiig (1990) in Appendix I.

Wilcoxon test a non-parametric test (*see* PARAMETRIC TESTS) used with the REPEATED MEASURES DESIGN for statistical analysis. The non-parametric equivalent test is the *t*-TEST for related samples. The scores should be ranked in an interval ranking scale. *See* Miller (1984).

Wilson Syntax Screening Test devised by Wilson, this SCREENING TEST is designed to identify signs of language impairment in nursery and reception children. There are 20 items which assess five grammatical constructions which are known to be problematic for children with specific language difficulty. It is suitable for children in the range of 4;00–5;11. *See* Wilson (2001) in Appendix I.

Windbag is a text-based communication system for Windows providing a means of communication for people with little or no speech. It allows a large number of messages to be stored and to be found quickly using abbreviation expansion and word prediction. It can speak pre-stored text by line, sentence or paragraph or speak selected text. Instant responses can be made with a single key and 26 instant messages with two keys. Chat boxes, as they are called, can be loaded and saved for future uses. There is also an extensive phrase bank. There is also a Winbag CE system for those who use the Windows CE operating system on their PC. *See* Appendix IV (Sensory Software International).

Windows

1. Used in icon software (*see* ICON) to show the choices on a menu. It can also be used in graphics where text can be written in a window to explain features of the graphics or as a bit of text referring to the graphic.
2. Users of IBM PCs and compatibles can use Microsoft Windows which is an OPERATING SYSTEM, allowing the operator to use a MOUSE to carry out various functions on the computer without having to type in command words as when using the DOS operating system. Each window has a menu bar with a number of pull-down menus which allow the operator to save, open, edit a file or change the fonts and size of print or choose the type of graphic to draw etc.
3. Operators of Apple Macintosh computers use a window in a similar way

although this type of operating system first appeared on an Apple Macintosh. There is a common menu bar with pull-down menus which changes according to the application being used at the particular time.

Winspeak is a dynamic screen communication software for Windows. It uses grids which are linked together in a logical way so that the person using Winspeak can select whole or parts of messages. It can be accessed using switches and can have text or graphics in the cells of the grids as well as allowing the person using it to continue using Windows menus and dialogue boxes. There are also ready-made vocabulary sets with hundreds of grids, thousands of symbols and printed workbooks. There is also Winspeak CE which can be loaded onto PCs which use the Windows CE operating system. *See* Appendix IV (Sensory Software International).

WISC-R *see* WECHSLER INTELLIGENCE SCALE FOR CHILDREN – REVISED.

WiViK 2.0 an on-screen keyboard, WiViK produces a movable, resizable window and offers a number of different keyboards. Keyboards can be customised to contain letters, numbers, short words, phrases and functions. Selections are made either through a puff switch or by holding the cursor on a character for an adjustable length of time. WiViK 2.0 can also be bundled with a Writing Rate Enhancement Package (WREP) to add word prediction and abbreviation expansion features. WiViK 2.0 requires the Windows 3.1 operating environment or later. *See* Appendix IV (Prentke Romich Company).

WiViK WREP a means of speeding up typing into WiViK, WiViK WREP (Writing Rate Enhancement Package) contains two methods of increasing speed of text entry: word prediction and abbreviation expansion. When the user types the first letter of a word, word prediction causes a group of words to be displayed. If the desired word appears, the user selects it and that word is immediately sent to the working application. If the desired word is not listed, typing an additional letter will refine the word list. Abbreviation expansion allows short sequences of letters such as N and A to stand for longer phrases such as 'Name and address'. WiViK WREP will only work if WiViK 2.0 is already installed on the computer. See Appendix IV (Prentke Romich Company).

word the basic unit used by people to express themselves in spoken and written forms. It is recognised intuitively (*see* INTUITION) by a native speaker but when examined more scientifically by linguists, 'what is a word?' becomes a more complex problem. For example, it is necessary to distinguish between individual word forms occurring in utterances such as 'scream', 'screams', 'screamed'. At a more abstract level, however, linguists would like to recognise all three as forms of a word 'scream'. The latter is sometimes referred to as a lexeme. *See* Lyons (1968); Fromkin and Rodman (2003).

word and paradigm (WP) *see* MORPHOLOGY.

word-final the description of a sound which occurs at the end of a word. For example, in the word /buk/ ('book'), the sound [k] is said to appear word-finally.

word-finding difficulty *see* LEXICAL SYNTACTIC DEFICIT.

Word-Finding Vocabulary Scale devised by Renfrew in 1968 (2nd edition 1972, 3rd edition 1988). It includes 45 pictures each line-drawn on a separate card and arranged in order of frequency of recognition. A guide is given as to which picture testing should start, relative to the child's age, and also guidance as to the number of failures made before discontinuing the test. It is useful for finding whether a child has difficulty retrieving words to which he would respond correctly when named. The test is standardised in the UK and norms are supplied for children of 3;6–8;0 years. *See* Renfrew (1988) in Appendix I.

word-form dyslexia *see* ACQUIRED DYSLEXIA.

word-initial the description of a sound which occurs at the beginning of a word. For example, in the word 'bin', the sound [b] is said to appear word-initially.

word-medial the description of a sound occurring in the middle of the word. For example, in the word /bʌtə/ 'butter', the sound [t] is said to appear word-medially.

word order the sequence of words used to construct phrases and sentences. In English the word order is fixed (*see* SYNTAGMATIC RELATIONS) while in German it is more variable with adverbial phrases and verbs floating around the sentence as long as the verb remains the second idea, not necessarily the second word, of the sentence. *See* Lyons (1968).

word prediction a way of reducing the number of keystrokes over regular spelling with a keyboard. Word prediction software works in such a way that the person using it hits a letter, for example, 'l' (as in the word 'lucky') and in the window appears a number of words starting with 'l' organised by frequency of use. The user then hits a number key or function key to access the word or uses a switch for scanning (if the software allows for switch access). If the word does not appear in the window, the next letter is typed and so on until it does appear. PREDICTIVE ADAPTIVE LEXICON, SOOTHSAYER, PROTOTYPE, Keyrep (see WiViK WREP)and EZ KEYS are some examples of word prediction software. *See* Glennen and DeCoste (1997); Beukelman and Mirenda (1998).

word processor a machine for typing any kind of document by the use of computer technology. It can also refer to the piece of software for use with a microcomputer. Some advantages in using a word processor instead of a manual or electronic typewriter include:

1. The text appears on the screen and can be edited before it is printed or saved on disk.

2. Corrections, which can be made quickly, can be carried out on text which is on disk and then resaved.

3. A letter format can be put on disk and used time after time.

See Bishop (1985).

WordCore a word-based programme designed to work on communication aids, PCs or Macintosh computers. It has 45 keys and the Core screen shows an overlay consisting of only four types of keys – single-hit words (colour-coded in purple); two-hit words or phrases accessed by hitting a green key followed by a second key to generate words like 'I', 'you', etc. and phrases like 'you will/will you'; shortcuts marked by keys with green stripes accessing groups of words like 'question words' or 'th-words' and finally tools designated as blue keys giving commands to the system WordCore is being used on rather than speaking out vocabulary. It has word prediction and a smart row for adding word endings e.g. changes 'decide' to 'decided' or 'deciding' and so on. *See* Cross (2002); Appendix IV (Prentke Romich Company).

Words Strategy devised by Bruce Baker in the late 1980s, it is a MINSPEAK APPLICATION PROGRAM (MAP) for use with the older child, adolescent or adult. Words Strategy has a large core vocabulary with over 2500 individual words and phrases. Almost all the vocabulary is coded by icons and grammatical labels. Some grammatical labels have only one form while others have many forms. The multiple forms are Words Strategy's greatest strengths. No selection requires more than three icon actuations, the majority only require two. In practical usage, Words Strategy has a 66–75 per cent reduction in actuation for spelling. The user does not need to know the grammatical concepts as a prerequisite to using the system. Many acquire vocabulary on an item-by-item basis and understand at a later date the grammatical categories. Words Strategy is not an end point. The preprogrammed vocabulary and grammatical functions can be deleted so that it can be customised for each client to reflect his personality and environment, etc. Grammatical labels on the overlay can be changed to graphic symbols or Minsymbols or even Blissymbols. *See* Baker (1989); Appendix IV (Prentke Romich Company).

WordWall a writing support tool, suitable for all ages. It includes extensive support for word finding, and includes a powerful word prediction engine and works as a specialised on-screen keyboard with standard applications. Word grids can be configured to give lists of words which are easily accessed. *See* Appendix IV (Sensory Software International).

working through *see* PSYCHOANALYSIS.

WP (word and paradigm) *see* MORPHOLOGY.

write the opposite process from read. Data are transferred to a storage device such as a disk. Data can be read from a disk, if they have been previously written to the disk.

wug an imaginary bird-like creature used in an experiment to find out the order of acquisition of grammatical morphemes. In 1958, Berko proposed that if a child had learnt the correct morphological affixes for nouns and verbs, then he could put the correct endings on imaginary words. She drew pictures of imaginary creatures, of which the 'wug' was one. The picture was presented to the child, who was told what it was, and then another picture of the same creature was presented. To the first one, the child was told 'This is a wug, here is another, we have two...', and usually the child replied correctly: 'wugs'. *See* Clark and Clark (1977).

X chromosome *see* CHROMOSOMES.

X-ray *see* RADIOGRAPHY.

xeroradiography a type of X-ray imaging system which enhances contrast in soft tissue by producing a high kilovolt X-ray. It produces an image on a xerographic plate from the effects of X-rays on an electrically charged plate. This technique has been used to examine the VOCAL TRACT during PHONATION. Information about the functioning of the PHARYNX can be assessed along with laryngographic recordings. See Greene and Mathieson (1989); Freeman and Fawcus (2001).

Y-cord hearing aid *see* HEARING AID.

yawn/sigh a technique advocated by Boone in 1977 for treating VOCAL NODULES, it is a means of producing voice without the hard glottal attack which produces vocal nodules. The person is advised to relax completely, take in a deep breath and let it out gradually as a yawn or a sigh and, during this stage, begin to phonate, thus preventing the VOCAL FOLDS from rubbing together harshly. *See* Freeman and Fawcus (2001).

yes/no questions the type of question which will require the answer 'yes' or 'no'. In general, these questions are formed by inversion of the verb and subject or first noun phrase, i.e. NP1:

(1)   He can play football.
(1') Can he play football?

Yes/no questions can be contrasted with WH- QUESTIONS. *See* Clark and Clark (1977); Glennen and DeCoste (1997).

Z scores a way of standardising a person's scores compared to the other scores in that group by converting the raw scores into Z scores. Z scores have a mean of 0 and a standard deviation of 1. So, by converting from a raw score to a Z score, all that has happened is a change of scale so that the raw score is now measured in terms of standard deviations. If a score is the same as the mean of its parent population, it must have a Z score of 0 because it is not different from the mean. If it is one standard deviation away from the mean, it must have a Z score of 1. *See* Miller (1984); Hole (2000).

zero hearing level *see* AUDIOMETRIC ZERO.

zygomatic arch the arch of bones which form the cheeks. The bones which form the arch and the protruding part of the cheek are the zygomatic bones. See Tortora and Grabowski (2000).

Appendix I
Assessments by age groups and client groups

Assessments for children

Acquired Aphasia Assessments

Whurr, R., Evans, S. (1999). *Children's Acquired Aphasia Screening Test (CAAST)*. London: Whurr.

Articulation Assessments

Anthony, A., Bogle, D., Ingram, T.T.S., McIsaac, M.W. (1971). *Edinburgh Articulation Test*. Edinburgh: Churchill Livingstone.
Goldman, R., Fristoe, M. (1972). *Goldman-Fristoe Test of Articulation*. Berks: NFER-Nelson.
Rees, O., Trythall, M. (1995). CWLWM (Welsh Phonetic Screening Assessment). Northumberland: Stass Publications.
Wilcox, K., Morris, S. (1999). *Children's Speech Intelligibility Measures (CISM)*. Kent: The Psychological Corporation.

Auditory Skills Assessments

Goldman, R., Fristoe, M., Woodcock, R.W. (1976). *Goldman-Fristoe-Woodcock Auditory Skills Test Battery*. Circle Pines, MN: American Guidance Service.
Keith, R.W. (1999). *SCAN-C: Test for auditory processing disorders in children – revised*. Kent: The Psychological Corporation.
Morgan-Barry, R. (1988). *Auditory Discrimination and Attention Test*. Berks: NFER-Nelson.
Parsloe, R., Morrell, J. (1996). *Graded Auditory Speech Perception Screen*. Northumberland: Stass Publications.
Renfrew, C.E. (1991). *The Bus Story* (3rd edn). Oxford: author.

Autism Assessments

Aarons, M., Gittens, T. (1992). *The Autistic Continuum: an assessment and intervention schedule*. Berks: NFER-Nelson.
Gilliam, J.E. (1995). *The Gilliam Autism Rating*. Berks: NFER-Nelson.

Cognitive Development

Goodenough, F.L., Harris, D.B. (1963). *Goodenough-Harris Drawing Test*. New York: The Psychological Corporation.

Dyslexia Assessments

Fawcett, A., Nicolson, R. (1996). *Dyslexia Screening Test (DST)*. Kent: The Psychological Corporation.

Miles, T.R. (1982). *Bangor Dyslexia Test*. Wisbech, Cambs: LDA.

Nicolson, R., Fawcett, A. (1996). *Dyslexia Early Screening Test (DEST)*. Kent: The Psychological Corporation.

Feeding/Oral Movement Assessments

Brindley, C., Cave, D., Crane, S., Lees, J., Moffat, V. (1996). *Paediatric Oral Skills Package (POSP)*. London: Whurr.

Jelm, J.M. (1990). *Oral-Motor/Feeding Rating Scale*. Kent: The Psychological Corporation.

Wolf, L.S., Glass, P. (1992). *Feeding and Swallowing Disorders in Infancy: Assessment and management*. Kent: The Psychological Corporation.

Hearing Assessments

Sheridan, M. (1973). *STYCAR Hearing Tests*. Berks: NFER-Nelson.

Language Assessments

Armstrong, S., Ainley, M. (1988). *South Tyneside Assessment of Syntactic Structures*. Northumberland: STASS.

Berry, P., Mittler, P. (1981). *Language Imitation Test*. Manchester: Manchester University Press.

Bishop, D.V.M. (1984). *Test for Reception of Grammar*. Manchester: Manchester University Press.

Blank, M., Rose, A.S., Berlin, L.J. (1988). *Preschool Language Assessment Instrument (PLAI)*. Kent: The Psychological Corporation.

Boehm, A.E. (1976). *Boehm Resource Guide for Basic Concept Teaching*. Kent: The Psychological Corporation.

Boehm, A.E. (1986a). *Boehm Test of Basic Concepts: Preschool version*. Kent: The Psychological Corporation.

Boehm, A.E. (1986b). *Boehm Test of Basic Concepts: Revised*. Kent: The Psychological Corporation.

Boehm, A.E. (2000). *Boehm Test of Basic Concepts 3rd Edition (Boehm-3)*. Kent: The Psychological Corporation.

Boehm, A.E. (2001). *Boehm-3 Preschool*. Kent: The Psychological Corporation.

Boucher, J., Lewis, V. (1997). *Preschool Language Scale-3 (UK)* (adapted for the UK). Kent: The Psychological Corporation.

Bracken, B.A. (1998). *Bracken Basic Concept Scale – Revised (BBCS-R)*. Kent: The Psychological Corporation.

Brimer, M.A., Dunn L.M. (1962). *English Picture Vocabulary Tests: Manual*. Awre, Glos: Education Evaluation Enterprises.

Brimer, M.A., Dunn L.M. (1973). *English Picture Vocabulary Tests: Administration manual*. Awre, Glos: Education Evaluation Enterprises.

Brownell, R. (2000). *Expressive and Receptive One-Word Picture Vocabulary Tests EOWPVT and ROWPVT*. Kent: The Psychological Corporation.

Bzoch, K., League, R. (2003). *Receptive-Expressive Emergent Language Scales: Third Edition – REELS*. Berks: NFER-Nelson.

Carrow-Woolfolk, E. (1974). *Carrow Elicited Language Inventory*. Berks: NFER-Nelson.

Carrow-Woolfolk, E. (rev 1985). *Test for Auditory Comprehension of Language*. Berks: NFER-Nelson.

Carrow-Woolfolk, E. (1998). *Test for Auditory Comprehension of Language: Third Edition – TACL-3.* Berks: NFER-Nelson.

Dean, E., Howell, J., Hill, A., Waters, D. (1990). *Metaphon Resource Pack.* Berks: NFER-Nelson.

Dewart, H., Summers, S. (1988). *Pragmatics Profile of Early Communication.* Berks: NFER-Nelson.

Dewart, H., Summers, S. (1995). *Pragmatics Profile of Everyday Communication Skill in Children – PPC.* Berks: NFER-Nelson.

DiSimoni, F. (1978). *The Token Test for Children.* Berks: NFER-Nelson.

Dodds, B., Crosbie, S., McIntosh, B., Teitzel, T., Ozanne, A. (2000). *Preschool and Primary Inventory of Phonological Awareness.* Kent: The Psychological Corporation.

Duncan, D., Gibbs, D., Singh Noor, N., Mohammed Whittaker, H. (1987). *Sandwell Bilingual Screening Assessment.* Berks: NFER-Nelson.

Dunn, L.M. (1969). *Peabody Picture Vocabulary Test.* Circle Pines, MN: American Guidance Service.

Dunn, L., Dunn, L., Whetton, C., Burley, J. (1997). *British Picture Vocabulary Scale: Second Edition – BPVS II.* Berks: NFER-Nelson.

Dunn, L., Dunn, L., Whetton, C., Pintilie, D. (1982). *British Picture Vocabulary Scales.* Berks: NFER-Nelson.

Edwards, S., Fletcher, P., Garman, M., Hughes, M., Letts, A., Sinka, I. (1997). *The Reynell Developmental Language Scales III: The University of Reading edition.* Berks: NFER-Nelson.

Fawcett, A., Nicolson, R., Lee, R. (2001) *Pre-School Screening Tests (PREST).* London: The Psychological Corporation.

Gutfreund, M. (1989). *Bristol Language Development Scales.* Berks: NFER-Nelson

Kiernan, C., Reid, B. (1987). *Pre-verbal Communication Schedule.* Berks: NFER-Nelson.

Lee, L.L. (1969). *The Northwestern Syntax Screening Test.* Evanston, Ill: Northwestern University Press.

Leiter, R.G. (1969). *The Leiter International Performance Scale.* Chicago: Stoeting & Co.

Locke, A., Beech, M. (1991). Teaching Talking. Berks: NFER-Nelson.

Masidlover, M., Knowles, W. (1987) (revised). *Derbyshire Language Scheme.* Educational Psychology Service, Derbyshire County Council, Ripley.

Newton, M., Thomson, M. (1976). *Aston Index.* London: LDA.

Phelps-Terasata, D., Phelps-Gunn, T. (1992). *Test of Pragmatic Language.* Kent: The Psychological Corporation.

Porch, B. (1971) *The Porch Index of Communicative Ability in Children.* Palo Alto: Consulting Psychologists Press.

Renfrew, C.E. (1971). *Renfrew Language Attainment Scales.* Oxford: Churchill Hospital.

Renfrew, C.E. (1988) *Word Finding Vocabulary* (3rd edn). Oxford: author.

Renfrew, C.E. (1989) *Action Picture Test* (2nd edn). Oxford: author.

Renfrew, C.E. (1991) *The Bus Story* (3rd edn). Oxford: author.

Reynell, J. (1985) *Reynell Developmental Language Scales.* (2nd rev, M. Huntley). Berks: NFER-Nelson.

Rinaldi, W. (1996). *Understanding Ambiguity: An assessment of pragmatic meaning.* Berks: NFER-Nelson.

Rinaldi, W. (2000). *Developing Language.* Berks: NFER-Nelson.

Semel, E., Wiig, E.H., Secord, W. (2000). *Clinical Evaluation of Language Fundamentals (3rd edn) (UK) (CELF-3^{UK}).* Kent: The Psychological Corporation.

Shaw, R. (2000). *Test of Word and Grammatical Awareness – TOWGA.* Berks: NFER-Nelson.

Sheridan, M. (1976). *STYCAR Language Test.* Berks: NFER-Nelson.

Wheldall, K., Mittler, B., Hobsbaum, A. (1987) (revised) *Sentence Comprehension Test.* Berks: NFER-Nelson.

Wiig, E.H. (1982a). *Let's Talk – Developing Prosocial Communication Skills*. Kent: The Psychological Corporation.

Wiig, E.H. (1982b). *Let's Talk – Inventory for Adolescents (LTIA)*. Kent: The Psychological Corporation.

Wiig, E.H. (1983). *Let's Talk - For Children.(LTC)*. Kent: The Psychological Corporation.

Wiig, E.H. (1984). *Let's Talk – Intermediate Level (LTIL)*. Kent: The Psychological Corporation.

Wiig, E.H. (1987). *Let's Talk – Inventory for Children (LTIC)*. Kent: The Psychological Corporation.

Wiig, E.H. (1988a). *CELF-R Scoring Assistant*. Kent: The Psychological Corporation.

Wiig, E.H. (1988b). *CELF-R Screening Test*. Kent: The Psychological Corporation.

Wiig, E.H. (1990). *Wiig Criterion Referenced Inventory of Language (Wiig CRIL)*. Kent: The Psychological Corporation.

Wiig E.H. (1994). *Clinical Evaluation of Language Fundamentals* (*Revised edn UK*) *Adaptation (CELF-R^{UK})*. Kent: The Psychological Corporation.

Wiig, E.H., Secord, W. (1989). *Test of Language Competence – Expanded Edition (TLC-Expanded)*. Kent: The Psychological Corporation.

Wiig, E.H., Secord, W. (1992). *Test of World Knowledge (TOWK)*. Kent: The Psychological Corporation.

Wiig, E.H., Secord, W., Semel, E. (2000). *Clinical Evaluation of Language Fundamentals Preschool* (UK edn). Kent: The Psychological Corporation.

Wilson, M.S. (2001). *Wilson Syntax Screening Test*. Kent: The Psychological Corporation.

Zimmerman, I.L., Steiner, V., Pond, R.E. (1997). *Preschool Language Scale – 3*. Kent: The Psychological Corporation.

Learning Disability/Special Needs Assessments

Douglas, J. (1990). *Special Needs Assessment Software*. Berks: NFER-Nelson.

Jones, S. (1989). *INTECOM*. Berks: NFER-Nelson.

Rinaldi, W. (1992). *Social Use of Language Programme – enhancing the social communication of children and teenagers with special educational needs*. Berks: NFER-Nelson.

Listening Skills Assessments

Lloyd, P., Peers, I., Foster, C. (2001). *The Listening Skills Test*. Kent: The Psychological Corporation.

Motor Skills Assessments

Hayden, D., Square, P. (1999). *Verbal Motor Production Assessment for Children (VMPAC)*. Kent: The Psychological Corporation.

Naming Assessments

German, D.J. (2000). *Test of Word Finding*. Kent: The Psychological Corporation.

Phonology Assessments

Armstrong, S., Ainley, M. (1988). *South Tyneside Assessment of Phonology*. Northumberland: STASS.

Frederickson, N., Frith, U., Reason, R. (1997). *Phonological Assessment Battery: Standardised Edition – PhAB*. Berks: NFER-Nelson.

Grunwell, P. (1985a). *Phonological Assessment of Child Speech*. Berks: NFER-Nelson.

Grunwell, P. (1985b). *PACS Pictures: Language elicitation materials*. Berks: NFER-Nelson.
Grunwell, P. (1995). *PACS Toys Screening Test*. Berks: NFER-Nelson.
Keeling, M., Keeling, J. (2001) *The CLEAR Phonology Screening Assessment*. Kent: Terracotta Design.
Muter, V., Hulme, C., Snowling M. (1997). *Phonological Abilities Test (PAT)*. Kent: The Psychological Corporation.
Shriberg L., Kwiatowski, J. (1980). *Natural Process Analysis*. New York: Wiley.
Torgesen, J.K., Bryant, B.R. (1997). *Test of Phonological Awareness (TOPA)*. Kent: The Psychological Corporation.
Weiner, F.F. (1979). *Phonological Process Analysis*. Baltimore, MD: University Park Press.

Play Assessments

Lewis, V., Boucher, J. (1997). *Test of Pretend Play (ToPP)*. Kent: The Psychological Corporation.
Lowe, M., Costello, A. (1988). *Symbolic Play Test* (2nd edn). Berks: NFER-Nelson.

Psycholinguistics

Kirk, S., McCarthy, J. Kirk, W. (1969) *Illinois Test of Psycholinguistic Abilities*. Berks: NFER-Nelson.
Paraskevopoulos, J. N. Kirk, S A. (1985) *The Development and Psychometric Characteristics of the Revised Illinois Text of Psycholinguistic Abilities*. Champaign: University of Illinois Press.

Stammering Assessments

Crowe, T.A., DiLollo, A.P., Crowe, B.T. (2000). *Crowe's Protocols: A comprehensive guide to stuttering assessment*. Kent: The Psychological Corporation.
Rustin, L. (1987). *Assessment and Therapy Programme for Dysfluent Children*. Berks: NFER-Nelson.
Rustin, L., Kelman, E., Botterill, W. (1996). *Assessment and Therapy for Young Dysfluent Children: Family interaction*. London: Whurr.

Adult assessments

Acquired Aphasia – Comprehension Assessments

DeRenzi, E., Faglioni, P. (1978). Normative data and screening power of a shortened version of the Token Test. *Cortex* **14**: 41–49.
DeRenzi, E., Ferrari, C. (1978). The Reporter's Test: a sensitive test to detect expressive disturbance in aphasics. *Cortex* **14**: 279–293.
DeRenzi, E., Vignolo, L.A. (1962). The Token Test: a sensitive test to detect receptive disturbances in aphasics. *Brain* **85**: 665–678.
McNeil, M. R., Prescott, T. E. (1978). *Revised Token Test*. Baltimore: University Park Press.
Spellacy, F.J., Spreen, O. (1969). A short form of the Token Test. *Cortex* **5**: 390.

Acquired Aphasia – Expressive Language and Comprehension Assessments

Bastiaanse, R., Edwards, S., Rispers, J. (2002) *Verb and Sentence Test*. Kent: The Psychological Corporation.
Enderby, P., Wood, V., Wade, D. (1987). *Frenchay Aphasia Screening Test*. Berks: NFER-Nelson.
Enderby, P., Wood, V., Wade, D. (1997). *Frenchay Aphasia Screening Test*. London: Whurr.

Goodglass, H., Kaplan, E., Barressi, B. (2000). *Boston Diagnostic Aphasia Examination*. Philadelphia: Lea and Febiger.

Kay, J., Lesser, R., Coltheart, M. (1992). *Psycholinguistic Assessments of Language Processing in Aphasia*. Hove: Erlbaum.

Kertesz, A. (1982). *Western Aphasia Battery*. New York: Psychological Corporation.

LaPointe, L.L. (1977) Base-10 programmed stimulation: Task specification, scoring and plotting performance in aphasia therapy. *Journal of Speech and Hearing Disorders* 42: 90–105.

Porch, B. (1967). *The Porch Index of Communicative Ability*. Palo Alto: Consulting Psychologists Press.

Schuell, H. (1973) (revised). *Minnesota Test for the Differential Diagnosis of Aphasia*. Berks: NFER-Nelson.

Syder, D., Body, R., Parker, M., Boddy, M. (1994). *Sheffield Screening Test for Acquired Language Disorders*. Berks: NFER-Nelson.

West, J.F., Sands, E., Ross-Swain, D. (1998). *Bedside Evaluation Screening Test – Second Edition (BEST-2)*. Kent: The Psychological Corporation.

Whurr, R. (1996). *The Aphasia Screening Test: Second edition*. London: Whurr.

Acquired Aphasia – Naming Assessments

Kaplan, E., Goodglass, H., Weintraub, S. (1983). *Boston Naming Test*. Philadelphia: Lea & Febiger.

McKenna, P., Warrington, E. (1983). *Graded Naming Test*. Berks: NFER-Nelson.

Acquired Aphasia – Reading Comprehension Assessments

LaPointe, L.L., Horner, J. (1979). *Reading Comprehension Battery for Aphasia*. Austin, TX: PRO-ED.

Acquired Apraxia Assessments

Dabul, B. (2000). *Apraxia Battery for Adults*. Kent: The Psychological Corporation.

Hickman, L.A. (1997). *The Apraxia Profile*. Kent: The Psychological Corporation.

Acquired Dysarthria Assessments

Drummond, S.S. (1993). *Dysarthria Examination Battery*. Kent: The Psychological Corporation.

Enderby, P. (1988). *Frenchay Dysarthria Assessment and Computer Differential Analysis*. Berks: NFER-Nelson.

Acquired Dysphagia

Avery-Smith, W., Rosen, A.B., Dellarosa, D. (1997). *Dysphagia Evaluation Protocol*. Kent: The Psychological Corporation.

Attention-Deficit Disorder

Brown, T.E. (1996) *Brown Attention-Deficit Disorder Scales*. Lutz, FL.: PAR Inc.

Auditory Processing Assessments

Keith, R.W. (1994). *SCAN-A: A Screening Test for Auditory Processing Disorders in Adolescents and Adults*. Kent: The Psychological Corporation.

Cognition

Helm-Estabrody (2000). *Cognitive Lingustic Quick Test*. Kent: The Psychological Corporation.
Mallall, D.J. (1989). *Functional Performance Record*. Berks: NFER-Nelson.

Dyslexia

Fawcett, A., Nichoson, R. (1998). *Dyslexia Adult Screening Test*. Kent: The Psychological Corporation.

Functional Communication Assessments

Baines, K.A., Heeringa, H.M., Martin, A.W. (1999). *Assessment of Language – Related Functional Activities*. Austin, TX: PRO-ED.
Holland, A.L., Frattali, C.M., Fromm, D. (1999). *Communicative Abilities in Daily Living – Second Edition*. Kent: The Psychological Corporation.
Skinner, C., Wirz, S., Thompson, I., Davidson, J. (1984). *Edinburgh Functional Communication Profile: An observation procedure of the evaluation of disordered communication in elderly patients*. Winslow, Bucks: Winslow Press.

Hearing

Hallam, R. (1997). *Tinnitus Questionnaire*. Kent: The Psychological Corporation.
Hallam, R. (1997). *Hearing Attitudes in Rehabilitation Questionnaires*. Kent: The Psychological Corporation.

Learning Disabilities

Bloomberg, K., West, D. (1999). *The Triple C: checklist of communication competencies*. Victoria, Australia: SCIOP.
Hitchings, A., Spence, R. (1991). *Personal Communication Plan*. Berks: NFER-Nelson.

Neuropsychology

Randolph, C. (1998). *Repeatable Battery for the Assessment of Neuropsychological Status*. Kent: The Psychological Corporation.

Psychological Assessments

Elliott, C.D., Smith, P., Mc Culloch, K (1996) *British Ability Scales. Second Edition*. Berks: NFER-Nelson
Statsman, R (1926–1931) *Merill-Palmer Pre-school Intelligence Test*. Berks: NFER-Nelson

261

Appendix II
Speech and language development

Age	Description
0;0–0;3	Cries and reflexive sounds.
0;3–1;0	Babbling begins; babbling and intonation sounds like human language, i.e. babbling drift.
1;3–2;6	Lexical overgeneralisation, i.e. protowords or vocables.
1;0–1;9	First word stage: later in this stage, intonation is used meaningfully.
1;9–2;3	Second word stage: the child begins to use semantic categories; his language begins to become more complex.

Acquisition of syntax

Verb phrase – tense, aspect, mood

(a) Simple present
(b) Progressive
(c) Past tense (use of 'did')
(d) Future (use of 'going to')
(e) Passive (develops between 6;0–9;0)

Auxiliary

(a) Can't ⎱ used as
(b) Don't ⎰ negatives
(c) No/not – alternatives
(d) Did
(e) Will
(f) Can

Negation

(a) No/not (used at start of sentence)
(b) Can't ⎱ used as
(c) Don't ⎰ negatives
(d) No/not – used as alternatives
    e.g. I no eat meat
    e.g. I not eat meat

Noun phrase – demonstratives/articles, pronouns, adjectives

Order of appearance in:

1. Demonstratives/articles
   (a) this/that
   (b) indefinite article
   (c) definite article
2. Pronouns
   (a)   (i) 1st person subject – I (me/mine)
         (ii) 3rd person inanimate – it (object)
   (b)   (i) 1st person object – me, mine
         (ii) 3rd person inanimate – it (subject)
   (c) he, she, him, her
   (d) remainder includes second person and plurals
3. Adjectives
   (a) adjectives of size
   (b) adjectives of affection
   (c) adjectives of colour

Some adjectives appear at two-word stage

Adverbials

(a) Location – two-word stage
(b) Time – 6 months after start of two-word stage
(c) Manner – end of first year of developing syntax
(d) Sentence adverbials – 4;0

Prepositions

(a) In, on, under
(b) Back, front, between (+featured object)
(c) Back, front (+unfeatured object)
(d) Left, right

Interrogative

(a) Yes/no questions   – marked by intonation and gesture
                       – auxiliaries added not necessarily correctly formed, e.g. does
                         lions walk?
                       – auxiliary-subject inversion correctly used
(b) Wh- questions   – wh- words without auxiliary or inversion, e.g. where me
                         sleep?
                       – wh- word with auxiliary but without inversion, e.g. where
                         me do sleep?
                       – wh- word used correctly with both auxiliary and inversion,
                         e.g. where do I sleep?

Acquisition of wh- words

(a) What
(b) Where – used for locatives in two-word stages
(c) Why   ⎫ large gap between the development
    What ⎬ of these three and first two seems
    Where ⎭ to reflect cognitive/social development

Conjunctions

(a) And, but (early)
(b) So, if, because, when ⎫ developed by
(c) Before, after   ⎬ almost 4;0

Acquisition of morphology

Inflectional morphology

1. The form of morpheme occurs as a free variant with the root form:
   (a) third person simple present
          [s] after voiceless C
   {z}⟷ [z] after voiced C
          [ɪz] after sibilants
   (b) past tense
          [t] after voiceless C
   {D}⟷ [d] after voiced C
          [ɪd] after /t,d/

2. The morpheme occurs correctly and consistently but is not always used where it would be obligatory in adult language.

3. The morpheme occurs correctly and consistently although the actual phonological form may vary.

Note: The transition between (2) and (3) may take several months so it is difficult to say when the morpheme is used correctly; it is best to say it is present when it occurs on 90 per cent of occasions where it would occur in adult language. Using such a criterion the order of inflectional morphemes is as follows:

(a) Present progressive {be...ing}
(b) Plural
(c) Past
(d) Third person singular present

Note: These forms are only acquired in this order, not necessarily with meaning (*see also* MEAN LENGTH OF UTTERANCE).

Acquisition of lexis

Comprehension of words is very likely to be ahead of their production.

1. Production averages (words):
   By 1;6   100–200
   By 2;6   500
   By 5;0   2000
   By 6;0–7;0 4000

2. Words learnt in order:
   (a)   names for classes of food
   (b)   body parts
   (c)   articles of clothing
   (d)   small household/garden objects
   (e)   animals
   (f)   vehicles
   (g)   toys
   (h)   pictures in picture books

3. Word meaning:
   (a)   reference – most words learnt this way; the object is present when named but could lead to mislearning.
   (b)   linguistic induction – at 3;0–4;0. The children begin to guess the meaning of the new word by knowing the meaning of the words in the immediate environment of the new one.
   (c)   learning by deduction – comes later, perhaps not until the child's early years at school.

Note: These have been found in research and are based on Cruttenden (1979). As there is variation in children's acquisition of speech and language, all ages given and the order of various items should be treated with caution.

Appendix III
The International Phonetic Alphabet (revised to 1989)

CONSONANTS

	Bilabial	Labiodental	Dental	Alveolar	Postalveolar	Retroflex	Palatal	Velar	Uvular	Pharyngeal	Glottal
Plosive	p b			t d		ʈ ɖ	c ɟ	k g	q ɢ		ʔ
Nasal	m	ɱ		n		ɳ	ɲ	ŋ	N		
Trill	ʙ			r					R		
Tap or Flap				ɾ		ɽ					
Fricative	ɸ β	f v	θ ð	s z	ʃ ʒ	ʂ ʐ	ç ʝ	x ɣ	χ ʁ	ħ ʕ	h ɦ
Lateral fricative				ɬ ɮ							
Approximant		ʋ		ɹ		ɻ	j	ɰ			
Lateral approximant				l		ɭ	ʎ	L			
Ejective stop	p'			t'		ʈ'	c'	k'	q'		
Implosive	ƥ ɓ			ƭ ɗ			ƈ ʄ	ƙ ɠ	ʠ ʛ		

Where symbols appear in pairs, the one to the right represents a voiced consonant. Shaded areas denote articulations judged impossible.

DIACRITICS

˳ Voiceless	n̥ d̥	ˏ More rounded	ɔ�హ	ʷ Labialised	tʷ dʷ	~ Nasalised	ẽ
ˬ Voiced	s̬ t̬	˛ Less rounded	ɔ̜	ʲ Palatalised	tʲ dʲ	ⁿ Nasal release	dⁿ
ʰ Aspirated	tʰ dʰ	˖ Advanced	u̟	ˠ Velarised	tˠ dˠ	ˡ Lateral release	dˡ
¨ Breathy voiced	b̤ a̤	ˍ Retracted	i̱	ˤ Pharyngealised	tˤ dˤ	˺ No audible release	d˺
~ Creaky voiced	b̰ a̰	¨ Centralised	ë	~ Verbalised or pharyngealised	ɫ		
ˌ Linguolabial	t̼ d̼	˟ Mid-centralised	e̽	ˌ Raised	e̝ (ɹ̝ = voiced alveolar fricative)		
̪ Dental	t̪ d̪	ˌ Syllabic	ɹ̩	ˎ Lowered	e̞ (β̞ = voiced bilabial approximant)		
ˡ Apical	t̺ d̺	ˆ Non-syllabic	e̯	ˌ Advanced tongue root	e̘		
˳ Laminal	t̻ d̻	˞ Rhoticity	ɚ˞	ˌ Retracted tongue root	e̙		

266

VOWELS

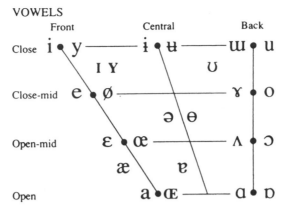

Where symbols appear in pairs, the one to the right represents a rounded vowel.

OTHER SYMBOLS

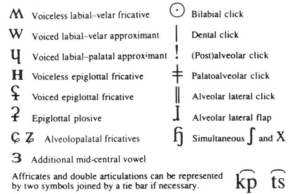

ʍ Voiceless labial–velar fricative	⊙ Bilabial click
w Voiced labial–velar approximant	ǀ Dental click
ɥ Voiced labial–palatal approximant	ǃ (Post)alveolar click
ʜ Voiceless epiglottal fricative	ǂ Palatoalveolar click
ʢ Voiced epiglottal fricative	‖ Alveolar lateral click
ʡ Epiglottal plosive	ɺ Alveolar lateral flap
ɕ ʑ Alveolopalatal fricatives	ɧ Simultaneous ʃ and X
ɜ Additional mid-central vowel	

Affricates and double articulations can be represented by two symbols joined by a tie bar if necessary. k͡p t͡s

SUPRASEGMENTALS

ˈ	Primary stress	ˌfoʊnəˈtɪʃən
ˌ	Secondary stress	
ː	Long	eː
ˑ	Half-long	eˑ
�‿	Extra-short	ĕ
.	Syllable break	ɹi.ækt
ǀ	Minor (foot) group	
‖	Major (intonation) group	
‿	Linking (absence of a break)	
↗	Global rise	
↘	Global fall	

TONES and WORD ACCENTS

LEVEL

e̋ or ˥	Extra high
é ˦	High
ē ˧	Mid
è ˨	Low
ȅ ˩	Extra low
↓	Downstep
↑	Upstep

CONTOUR

ě or ˄	Rising
ê ˅	Falling
e᷄ ˧˥	High rising
e᷅ ˩˨	Low rising
e᷈ ˧˦	Rising-falling etc.

267

Appendix IV
Acknowledgements

Acknowledgements of trademarks and UK suppliers of AAC devices, computer hardware, peripherals and software

Ability Net is an organisation which provides asssessments, advice and information about technology for people with disabilities.

AbleNet holds the trademarks for BIGmack, Big Red Switches, Jelly Bean Switches, One Step Communicator, Speak Easy, Step-by-Step Communicator, and Step-by-Step Communicator with Levels, TalkTrac and is supplied in the UK by various companies: Inclusive Technology website: www.inclusive.co.uk; Liberator Ltd. website: www.liberator.co.uk; Don Johnston Special Needs Ltd. website: www.donjohnston.com/uk; QED Ltd. website: www.qedltd.com; SEMERC website: www.semerc.com; SpaceKraft website: www.SpaceKraft.co.uk; Prentke Romich International website: www.prentromint.com

Active holds the trademarks for DigiVox, DigiVox 2 and Digimax.

AdamLab holds the trademarks for Black Hawk, Hawk II, Hawk III, Light Hawk and SuperHawk which are supplied in Europe by Techcess. Website: www.techcess.co.uk

Applied Human Factors holds the trademarks for JoystickBuddy, REACH Interface Author, REACH Smart Key Technology, ScanBuddy, SoothSayer. These products are supplied by ITAbility in the UK and Ireland. Website: www.chatability.co.uk/ITAbility

Bostock holds the trademark for IconSpeak. http://www.bostock.com/IconSpeak International.htm

Cambridge Adaptive Communication holds the trademarks for all models of the Cameleon. Website: www.cameleon-web.com

Canon holds the trademark for the Canon Communicator which is supplied in the UK by EasiAids. Website: www.easiaids.co.uk

Digital Corporation (see Digital Equipment Company)

Digital Equipment Company holds the trademark for DECtalk.

Don Johnston Development Equipment Inc. holds the registered trademark of Kn:ex and it is supplied in the UK by Don Johnston Special Needs Ltd. Website: www. donjohnston.com/uk

DynaVox Systems Inc. holds the trademarks for DynaCards, DynaMo, DynaMyte, DynaSyms, DynaVox, DynaVox System Software and DynaWrite which are all supplied in the UK by Sunrise Medical. Website: www.sunrisemedical.co.uk

Eye Tracking Systems holds the trademark for the Quick Glance Eye Tracking System.

Falck holds the trademarks for VocaFlex and Spokesman which are supplied in the UK and Ireland by Toby Churchill. Website: www.toby-churchill.com

Hartana Developments Ltd. holds the trademark for Tana Talker which is manufactured by Masterswitch (UK) Ltd.

Hugh MacMillan Rehabilitation Centre holds the trademarks for WiViK2, WiVox and KeyREP which are supplied in the UK by Prentke Romich International. Website: www.prentromint.com

Ingfield Manor designed a vocabulary system for the Cameleon communication aids.

Madentec holds the trademarks for ScreenDoors, Tracker and Wisp.

Maltron holds the trademarks for its various ergonomic keyboards.

Metrovision holds the trademark for VisioBoard. Website: www.chatability.co.uk/ITAbility

Morphonics Ltd. is the manufacturer and supplier of the Eclipse communication aid.

Origin Systems holds the trademark for HeadMouse and is supplied in the UK by Don Johnston Special Needs Ltd.

Possum holds the trademarks for Compact, Companion and Freeway environmental controllers. Website: www.possum.co.uk

Prentke Romich Company holds the registered trademarks for AlphaTalker II, AXS-1600, BUILLD, DeltaTalker, Director, HeadMaster, IntroTalker, Liberator, LightTalker, M.I.K.E., Pathfinder, Scanning Director, SideKick, Springboard, TouchTalker, Vanguard, Vanguard for Windows, Vantage and Words Strategy which are all supplied by Prentke Romich International. Website: www.prentromint.com

Richard Hill and Associates is the supplier of TouchSpeak.

RSL Steeper supplies the Fox, Lynx and Persona environmental controls. Website: http://www.rslsteeper.com/

Saltillo Corp. holds the registered trademarks for ChatBox, ChatBox DX and ChatPC which are supplied by Liberator Ltd. and Prentke Romich International. Websites: www. liberator.co.uk and www.prentromint.com

Sandwell Special Projects manufactures the Echo4.

Semantic Compaction Systems holds the registered trademarks for Minspeak, Unity and AQLS which are supplied by Prentke Romich International. Website: www.prentromint.com

Sensory Software International holds the copyright for AllWrite, InGrid, HandsOff, Prototype, Windbag, Winspeak and WordWall. Website: www.sensorysoftware.com

TASH holds the trademark for Buddy Button.

Technology and Integration holds the trademarks for Tellus 2, Mind Express and Feelix which are supplied in the UK by Techcess Ltd. Website: www.techcess.co.uk

Toby Churchill holds the trademarks for all models of Lightwriter and adVOCAte. Website: www.toby-churchill.com

Vocab Voice Systems Ltd. holds the trademark for the Vocab+ software which is supplied by Liberator Ltd. in the UK and Ireland. Website: www.liberator.co.uk

Words+ holds the trademarks for MessageMate, EZ Keys for Windows and Talking Screen for Windows which are supplied by Cambridge Adaptive Communication. Website: www.cameleon-web.com

Zygo holds the trademarks for Macaw, Parakeet, Parrot and IconsLink. They are supplied in the UK by Toby Churchill. Website: www.toby-churchill.com

Bibliography

Abercrombie, D. (1967). *Elements of General Phonetics*. Edinburgh: Edinburgh University Press.

Adams, C. (1997). Facilitated communication training: an evaluation. *European Journal of Communication Disorders* **32**: 70–75.

Adams, C. (2001). Clinical diagnostic and intervention studies of children with semantic-pragmatic language disorder. *International Journal of Language and Communication Disorders* **36**: 289–306.

Adams, C., Bishop, D.V.M. (1989). Conversational characteristics of children with semantic-pragmatic disorder. I: Exchange structure, turntaking, repairs, cohesion. *British Journal of Disorders of Communication* **24;3**: 211–239.

Adams, C., Byers Brown, B., Edwards, M. (1997). *Developmental Disorders of Language* (2nd edn). London: Whurr.

Adams, S.G., Lang, A.E. (1992). Can the Lombard effect be used to improve voice intensity in Parkinson's disease? *European Journal of Communication Disorders* **27;2**: 121–128.

Adamson, C., Byers Brown, B., Edwards, M. (1997). *Developmental Disorders of Language*. London: Whurr.

Adamson, L.B., Dunbar, B. (1991). Communication development of young children with tracheostomies. *Augmentative and Alternative Communication* **7;4**: 275–283.

Aiken, L.R. (1988) *Psychological Testing and Assessment* (6th edn). Massachusetts: Allyn and Bacon.

Ainsworth, M.D.S. (1979). Infant–mother attachment. *American Psychologist* **34**: 932–937.

Allen, D.A. (1988). Autistic spectrum disorders: clinical presentation in preschool children. *Journal of Child Neurology* **3**: S48–S56.

Allen, D.A. (1989). Developmental language disorders in preschool children: clinical subtypes and syndromes. *School Psychology Review* **18**: 442–451.

Allerton, D.J. (1979). *Essentials of Grammatical Theory: A consensus of syntax and morphology*. London: Routledge and Kegan Paul.

Allum-Mecklenberg, D.J. (1996). *Cochlear Implant Rehabilitation in Children and Adults*. London: Whurr.

American Psychiatric Association (1991). *Diagnostic and Statistical Manual of Mental Disorders* (4th edn) (DSM-IV). Washington DC: American Psychiatric Association.

Anderson, R.T. (2001). Learning an invented inflectional morpheme in Spanish by children with typical language skills and with specific language impairment (SLI). *International Journal of Language and Communication* **36;1**: 1–19.

Argyle, M. (1994). *The Psychology of Interpersonal Behaviour*. London: Penguin.

Armstrong, L., Jans, D., MacDonald, A. (2000). Parkinson's disease and aided AAC: some evidence from practice. *International Journal of Language and Communication Disorders* **35;3**: 377–389.

Aten, J.L. (1991). Group therapy for aphasic patients: let's show it works. *Aphasiology* **5;6**: 559–561.

Badman, A.L., Baker, B., Banajee, M., Cross, R., Lehr, J.S., Maro, J., Zucco, M. (1995). *Unity/128*. Wooster, Ohio: Prentke Romich Company.

Bailey, P., Jenkinson, J. (1982). The application of Blissymbols. In M. Peter, B. Baker (eds) Minspeak: A Semantic Compaction System that Makes Self-expression Easier for Communicatively Disabled Individuals. *Byte* Sept.

Baker, B. (1982) Minspeak: A Semantic Compaction System that Makes Self-expression Easier for Communicatively Disabled Individuals. *Byte* Sept.

Baker, B. (1989). Words strategy. *Proceedings of 1st UK Minspeak Conference*. Sept.

Balandin, S., Morgan, J. (2001). Preparing for the future: aging and Alternative and Augmentative Communication. *Augmentative and Alternative Communication* **17;2:** 99–100.

Ball, M.J. (1999). Reynell Developmental Language Scales III: a quick and easy LARSP. *International Journal of Language and Communication Disorders* **34;2:** 171–174.

Ball, M., Lowry, O. (2001). *Methods in Clinical Phonetics*. London: Whurr.

Ballantyne, D., Martin, M. (2001) Subjective audiometry. In J. Graham, M. Martin, (eds) *Ballantyne's Deafness* (6th edn). London: Whurr.

Bandura, A. (1969). *Principles of Behavior Modification*. New York: Holt, Rinehart and Winston.

Barker, P. (1981). *Basic Family Therapy*. London: Granada.

Barlow, D.H., Hersen, M. (1984). *Single Case Experimental Designs: Strategies for studying behaviour change*. Oxford: Pergamon Press.

Baron-Cohen, S. (1987). Autism and symbolic play. *British Journal of Developmental Psychology* **5:** 139–148.

Barr, M.L. (1988). *The Human Nervous System: An anatomical viewpoint* (5th edn). Philadelphia PA: Lippincott.

Basso, A. (1992). Prognostic factors in aphasia. *Aphasiology* **6;4:** 337–348.

Bayles, K.A. (1984). Language and dementia. In H.A. Holland (ed.) *Language in Adults*, pp. 209–244. San Diego: College-Hill Press.

Beard, R.M. (1969). *An Outline of Piaget's Developmental Psychology*. London: Routledge and Kegan Paul.

Beck, A.R., Fritz, H. (1998). Can people who have aphasia learn iconic codes? *Augmentative and Alternative Communication* **14;3:** 184–195.

Beckwith, J.B. (1963). Extreme cytomegaly of the fetal adrenal cortex, omphalocele, hyperplasia of kidneys and pancreas, and Leydig-cell hyperplasia: another syndrome? *Presented at the Annual Meeting of Western Society for Paediatric Research*, Los Angeles, California, November 11.

Bedrosian, J.L. (1997). Language acquisition in young AAC system users: issues and directions for future research. *Augmentative and Alternative Communication* **13;3:** 179–185.

Beech, J.R., Harding, L., Hilton-Jones, D. (1993). *Assessments in Speech and Language Therapy*. London: Routledge.

Beeghly, M., Benigni, L., Bretherton, I., Camaioni, L., Volterra, V. (1990). Beyond sensori-motor functioning: early communicative and play development of children with Down syndrome. In D. Cicchetti, M. Beeghly (eds) *Children with Down Syndrome: A developmental perspective*, p. 329. Cambridge: Cambridge University Press.

Beliveau, C., Hodge, M.M., Hagler, P.H. (1995). Effects of supplemental linguistic cues on the intelligibility of severely dysarthric speakers. *Augmentative and Alternative Communication* **11;3:** 176–186.

Bench, J. (1992). *Communication Skills in Hearing-Impaired Children*. London: Whurr.

Benson, D.F. (1979). Neurologic correlates of anomia. In H.A. Whitaker, H. Whitaker (eds) *Studies in Neurolinguistics*, vol. 4. London: Academic Press.

Benson, D.F., Geschwind, N. (1969). The Alexias. In P.J. Vinken, G.W. Bruyn (eds) *Handbook of Clinical Neurology,* vol. 4, pp. 112–140. Amsterdam: North Holland Publishing Company.

Berko, J., Brown, R. (1960). Psycholinguistic research in children's language. In P.H. Mussen (ed.) *Handbook of Research Methods in Child Development.* New York: John Wiley and Sons.

Berry, P. (ed.) (1976). *Language and Communication in the Mentally Handicapped.* London: Edward Arnold.

Best, W., Bryan, K., Maxim, J. (2000). *Semantic Processing: Theory and practice.* London: Whurr.

Beukelman, D.R., Mirenda, P. (1998) *Augmentative and Alternative Communication: Management of severe communication disorders in children and adults* (2nd edn). Baltimore: Paul H. Brookes Publishing Co.

Beukelman, D.R., Yorkston, K.M. (1989). Alternative and Augmentative Communication for persons with severe acquired communication disorders: an introduction. *Augmentative and Alternative Communication* **5;1:** 42–48.

Bishop, D.V.M. (1979). Comprehension in developmental language disorders. *Developmental Medical Child Neurology* **21:** 225–238.

Bishop, D.V.M. (1982). Comprehension of spoken, written and signed sentences in childhood language disorders. *Journal of Child Psychology Psychiatry* **23;1:** 1–20.

Bishop, D.V.M. (1984). Automated LARSP: computer-assisted grammatical analysis. *British Journal of Disorders of Communication* **19;1:** 78–87.

Bishop, D.V.M. (2000). What's so special about Asperger's syndrome? The need for further exploration of the borderlands of autism. In A. Klin, F.R. Volkmar, S.S. Sparrow (eds) *Asperger Syndrome* (pp. 254–277). New York: Guilford.

Bishop, D.V.M., Adams, C. (1989). Conversational characteristics of children with semantic-pragmatic disorders. II: What features lead to a judgement of inappropriacy? *British Journal of Disorders of Communication* **24;3:** 241–263.

Bishop, D.V.M., Chan, J., Adams, C., Hartley, J., Weir, F. (2000). Conversational responsiveness in specific language impairment: disproportionate pragmatic difficulties in a subset of children. *Development and Psychopathology* **12:** 177–197.

Bishop, D.V.M., Mogford, K. (1993). *Language Development in Exceptional Circumstances.* Hove: Lawrence Erlbaum Associates.

Bishop, P. (1985). *Comprehensive Computer Studies* (4th impression 1989). London: Hodder & Stoughton.

Blackburn, D., Bonvillian, J., Ashby, R. (1984). Manual communication as an alternative mode of language instruction for children with severe reading disabilities. *Language, Speech and Hearing Services in Schools* **15:** 22–31.

Blanken, G. (1991). The functional basis of speech automatisms (recurring utterances). *Aphasiology* **5;2:** 103–128.

Bliss, C. (1965). *Semantography.* Sydney, Australia: Semantography Publications.

Blomert, L., Kean, M.L., Koster, Ch., Schokker, J. (1994). Amsterdam-Nijmeyer Everyday Language Test: Construction, reliability and validity. *Aphasiology* **8;4:** 381–407.

Bloomberg, K., Karlan, G., Lloyd, L. (1990). The comparative translucency of initial lexical items represented by five graphic symbol systems and sets. *Journal of Speech and Hearing Research* **33:** 717–725.

Bloomberg, K., West, D. (1999). *The Triple C: Checklist of communication competencies.* Victoria, Australia: SCIOP

Boden, M.A. (1994) *Piaget* (2nd edn). London: Fontana Press.

Bollinger, R.L., Musson, N.D., Holland, A.L. (1993). A study of group communication intervention with chronic aphasic persons. *Aphasiology* **7;3**: 301–314.

Bolton, S.O., Dashiell, S.E. (1984). *Interacion Checklist for Augmentative Communication*. California: Imaginative Communication Products.

Bondy, A.S., Frost, L.A. (1993). Mands across the water: A report on the application of the picture-exchange communication system in Peru. *The Behaviour Analyst* **16**: 123–128.

Bondy, A., Frost, L. (1995a). Hands across the water: A report on the application of the picture-exchange communication system in Peru. *The Behaviour Analyst* **16**: 123–128.

Bondy, A., Frost, L. (1995b). Educational approaches in preschool: behaviour techniques in a public school setting. In E. Schopler, G. Mesibov (eds) *Learning and Cognition in Autism* (pp. 331–333). New York: Plenum.

Bonvillian, J., Friedman, R. (1978). Language development in another mode: The acquisition of signs by a brain-damaged adult. *Sign Language Studies* **19**: 111–120.

Bornstein, H., Hamilton, L.B. (1978). *Signed English*. Ways and Means. Globe Education.

Botting, N. (1998). Semantic-Pragmatic disorder (SPD) as a distinct diagnostic entity: making sense of the boundaries. *International Journal of Disorders of Communication* **33;1**: 87–90.

Botting, N., Conti-Ramsden, G. (2001). Non-words repetition and language development with specific language impairment (SLI). *International Journal of Disorders of Communication* **36;4**: 421–432.

Botting, N., Conti-Ramsden, G., Crutchley, A. (1998a). Educational transitions from a clinical perspective: a reply to commentaries. *International Journal of Disorders of Communication* **33;2**: 215–220.

Botting, N., Crutchley, A., Conti-Ramsden, G. (1998b) Educational transitions of 7-year-old children with SLI in language units: a longitudinal survey. *International Journal of Disorders of Communication* **33;2**: 177–197.

Boucher, J. (1998a). SPD as a distinct diagnostic entity: logical consideration and directions for future research. *International Journal of Disorders of Communication* **33;1**: 71–81.

Boucher, J. (1998b). Some issues in the classification of developmental disorders. *International Journal of Disorders of Communication* **33;1**: 95–108.

Bourgeois, M.S. (1992). Evaluating memory wallets for adults with dementia. *Journal of Speech and Hearing Research* **34**: 831–844.

Bourgeois, M.S., Dijkstra, K., Burgio, L., Allen-Burge, R. (2001). Memory aids as an Augmentative and Alternative Communication strategy for nursing home residents with dementia. *Augmentative and Alternative Communication* **17;3**: 196–210.

Bowen, C., Cupples, L. (1999a). Parents and children together (PACT): a collaborative approach to phonological therapy. *International Journal of Language and Communication Disorders* **34;1**: 35–55.

Bowen, C., Cupples, L. (1999b). A phonological therapy in depth: a reply to commentaries. *International Journal of Language and Communication Disorders* **34;1**: 65–83.

Bowler, D.M., Lister Brook, S. (1998). SPD and autistic spectrum disorder. *International Journal of Disorders of Communication* **33;1**: 91–95.

Bromley, D.B. (1988). *Human Ageing: An introduction to gerontology*. London: Penguin.

Brookshear, J.G. (1991). *Computer Science: An overview*. California: Benjamin Cummings Publishing Company, Inc.

Brosnahan, L.F., Malmberg, B. (1976). *Introduction to Phonetics*. Cambridge: Cambridge University Press.

Brown, K., Miller, J. (1991) *Syntax: A Linguistic Introduction to Sentence Structure* (2nd edn). London: Routledge.

Brown, R. (1973). *A First Language: The early stages*. Cambridge, MA: Harvard University Press.

Bruno, J. (1989a). Interaction, Education and Play. *Proceedings of 1st UK Minspeak Conference*. Swinstead: Liberator Ltd.

Bruno, J. (1989b). Customizing a Minspeak system for a preliterate child: A case example. *Augmentative and Alternative Communication* **5;2**: 89–100.

Burden, V., Stott, C.M., Forge, J., Goodyer, I. (1996). The Cambridge Language and Speech Project (CLASP). I. Detection of language difficulties at 36 to 39 months. *Developmental Medicine and Child Neurology* **38**: 613–631.

Burroughs, J., Albritton, E., Eaton, B., Montague, J. (1990). A comparative study of language delayed preschool children's ability to recall symbols from two symbol systems. *Augmentative and Alternative Communication* **11**: 37–48.

Burton, M. (2001). Acquired sensorineural hearing loss. In J. Graham, M. Martin (eds) *Ballantyne's Deafness* (6th edn). London: Whurr.

Butterworth B. (1984). Jargon aphasia: processes and strategies. In S.K. Newman, R. Epstein (eds) *Current Perspectives in Dysphasia*. Edinburgh: Churchill Livingstone.

Byers Brown, B. (1976). Language vulnerability, speech delay and therapeutic intervention. *British Journal of Disorders of Communication* **11**: 43–56.

Byers Brown, B. (1981). *Speech Therapy: Principles & practice*. Edinburgh: Churchill Livingstone.

Byrne, K., Abbeduto, L., Brooks, P. (1990). The language of children with spina bifida and hydrocephalus meeting task demands and mastering syntax. *Journal of Speech and Hearing Disorders* **55;1**: 118–123.

Calculator, C.N. (1997). Fostering early language acquisition and AAC use: exploring reciprocal influences between children and their environments. *Augmentative and Alternative Communication* **13;3**: 149–157.

Cameron, R.J., White, M.E. (1987). *Portage Early Education Programme*. Berks: NFER-Nelson.

Canning, B.A., Rose, M.F. (1974). Clinical measurements of the speed of tongue and lip movements in British children with normal speech. *British Journal of Disorders of Communication* **9;1**: 45–50.

Carlson, F. (1985). *Picsyms Categorical Dictionary*. Lawrence, KS: Baggeboda Press.

Carmeli, S., Shen, Y. (1998). Semantic transparency and translucency in compound Blissymbolics. *Augmentative and Alternative Communication* **14;3**: 162–170.

Carr, P. (1993). *Phonology*. London: MacMillan Press.

Catford, J.C. (1977). *Fundamental Problems in Phonetics*. Edinburgh: Edinburgh University Press.

Catford, J.C. (1989). *Practical Introduction to Phonetics*. Oxford: Clarendon Press.

Chan, J.B., Iacono, T. (2001). Gesture and word production in children with Down syndrome. *Augmentative and Alternative Communication* **17;2**: 73–87.

Chandor, A., Graham, J., Williamson, R. (1985). *The Penguin Dictionary of Computers*. London: Penguin.

Chapman, R., Kay-Raining, E., Schwartz, S. (1990). Fast mapping in event contexts by children with Down syndrome. *Journal of Speech and Hearing Disorders* **55**: 761–770.

Chomsky, N. (1957). *Syntactic Structures*. The Hague: Mouton.

Chomsky, N. (1965). *Aspects of the Theory of Syntax*. Cambridge, MA: M.I.T. Press.

Chomsky, N. (1972). *Language and Mind*. New York: Harcourt Brace Jovanovich.

Chomsky, N. (1982). *Some Concepts and Consequences of the Theory of Government and Binding*. Cambridge, MA: M.I.T. Press.

Chomsky, N., Halle, M. (1968). *The Sound Pattern of English*. New York: Harper and Row.

Clark, C., Davies, C., Woodcock, R. (1974). *Standard Rebus Glossary*. Circle Pines, MN: American Guidance.

Clark, H.H., Clark E.V. (1977). *Psychology and Language: An Introduction to Psycholinguistics*. New York: Harcourt Brace Jovanovich.

Clark, L.W., Witte, K. (1995). Nature and efficacy of communication management in Alzheimer's disease. In R. Lubinsky (ed.) *Dementia and Communication* (3rd edn). Radnor, PA: Chilton Book Co.

Clarke, A.M., Clarke, A.D.B. (1974). *Readings in Mental Deficiency: The changing outlook*. London: Methuen.

Clarke, G.M., Cooke, D. (1992). *A Basic Course in Statistics*. London: Edward Arnold.

Clibbens, J., Powell, G.G., Atkinson, E. (2002). Strategies for achieving joint attention when signing to children with Down syndrome. *International Journal of Language and Communication Disorders* 37;3: 309–323.

Code, C., Müller, D.J. (1989). *Aphasia Therapy*. London: Whurr.

Code, C., Müller, D.J. (1992). *The Code-Müller Protocols: Assessing Perceptions of Psychosocial Adjustment to Aphasia and Related Disorders*. London: Whurr.

Code, C., Müller, D.J. (1995). *Treatment of Aphasia: From Theory to Practice*. London: Whurr.

Code, C., Müller, D.J. (1996). *Forums in Clinical Aphasiology*. London: Whurr.

Code, C., Müller, D.J., Hogan, A., Herrmann, M. (1999). Perceptions of psychosocial adjustment to acquired communication disorders: applications of the Code-Müller Protocols. *International Journal of Language and Communication Disorders* 34;2: 193–207.

Cohen, M.M., Jr., Kreiborg, S., Ordont, D.D.S. (1993). An updated paediatric perspective on the Apert syndrome. *American Journal of Diseases of Childhood* 147: 989–993.

Coles, R. (2001). Noise and hearing. In J. Graham, M. Martin (eds) *Ballantyne's Deafness*. (6th edn). London: Whurr.

Coltheart, M. (1983). Aphasia therapy research: a single case study approach. In C. Code, D.J. Müller (eds) *Aphasia Therapy*. London: Whurr.

Connery, V., Henry, C., Hammond, C., Williams, P., Riley, J. (1992). *Nuffield Centre Dyspraxia Programme*. London: Nuffield Hearing and Speech Centre.

Cook, F., Rustin, L. (1997). Commentary on the Lidcombe Programme of early stuttering intervention. *European Journal of Communication Disorders* 32: 250–258.

Cooper, H. (2001). Cochlear implant. In J. Graham, M. Martin (eds) *Ballantyne's Deafness*. (6th edn). London: Whurr.

Corrigan, R. (1982). The control of animate and inanimate components in pretend play and language. *Child Development* 53: 1348–1353.

Crabtree, M., Mirenda, P., Beukelman, D.R. (1990). Age and gender preferences for synthetic and natural speech. *Augmentative and Alternative Communication* 6;4: 256–261.

Creedon, M. (1973). Language development in nonverbal autistic children using a simultaneous communication system. *Paper presented at the meeting of the Society for Research in Child Development, Philadelphia*.

Cress, C.J., King, J.M. (1999). AAC strategies for people with primary progressive aphasia without dementia: two case studies. *Augmentative and Alternative Communication* 15;4: 248–259.

Crockford, C., Lesser, R. (1994). Assessing functional communication in aphasia: clinical utility and time demands of three methods. *European Journal of Communication Disorders* 29;2: 165–182.

Cross, R.T. (1991). *Intro Talker IEP+*. Wooster, OH: Prentke Romich Company.

Cross, R.T. (2002). *WordCore*. Wooster, OH: Prentke Romich Company.

Cross, R.T., Jones, T., Morris, D. (1994). A reply to Woltosz: re-reading the literature. *Communication Matters Journal* 8;1: 10–15.

Crossley, R. (1988). Unexpected communication attainment by persons diagnosed as autistic and intellectually impaired. *Proceedings 5th ISAAC Conference*, Anaheim, C.A.

Crossley, R. (1997a). Remediation of communication problems through facilitated communication training: a case study. *European Journal of Communication Disorders* 32: 61–70.

Crossley, R. (1997b). Response to commentaries. *European Journal of Communication Disorders* 32: 83–87.

Crossley, R., McDonald, A. (1984). *Annie's Coming Out.* New York: Viking Penguin.

Cruttenden, A. (1970). A phonetic study in babbling. *British Journal of Disorders of Communication* 5: 110–117.

Cruttenden, A. (1972). Phonological procedures for child language. *British Journal of Disorders of Communication.* 7: 30–37.

Cruttenden, A. (1979). *Language in Infancy and Childhood.* Manchester: Manchester University Press.

Cruttenden, A. (1986). *Intonation.* Cambridge: Cambridge University Press.

Cruttenden, A. (1994). *Gimson's Pronunciation of English* (5th edn revised). London: Edward Arnold.

Crystal, D. (1981). *Clinical Linguistics.* London: Whurr.

Crystal, D. (1984). *Linguistic Encounters with Language Handicap.* London: Blackwell.

Crystal, D. (1992). *Profiling Linguistic Disability.* London: Whurr.

Crystal, D., Davy, D. (1969). *Investigating English Style.* London: Longman.

Crystal, D., Fletcher, P., Garman, M. (1989). *The Grammatical Analysis of Language Disability.* London: Whurr.

Crystal, D., Varley, R. (1998) *Introduction to Language Pathology* (4th edn). London: Whurr.

Culler, J. (1986) *Saussure* (2nd edn). London: Fontana.

Culp, D.M. (1989). Developmental apraxia and augmentative and alternative communication. *Augmentative and Alternative Communication* 5;1: 27–34.

Culp, D.M., Ladtkow, M. (1992). Locked-in syndrome and augmentative communication. In K. Yorkston (ed.) *Augmentative Communication in the Medical Setting* (pp. 59–138). San Antonio, TX: The Psychological Corporation.

Cumley, G.D., Swanson, S. (1999). Augmentative and Alternative Communication options for children with developmental apraxia of speech: three case studies. *Augmentative and Alternative Communication* 15;2: 110–125.

Cunningham, C. (1982). *Down Syndrome: An introduction for parents.* London: Souvenir Press.

Dalton, P. (1983). *Approaches to the Treatment of Stuttering.* Kent: Croom Helm.

Dalton, P. (1994). *Counselling People with Communication Problems.* London: Sage Publications.

Dalton, P., Hardcastle, W.J. (1989). *Disorders of Fluency and their Effect on Communication.* London: Whurr.

Daniloff, J., Lloyd, L., Fristoe, M., (1983). Amer-Ind transparency. *Journal of Speech and Hearing Disorders* 48: 103–110.

Daniloff, J., Noll, J., Fristoe, M. Lloyd, L. (1982). Gesture recognition in patients with aphasia. *Journal of Speech and Hearing Disorders* 47: 43–56.

Daniloff, J., Shafer, A. (1981). A gestural communication program for severe-profoundly handicapped children. *Language, Speech and Hearing Services in Schools* 12: 258–268.

Daniloff, J., Vergara, D. (1984). Comparison between the motoric constraints for Amer-Ind and ASL sign formation. *Journal of Speech and Hearing Research* 27: 76–88.

Darley, F.L., Aranson, A.E., Brown, J.R. (1975). *Motor Speech Disorders.* Philadelphia: Saunders.

Davison, G.C., Neale, J.M., Kring A. (2004). *Abnormal Psychology* (9th edn). New York: John Wiley and Sons.

De Meyer, W. (1972). Megalencephaly in children. *Neurology* 22: 634–643.

Decker-McCune, L. (1995). A normative study of representational play at the transition to language. *Developmental Psychology* 31: 198–206.

Denes, P.B., Pinson, E.N. (1993) *The Speech Chain: The physics and biology of spoken language* (2nd edn). New York: Freeman and Co.

Derbyshire, P. (1997). Facilitated communication training: comments from a head teacher. *European Journal of Communication Disorders* 32: 83.

Dockrell, J.E., Sterling, C. (1997). The contribution of psychology to understanding the remediation of communication problems through facilitated communication. *European Journal of Communication Disorders* 32: 75–81.

Doherty, J., Daniloff, J., Lloyd, L. (1985). The effect of categorical presentation on Amer-Ind transparency. *Augmentative and Alternative Communication* 1: 10–16.

Doherty, J.K., Lloyd, L.L. (1985). The effect of categorical presentation on Amer-Ind transparency. *Augmentative and Alternative Communication* 1;1: 5–9.

Donaldson, M. (1987). *Children's Minds.* Glasgow: Fontana/Collins.

Donlan, C. (1998). The importance of education transitions. *International Journal of Disorders of Communication* 33;2: 212–215.

Doyle, M., Phillips, B. (2001). Trends in Augmentative and Alternative Communication use by individuals with amyotrophic lateral sclerosis. *Augmentative and Alternative Communication* 17;2: 167–178.

Drager, K.D.R., Reichie, J.E. (2001). Effects of age and divided attention on listeners' comprehension of synthesized speech. *Augmentative and Alternative Communication* 17;2: 109–119.

Duckworth, M. (1990). A report on changes to the IPA symbols. *The Bulletin* 462: 5–7 Royal College of Speech and Language Therapy.

Ecklund, S., Reichle, J. (1987). A comparison of normal children's ability to recall symbols from two logographic systems. *Language, Speech and Hearing Services in Schools* 18: 34–40.

Edels, Y. (ed.) (1984). *Laryngectomy: Diagnosis to Rehabilitation.* Kent: Croom Helm.

Edwards, A.D.N. (1990). *Speech Synthesis – Technology for Disabled People.* Paul Chapman Publishing.

Edwards, S., Fletcher, P., Garman, M., Hughes, M., Letts, A., Sinka, I. (1999a). Assessing the comprehension and production of language on young children: an account of the Reynell Developmental Language Scales III. *International Journal of Language and Communication Disorders* 34;2: 151–171.

Edwards, S., Fletcher, P., Garman, M., Hughes, M., Letts, A., Sinka, I. (1999b). Reply: Moving on. *International Journal of Language and Communication Disorders.* 34;2: 184–191.

Eisenson, J. (1984). *Adult Aphasia.* New Jersey: Prentice Hall.

Ellis, A.W. (1993). *Reading, Writing and Dyslexia: A Cognitive Analysis.* Hove: Lawrence Erlbaum Associates.

Ellis, A., Beattie, G. (1986). *The Psychology of Language and Communication.* Hove: Lawrence Erlbaum Associates.

Ellis, K. (ed.) (1990). *Autism: Professional perspectives and practice.* London: Chapman and Hall.

Enderby, P. (1987). *Assistive Communication Aids for the Speech Impaired.* Edinburgh: Churchill Livingstone.

Erikson, E.H. (1963). *Childhood and Society.* New York: Norton.

Erickson, R.L. (1969). Assessing communication attitudes among stutterers. *Journal of Speech and Hearing Research* 12: 711–724.

Evans, J.L. (2002). Variability in comprehension strategy use in children with SLI: a dynamical systems account. *International Journal of Language and Communication Disorders* **37;2**: 95–116.

Fawcus, M. (1989). Group therapy: a learning situation. In C. Code, D.J. Müller (eds) *Adult Aphasia*. London: Whurr.

Fawcus, M. (1991). Managing group therapy: further considerations. *Aphasiology* **5;6**: 555–557.

Fawcus, M. (ed.) (1992). *Group Encounters in Speech and Language Therapy*. London: Whurr.

Fay, W.H. (1993). Infantile autism. In D. Bishop, K. Mogford (eds) *Language Development in Exceptional Circumstances*. Hove: Lawrence Erlbaum Associates.

Ferm, U., Amberntson, B., Thunberg, G. (2001). Development and evaluation of a Minspeak application using Blissymbols: experiences from two case studies. *Augmentative and Alternative Communication* **17;4**: 233–243.

Ferrier, L.J. (1991). Clinical study of a dysarthric adult using a TouchTalker with Words Strategy. *Augmentative and Alternative Communication* **7;4**: 266–274.

Fey, M.E. (1999). PACT: some comments and consideration. *International Journal of Language and Communication Disorders*. **34;1**: 55–59.

Fishman, S., Timlan, G., Yoder, D.E. (1985). Strategies for the prevention and repair of communication breakdown with communication board users. *Augmentative and Alternative Communication* **1;1**: 38–51.

Fitch, J.L. (1986). *Clinical Applications of Microcomputers in Communication Disorders*. London: Academic Press.

Fox, L.E., Fried-Oken, M. (1996). AAC aphasiology: partnership for future research. *Augmentative and Alternative Communication* **12;4**: 257–271.

Fox, L.E., Rau, M.T. (2001). Augmentative and Alternative Communication for adults following glossectomy and laryngectomy surgery. *Augmentative and Alternative Communication* **17;2**: 161–166.

Fransella, F. (1972). *Personal Change and Reconstruction*. London & New York: Academic Press.

Freeman, M., Fawcus, M. (2001). *Voice Disorders and their Management* (3rd edn). London: Whurr.

Fried-Oken, M. (2001). Been there, done that: a very personal introduction to the special issue on Augmentative and Alternative Communication and acquired disorders. *Augmentative and Alternative Communication* **17;2**: 138–140.

Fromkin,V., Rodman, R. (2003). *An Introduction to Language* (6th edn). New York: Holt-Saunders International Editions.

Frost, L., Bondy, A. (1994). *PECS: The Picture Exchange Communication System Training Manual*. Cherry Hill, NJ: Pyramid Educational Consultants.

Fry, D.B. (1979). *The Physics of Speech*. Cambridge: Cambridge University Press.

Fucci, D., Reynolds, M.E., Bettagere, R., Gonzales, M.D. (1995). Synthetic speech intelligibility under several experimental conditions. *Augmentative and Alternative Communication* **11;2**: 113–117.

Fuller, D.R. (1997). Initial study into the effects of translucency and complexity on the learning of Blissymbols by children and adults with normal cognitive abilities. *Augmentative and Alternative Communication* **13;1**: 30–39.

Fuller, D., Lloyd, L. (1991). Toward a common usage of iconicity terminology. *Augmentative and Alternative Communication* **8**: 67–74.

Gardner, H. (1993). *Frames of Mind: the theory of multiple intelligences*. New York: Basic Books.

Gardner, H. (1999). *Intelligences Reframed: Multiple intelligences for the 21st century*. New York: Basic Book.

Garnham, A. (1985). *Psycholinguistics: Central topics*. London: Routledge.

Garrett, K.L. (1998). Adults with severe aphasia. In D. Beukelman, P. Mirenda (eds) *Augmentative and Alternative Communication: Management of severe communication disorders in children and adults* (2nd edn, pp. 465–499). Baltimore: Paul H. Brookes Publishing Co.

Garrett, K.L., Beukelman, D.R., Low-Morrow, D. (1989). Comprehensive augmentative communication system for an adult with Broca's aphasia. *Augmentative and Alternative Communication* **5;1**: 55–61.

Garvey, C. (1990). *Play: The developing child*. Mass: Harvard University Press.

Gillham, W. (1979). *The First Words Language Programme*. London: George Allen & Unwin and Beaconsfield Publishers.

Gilman, L. (2001) The |Theory of Multiple Intelligences. Retrieved (12.03) from http://www.indiana.edu/~intell/mitheory.shtml

Gilroy, J., Holliday, P.L. (1982). *Basic Neurology*. New York: Macmillan.

Ginsberg, I.A., White, T.P. (1985). Otologic considerations in audiology. In J. Katz (ed.) *Handbook of Clinical Audiology*. Baltimore: Williams & Wilkins.

Ginsbergh, L. (1999) *Lecture Notes on Neurology* (7th edn). Oxford: Blackwell.

Glennen, S.L., Calculator, S.N. (1985). Training functional communication board use: a pragmatic approach. *Augmentative and Alternative Communication* **1;4**: 134–142.

Glennen, S.L., DeCoste, D.C. (1997). *Handbook of Augmentative and Alternative Communication*. San Diego, CA: Singular Publishing Group, Inc.

Goodglass, H., Kaplan, E. (2000). *The Assessment of Aphasia and Related Disorders*. Philadelphia: Lea & Febiger.

Goodman, R.M., Gorlin, R.J. (1983). *The Malformed Infant: An illustrated guide*. Oxford: Oxford University Press.

Goossens, C. (1989). Aided communication intervention before assessment: a case study of a child with cerebral palsy. *Augmentative and Alternative Communication* **5**: 14–26.

Goossens, C., Crain, S., Elder, P. (1994). *Communication Displays for Engineered Preschool Environments: Books 1 and 2*. Solana Beach, CA: Mayer-Johnson Co.

Goren, A.R., Tucker, G., Ginsberg, G.M. (1996). Language dysfunction in schizophrenia. *European Journal of Disorders of Communication* **32**: 153–170.

Gordon, N., McKinley, I. (1980). *Helping Clumsy Children*. Edinburgh: Churchill Livingstone.

Gorenflo, D.W., Gorenflo, C.W. (1997). Effects of synthetic speech, gender, and perceived similarity on attitudes toward the augmented communicator. *Augmentative and Alternative Communication* **13;2**: 87–91.

Graham, J., Martin, M. (eds) (2001). *Ballantyne's Deafness* (6th edn). London: Whurr.

Green, D.S. (1978). Pure tone air conduction testing. In J. Katz (ed.) *Handbook of Clinical Audiology*. Baltimore: Williams & Wilkins.

Green, G. (1984). Communication in therapy: some of the procedures and issues involved. *British Journal of Disorders of Communication* **19**: 35–46.

Green, J.H. (1982). *Basic Clinical Physiology*. Oxford: Oxford University Press.

Greenbaum, S., Quirk, R. (1990). *A Student's Grammar of the English Language*. (8th impression 1995). Essex: Longman.

Greene, M.C.L., Mathieson, L. (1989). *The Voice and its Disorders*. London: Whurr.

Greenhalgh, D., Mason, A. (1998). Educational transitions: what do they mean to our language unit? *International Journal of Disorders of Communication* **33;2**: 210–211.

Greven, A.J., Meijer, M.F., Tiwari, R.M. (1994). Articulation after total glossectomy: A clinical study of six patients. *European Journal of Disorders of Communication* **29;1**: 85–94.

Grove, N., Walker, M. (1990). The Makaton Vocabulary: using manual signs and graphic symbols to develop interpersonal communication. *Alternative and Augmentative Communication* 6: 15–28.

Grundy, K. (1999). Phonological therapy: a collaborative approach. *International Journal of Language and Communication Disorders* 34;1: 62–65.

Grunwell, P. (1987). *Clinical Phonology*. Kent: Croom Helm.

Grunwell, P. (ed.) (1993). *Analysing Cleft Palate Speech*. London: Whurr.

Grunwell, P., Harding, A. (1995). A note on describing types of nasality. *Journal of Clinical Linguistics and Phonetics*.

Haas, W. (1963). Phonological analysis of a case of dyslalia. *Journal of Speech and Hearing Disorders* 28;3: 239–246.

Haines, R.W., Mohiuddin, A. (1972). *Handbook of Embryology*. Edinburgh: Churchill Livingstone.

Halliday, M. (1994). *An Introduction to Functional Grammar* (2nd edn). London: Edward Arnold.

Hamilton, B., Snell, M. (1993). Using the milieu approach to increase spontaneous communication book use across environments by an adolescent with autism. *Augmentative and Alternative Communication* 9: 259–272.

Hammer, C.S., Tomblin, J., Zhang, X., Weiss, A.L. (2001). Relationship between parenting behaviours and specific language impairment in children. *International Journal of Language Communication Disorders* 36;2: 185–205.

Harding, A., Grunwell, P. (1996). Characteristics of cleft palate speech. *European Journal of Disorders of Communication* 31;4: 331–357.

Harding, A., Grunwell, P. (1998). Active versus passive cleft-type speech characteristics. *International Journal of Disorders of Communication* 33;3: 329–352.

Hass, U., Andersson, A., Brodin, H., Persson, J. (1997). Assessment of computer-aided assistive technology: analysis of outcomes and costs. *Augmentative and Alternative Communication* 13;2: 125–135.

Hayhow, R. (1997). Commentary on Onslow, O'Brian, Harrison [Lidcome Programme of early stuttering]. *European Journal of Communication Disorders* 32: 258–261.

Haynes, C. (1992). A longitudinal study of language-impaired children from a residential school. In *Proceedings of the Second International Symposium for Speech and Language Impaired Children* (pp. 166–182). London: AFASIC.

Hazan, V. (2001). Introduction to acoustics and speech perception. In J. Graham, M. Martin (eds) *Ballantyne's Deafness* (6th edn). London: Whurr.

Hazan, V., Wison, G., Howells, D., Miller, D., Abberton, E., Fourcin, A. (1995). Speech pattern audiometry for clinical use. *European Journal of Communication Disorders* 30: 116–123.

Hazell, J. (2001). Tinnitus and hyperacusis: mechanisms and retraining therapy. In J. Graham, M. Martin (eds) *Ballantyne's Deafness* (6th edn). London: Whurr.

Heller, K., Allgood, M., Ware, S., Arnold, S., Castelle, M. (1996). Initiating requests during community-based vocational training by students with mental retardation and sensory impairments. *Research in Developmental Disabilities* 17: 173–184.

Hetzroni, O.E., Belfiore, P.J. (2000). Preschoolers with communication impairments play Shrinking Kim: an interactive computer storytelling intervention for teaching Blissymbolics. *Augmentative and Alternative Communication* 16;4: 260–269.

Hetzroni, O.E., Lloyd, L.L. (2000). Shrinking Kim: Effects of active versus passive computer instruction on the learning of element and compound Blissymbols. *Augmentative and Alternative Communication* 16;2: 95–106.

Higgenbotham, D.J., Baird, E. (1995). Analysis of listeners' summaries of synthesized speech passages. *Augmentative and Alternative Communication* 11;2: 93–100.

Higgenbotham, D.J., Drazek, A.L., Kowarsky, K., Scally, C., Segal, E. (1994). Discourse comprehension of synthetic speech delivered at normal and slow presentation rates. *Augmentative and Alternative Communication* **10;3**: 184–190.

Hill, E.L. (2001). Non-specific nature of specific language impairment: a review of the literature with regard to concomitant motor impairments. *International Journal of Disorders of Communication* **36;2**: 149–171.

Hjelmquist, E., Sandberg, A.D., Hedelin, L. (1994). Linguistics, AAC, metalinguistics in communicatively handicapped adolescents. *Augmentative and Alternative Communication* **10;3**: 169–183.

Hodgson, W.R. (1985). Testing infants and young children. In J. Katz (ed.) *Handbook of Clinical Audiology.* Baltimore: Williams & Wilkins.

Hole, G. (2000). The Normal Curve and "Z" Scores. Retrieved (12.03) from http://www.cogs.susx.ac.uk/users/grahamh/sthand2.pdf

Honsinger, M.J. (1989). Midcourse intervention in multiple sclerosis: an inpatient model. *Augmentative and Alternative Communication* **5;1**: 71–73.

Hood, J.D. (1981). Speech audiometry. In H.A. Beagley (ed.) *Audiology and Audiological Medicine* (vol. 1. ch. 7). Oxford: Oxford University Press.

Hopkins, H.L., Smith H.D. (1993). *Willard and Spackman's Occupational Therapy* (8th edn). Philadelphia: Lippinott Co.

Hornsby, B. (1995). *Overcoming Dyslexia.* London: Optima.

Hornstein, N., Lightfoot, D. (eds) (1981). *Explanation in Linguistics: The logical problem of language acquisition.* London: Longman.

Hosking, G. (1982). *An Introduction to Paediatric Neurology.* London: Faber & Faber.

Huddleston, R. (1976). *An Introduction to English Transformational Syntax.* London: Longman.

Hurlbut, B., Iwata, B., Green, J. (1982). Nonvocal language acquisition in adolescents with severe physical disabilities: Blissymbol versus iconic stimulus formats. *Journal of Applied Behaviour Analysis* **15**: 241–258.

Hustad, K.C. (2001). Unfamiliar listeners' evaluation of speech supplementation strategies for improving the effectiveness of severely dysarthric speech. *Augmentative and Alternative Communication* **17;4**: 213–220.

Hyman, L.M. (1975). *Phonology, Theory and Analysis.* London: Holt Rinehart and Winston.

Illingworth, R.S. (1987). *The Development of the Young Infant and Young Child: Normal and abnormal.* Edinburgh: Churchill Livingstone.

Ingram, D., Ingram K. (1999). An innovative phonological therapy programme. *International Journal of Language and Communication Disorders* **34;1**: 60–61.

Jacobson, J.T., Hyde M.L. (1985). An introduction to auditory evoked potentials. In J. Katz (ed.) *Handbook of Clinical Audiology.* Baltimore: Williams & Wilkins.

Jakobson, R., Halle, M. (1956). *Fundamentals of Language.* The Hague: Mouton.

Jennings, A.A. (1984). What do I get for my money? *The Bulletin* **382**. Royal College of Speech and Language Therapists.

Jensema, C. (1982). Communication methods and devices for deaf-blind persons. *Directions* **3**: 60–69.

Johns, D.F. (1981). *Clinical Management of Neurogenic Communicative Disorders.* Boston: Little, Brown & Company.

Johnston J.R., Miller, J., Tallal, P. (2001). Use of cognitive state predicates by language-impaired children. *International Journal of Language and Communication Disorders* **36;3**: 349–370.

Jones, A.P. (1989). Language, Learning and Living. *Proceedings of 1st UK Minspeak Conference,* Sept. (pp. 70–91). Swinstead: Liberator Ltd.

281

Jones, A.P. (1991). *Language, Learning & Living*. Wooster, Ohio: Prentke Romich Company.

Jones, A.P. (1992). *Teaching Language, Learning & Living*. Swinstead: Liberator Ltd.

Jones, A.P. (1995a). *IMPACT: Implementing Augmentative Communication Training – A manual for staff training*. Swinstead: Liberator Ltd.

Jones, A.P. (1995b). *PATHWAYS: 'Language, Learning and Living' for beginners*. Swinstead: Liberator Ltd.

Jones, F., Pring, T., Grove, N. (2002). Developing communication in adults with profound and multiple learning difficulties using objects of reference. *International Journal of Language and Communication Disorders* **37;2**: 173–184.

Jones, K.L. (1997). *Recognizable Patterns of Human Malformation* (5th edn). Philadelphia: W.B. Saunders.

Joseph, J. (1979). *Essential Anatomy*. Lancaster: M.T.P. Press.

Josey, A.F. (1985). Auditory brainstem response in site of lesion testing. In J. Katz (ed.) *Handbook of Clinical Audiology*. Baltimore: William & Wilkins.

Kallen, D., Marshall, R.C., Casey, D.E. (1986). Atypical dysarthria in Munchausen syndrome. *British Journal of Disorders of Communication* **21;3**: 377–380.

Katz, J. (1985). *Handbook of Clinical Audiology*. Baltimore: William & Wilkins.

Katz, J. (1994). *Handbook of Clinical Audiology*. (4th edn). Baltimore: William & Wilkins.

Katz, R.C. (1986). *Aphasia Treatment and Microcomputers*. London: Taylor and Francis.

Kaye, A. (1991). *Essential Neurosurgery*. Edinburgh: Churchill Livingstone.

Kazdin, A. (1981). The token economy. In G. Davey (ed.) *Applications of Conditioning Theory*. London: Methuen.

Keller, E. (1994). *Fundamentals of Speech Synthesis and Speech Recognition*. New York: Wiley.

Kelly, G.A. (1955). *The Psychology of Personal Constructs*. New York: Norton.

Kempe, R.S., Kempe, C.H. (1978). *Child Abuse*. Suffolk: Fontana/Open Books.

Kennedy, M., Murdoch, B.E. (1994). Thalamic aphasia and striato-capsular aphasia as independent aphasic syndromes: a review. *Aphasiology* **8;4**: 303–313.

Kenstowicz, M. (1994). *Phonology in Generative Grammar*. Massachusetts: Blackwell Publishers.

Kersner, M. (1992). *Tests of Voice, Speech and Language*. London: Whurr.

Kiernan, C., Reid, B., Jones, L. (1982). *Signs and Symbols*. London: Heinemann Educational Books.

King, J.M., Hux, K. (1995). Intervention using talking word processing software: an aphasia case study. *Augmentative and Alternative Communication* **11;3**: 187–192.

Klasner, E.R., Yorkston, K.M. (2001). Linguistic and cognitive supplementation strategies as Augmentative and Alternative Communication techniques in Huntington's disease: case report. *Augmentative and Alternative Communication* **17;2**: 154–160.

Kleppe, S.A., Katayama, K.C., Shipley, K.G., Foushee, D.R. (1990). The speech and language characteristics of children with Prader-Willi syndrome. *Journal of Speech and Hearing Disorders* **55;2**: 300–309.

Koehler, L., Lloyd, L., Swanson, L. (1994). Visual similarity between manual and printed alphabet letters. *Augmentative and Alternative Communication* **10**: 87–95.

Kolb, B., Whishaw, I.Q. (1996). *Fundamentals of Human Neuropsychology*. New York: W.H. Freeman and Co.

Koul, R.K., Hanners, J. (1997). Words identification and sentence verification of two synthetic speech systems by individuals with intellectual disabilities. *Augmentative and Alternative Communication* **13;2**: 99–107.

Koul, R.K., Harding, R. (1998). Identification and production of graphic symbols by individuals with aphasia: efficacy of a software application. *Augmentative and Alternative Communication* **14;1**: 11–24.

Ladefoged, P. (1962). *Elements of Acoustic Phonetics*. Chicago: Chicago University Press.

Ladefoged, P. (1971). *Preliminaries to Linguistic Phonetics*. Chicago: Chicago University Press.

Ladefoged, P. (1993). *A Course in Phonetics*. New York: Harcourt Brace Jovanovich.

Ladefoged, P. (2001). *A Course in Phonetics* (4th edn). MA: Heinle and Heinle.

Langley, J. (1987). *Working with Swallowing Disorders*. London: Winslow Press.

Lasker, J.P., Bedrosian, J.L. (2001). Promoting acceptance of Augmentative and Alternative Communication by adults with acquired communication disorders. *Augmentative and Alternative Communication* 17;2: 141–153.

Lasker, J., Hux, K., Garrett, K.L., Moncrief, E.M., Eischeid, T.J. (1997). Variations on the written choice communication strategy for individuals with severe aphasia. *Augmentative and Alternative Communication* 13;2: 108–116.

Law, J. (1999). It's not just the pigs... a comment on the RDLS III. *International Journal of Language and Communication Disorders* 34;2: 181–184.

Le Dorze, G., Dionne, L., Ryalls, J., Julien, M.O. (1992). The effects of speech and language therapy for a case of dysarthria associated with Parkinson's Disease. *European Journal of Communication Disorders* 27: 313–324.

Lebrun, Y. (1988). Language and epilepsy. *British Journal of Disorders of Communication* 23;2: 97–110.

Lebrun, Y., Fabbro, F. (2002). *Language and Epilepsy*. London: Whurr.

Lees, J. (1993). *Children with Acquired Aphasias*. London: Whurr.

Lees, J. (1999). From 'Which pig is not outside the field?' to 'Which horse is not outside the field?': commentary on the Reynell Developmental Language Scales III (RDLS III). *International Journal of Language and Communication Disorders* 34;2: 174–180.

Leeson, T.S., Leeson, C.R., Papano, A.A. (1985). *Textbook of Histology*. Philadelphia: W.B. Saunders.

Lepschy, G.C. (1982). *A Survey of Structural Linguistics*. London: Andre Deutsch.

Lesser, R. (1988). *Linguistic Investigations of Aphasia*. London: Whurr.

Lesser, R., Perkins, L. (2000). *Cognitive Neuropsychology and Conversation Analysis in Aphasia*. London: Whurr.

Lewis, V., Boucher, J., Astell, A. (1992). The assessment of symbolic play in young children: a prototype test. *European Journal of Disorders of Communication* 27: 231–245.

Lewis, V., Boucher, J., Lupton, L., Watson, S. (2000) Relationships between symbolic play, functional play, verbal and non-verbal ability in young children. *International Journal of Disorders of Communication* 35;1: 117–127.

Light, J. (1997). 'Let's go star fishing': reflections on the context of language learning for children who use aided AAC. *Augmentative and Alternative Communication* 13;3: 158–171.

Lindsay, G., Dockrell, J.E. (1998). What's in a transition? A reply to Botting, Cructchley and Conti-Ramsden. *International Journal of Disorders of Communication* 33;2: 198–207.

Lloyd, L.L., Blischak, D. (1992). AAC terminology policy and issues update. *Augmentative and Alternative Communication* 8: 104–109.

Lloyd, L.L., Quist, R.W., Windsor, J. (1990). A proposed augmentative and alternative communication model. *Augmentative and Alternative Communication* 6;3: 172–183.

Lloyd, L.L., Quist, R.W., Windsor, J. (1993). AAC model explicated: response to Panton (1993). *Augmentative and Alternative Communication* 9;3: 193–195.

Locke, A. (1985). *Living Language*. Berks: NFER-Nelson.

Lombardino, L.J., Morris, D., Mercado, L., DeFillipo, F., Sarisky, C., Montgomery, A. (1999). The Early Reading Screening Instrument: a method for identifying kindergarteners at risk for learning to read. *International Journal of Disorders of Communication.* 34;2: 135–150.

Loncke, F.T., Clibbens, J., Arvidson, H.H., Lloyd, L. (1999). *Augmentative and Alternative Communication: New directions in research and practice.* London: Whurr.

Loverso, F.L. (1991). Aphasia group treatment, a commentary. *Aphasiology* **5;6**: 567–569.

Luftig, R.L., Beersani Jr., H.A. (1985). An investigation of two variables influencing Blissymbols learnability with non-handicapped adults. *Augmentative and Alternative Communication* **1;1**: 33–37.

Lyons, J. (1968). *Introduction to Theoretical Linguistics.* Cambridge: Cambridge University Press.

Lyons, J. (1981). *Language and Linguistics.* Cambridge: Cambridge University Press.

Lyons, J. (1991). *Chomsky* (3rd edn). London: Fontana.

Lysons, K. (1978). *Your Hearing Loss and How to Cope with it.* Vancouver, BC: David & Charles.

McCane, L. (1995). A normative study of representational play at the transition to language. *Developmental Psychology* **31**: 198–206.

McCune-Nicolich, L. (1981). Toward symbolic functioning: Structure of early pretend games and potential parallels with language. *Child Development* **52**: 785–797.

McDonald, E., Schultz, A. (1973). Communication boards for cerebral palsied children. *Journal of Speech and Hearing Disorders* **38**: 73–88.

MacKay, D. (1975). *Clinical Psychology: Theory and Therapy.* London: Methuen.

McLarty, M. (1995). Objects of reference. In D. Etheridge (ed.) *The Education of Dual Sensory Impaired Children: Recognising and developing ability.* London: David Fulton.

McLarty, M. (1997). Putting objects of reference in context. *European Journal of Special Needs Education* **12**: 12–20.

McLean, J., Snyder-McLean, L. (1987). Form and function of communicative behaviour among persons with severe developmental disabilities. *Australia and New Zealand Journal of Developmental Disabilities* **13**: 83–98.

MacMahon, M.K.C. (1990). *Basic Phonetics.* Unpublished.

McManamny, D.S., Barnett, J.S. (1985). Macroglossia as a presentation of the Beckwith-Wiedemann syndrome. *Plastic and Reconstructive Surgery* **75**: 170–176.

McNaughton, D., Fallon, K., Tod, J., Weiner, F., Neisworth, J. (1994). Effect of repeated listening experiences on the intelligibility of synthesized speech. *Augmentative and Alternative Communication* **10;3**: 161–168.

McNaughton, D., Light, J., Groszyk, L. (2001). 'Don't give up': employment experiences of individuals with amyotrophic lateral aclerosis who use Augmentative and Alternative Communication. *Augmentative and Alternative Communication* **17;2**: 179–195.

McNaughton, S. (1992). *Blissymbol Component Minspeak Words Strategy.* Wooster, OH: Prentke Romich Company.

McTear, M.F. (1985). Pragmatic disorders: a case of conversational disability? *British Journal of Disorders of Communication* **20;2**: 129–142.

McWilliams, B.J., Morris, H.L., Shelton, R.L. (1990). *Cleft Palate Speech.* Philadelphia, Toronto: B.C.

Maharaj, S. (1980). *Pictogram ideogram communication.* Regina, Saskatchewan, Canada: The George Reed Foundation for the Handicapped.

Manolson, A. (1992). *It Takes Two to Talk: A Parent's Guide to Helping Children Communicate.* Toronto: Hanen Centre.

Mark, V.W., Thomas, B.E., Berndt, R.S. (1992). Factors associated with improvement in global aphasia. *Aphasiology* **6;2**: 121–134.

Martin, M. (ed.) (1997). *Speech Audiometry.* (2nd edn). London: Whurr.

Martin, M. (2001). Hearing aids. In J. Graham, M. Martin (eds) *Ballantyne's Deafness* (6th edn). London: Whurr.

Martin, M., Summers, I. (1999). *Dictionary of Hearing.* London: Whurr.

Martins, I.P., Ferro, J.M. (1992). Recovery of acquired aphasia in children. *Aphasiology* **6;4:** 431–438.

Mathieson, L. (2001). *Greene and Mathieson's The Voice and its Disorders* (6th edn). London: Whurr.

Mathy-Laikko, P., Ratcliff, A.E., Villaruel, F., Yoder, D.E. (1987). Augmentative communication systems. In M. Bullis (ed.) *Communication Development in Children with Deaf-Blindness: III. Literature review* (pp. 205–241). Monmouth: Communication Skills Center for Younger Children with Deaf-Blindness, Teaching Research Division, Oregon State System of Higher Education.

Matthews, P.H. (1974). *Morphology: An introduction to the theory of word-structure.* Cambridge: Cambridge University Press.

Max, L., De Bruyn, W., Steurs, W. (1997). Intelligibility of oesophageal and tracheo-oesophageal speech: preliminary observations. *European Journal of Disorders of Communication* **32;4:** 429–440.

Meadow, K. (1980) *Deafness and Child Development.* London: Edward Arnold.

Meichenbaum, D. (1977). *Cognitive Behavior Modification.* New York: Plenum Press.

Miller, M.H. (1972). *Hearing Aids.* Indianapolis: Bobbs-Merrill.

Miller, N. (1986). *Dyspraxia and its Management.* Beckenham: Croom-Helm.

Miller, N. (1990). Review of the Pragmatics Profile by Dewart and Summers. *Clinical Linguistics and Phonetics* **4:** 179–182.

Miller, S. (1984). *Experimental Design and Statistics.* London: Methuen.

Mirenda, P. (1997). Supporting individuals with challenging behaviour through functional communication training and AAC: research review. *Augmentative and Alternative Communication* **13;4:** 207–227.

Mirenda, P. (1998a). Perspective on AAC: past, present and future. *Augmentative and Alternative Communication* **14;1:** 1.

Mirenda, P. (1998b). AAC: coming of age or over the hill? *Augmentative and Alternative Communication* **14;4:** 197–199.

Mirenda, P., Beukelman, D.R. (1987). A comparison of speech synthesis with listeners from three age groups. *Augmentative and Alternative Communication* **3;3:** 120–128.

Mirenda, P., Beukelman, D.R. (1990). A comparison of intelligibility among natural speech and seven synthesizers with listeners from three age groups. *Augmentative and Alternative Communication* **6;1:** 61–68.

Mirenda, P., Locke, P. (1989). A comparison of symbol transparency in nonspeaking persons with intellect disabilities. *Journal of Speech and Hearing Research* **54:** 131–140.

Mirenda, P., Santagrossi, J. (1985). A prompt free strategy to teach pictorial communication system use. *Augmentative and Alternative Communication* **1:** 143–150.

Mizuko, M. (1987). Transparency and ease of learning of symbols represented by Blissymbols, PCS, and Picsyms. *Augmentative and Alternative Communication* **3:** 129–136.

Molloy, D.W., Lubinsky, R. (1995). Dementia: impact and clinical perspectives. In R. Lubinsky (ed.) *Dementia and Communicating* (pp. 2–21). San Diego: Singular Publishing Group.

Money, D. (1997). A comparison of three approaches to delivering a speech and language therapy service to people with learning disabilities. *European Journal of Disorders of Communication* **32;4:** 449–466.

Morris, D. (1992). What constitutes at-risk: screening children for first grade reading intervention. In W.A. Secord, J.S. Damico (eds) *Best Practices in School Speech Pathology* (pp. 43–51). Orlando: Harcourt Brace Jovanovich.

Morris, D.W.H. (1994). Speech and language therapy in the United Kingdom in the 1990s. *Logopedie* **7;4:** 18–21.

Morris, D.W.H. (1995a). AAC & aphasia: does Minspeak have a role to play? *Communication Matters Journal* (ISAAC UK) **9;1**: 5–7.

Morris, D.W.H. (1995b). AAC & aphasia II: treatment, technology and language. *Proceedings of 9th Annual Minspeak Conference* July 1995. Wooster, Ohio: Prentke Romich Company.

Morris, D.W.H. (1998). *Language, Learning and Living for the Vanguard*. Swinstead: Liberator Ltd.

Morris, D.W.H. (2000). *Language, Learning and Living for the Pathfinder*. Swinstead: Liberator Ltd.

Mundy, P., Sigman, M., Ungerer, J., Herman, T. (1987). Nonverbal communication and play correlates of language development in autistic children. *Journal of Autism and Developmental Disorders* **17**: 349–364.

Murdoch, B.E., Hudson-Tennent, L.J. (1994). Speech disorders in children treated for posterior fossa tumours: ataxic and developmental features. *European Journal of Disorders of Communication* **29;4**: 379–397.

Murdoch, B., Theodoras, D. (2000). *Speech and Language Disorders in Multiple Sclerosis*. London: Whurr.

Murphy, J., Block, S. (2002). Motor neurone disease: AAC and everyday conversation. *Communication Matters* **16;1**: 3–7.

Murphy, J., Scott, J. (1995). *Attitudes and Strategies towards AAC: A training package for AAC users and carers*. Stirling: University of Stirling.

Musselwhite, C., Ruscello, D. (1984). Transparency of three symbol communication systems. *Journal of Speech and Hearing Research* **27**: 436–443.

Musselwhite, C., St. Louis, K. (1988). *Communication Programming for Persons with Severe Handicaps* (2nd edn). Austin: TX: PRO-ED.

Nelson, K.E. (1998). Processes of facilitating progress by language-delayed children in special language-centred school units. *International Journal of Disorders of Communication* **33;2**: 208–210.

Nelson, N.W. (1992). Performance is the prize: language competence and performance among AAC users. *Augmentative and Alternative Communication* **8;1**: 3–18.

Nelson-Jones, R. (1982). *The Theory and Practice of Counselling Psychology*. London: Holt, Rinehart and Winston.

Nelson-Jones, R. (1997). *Practical Counselling Skills and Helping Skills* (4th edn). London: Holt, Rinehart and Winston.

Nelson-Jones, R. (2000). *Introduction to Counselling Skills*. London: Holt, Rinehart and Winston.

Nelson-Jones, R. (2001). *The Theory and Practice of Counselling and Therapy* (3rd edn). London: Holt, Rinehart and Winston.

Neugarten, B.L. (ed.) (1968). *Middle Age and Aging*. Chicago: Chicago University Press.

Newell, A.F., Arnott, J.L., Booth, L., Beattie, W., Brophy, B., Ricketts, W. (1992). Effect of the 'PAL' word prediction system on the quality and quantity of text generation. *Augmentative and Alternative Communication* **8;4**: 304–311.

Nickels, L. (1995). Reading too little into reading?: strategies in the rehabilitation of acquired dyslexia. *European Journal of Disorders of Communication* **30;1**: 37–50.

Northern, J., Downs, M. (1991). *Hearing in Children*. (4th edn). Baltimore: Williams and Wilkins.

O'Hara, M., Johnston, J. (1997). Syntactic bootstrapping in children with specific language impairment. *European Journal of Disorders of Communication* **32;2**: 189–205.

Obler, L.K., Albert, M.L. (1981) Language in the elderly aphasic and in the dementing patient. In M.T. Sarno (ed.) *Acquired Aphasia*. London: Academic Press.

Ockleford, A. (1994). *Objects of Reference*. London: RNIB.

Onslow, M., O'Brian, S., Harrison, E. (1997a). The Lidcombe Programme of early stuttering intervention: methods and issues. *European Journal of Communication Disorders* **32**: 231–250.

Onslow, M., O'Brian, S., Harrison, E. (1997b). The Lidcombe Programme: maverick or not? *European Journal of Communication Disorders* **32**: 261–266.

Orsolini, M., Sechi, E., Maronato, C., Bonvino, E., Corcelli, A. (2001). Nature of phonological delay in children with specific language impairment. *International Journal of Language and Communication Disorders* **36;1**: 63–90.

Pachalska, M. (1991a). Group therapy: a way of reintegrating patients with aphasia. *Aphasiology* **5;6**: 573–577.

Pachalska, M. (1991b). Group therapy for aphasia patients. *Aphasiology* **5;6**: 541–554.

Palmer, F.R. (1976). *Semantics: A new outline*. Cambridge: Cambridge University Press.

Palmer, L.R. (1978). *Descriptive and Comparative Linguistics: A critical introduction*. London: Faber.

Panton, L. (1993). AAC model: comments on Lloyd, Quist, Windsor (1990). *Augmentative and Alternative Communication* **9;3**: 191–193.

Park, K. (1997). How do objects become objects of reference? A review of the literature on objects of reference and a proposed model for the use of objects in communication. *British Journal of Special Education* **24**: 108–114.

Patel, P.G., Satz, P. (1994). The language production system and senile dementia of Alzheimer's type: neuropathological implications. *Aphasiology* **8;1**: 1–18.

Patterson, K., Kay, J. (1982). Letter-by-letter reading: psychological descriptions of a neurological syndrome. *Quarterly Journal of Experimental Psychology* **34A**: 411–441.

Paul, R. (1997a). Introduction: special section on language development in which children who use AAC. *Augmentative and Alternative Communication* **13;3**: 139–140.

Paul, R. (1997b). Facilitating transitions in language development for children using AAC. *Augmentative and Alternative Communication* **13;3**: 141–148.

Pennington, L., Jolleff, N., McConachie, H., Wisbeach, A., Price, K. (1993) *'My Turn to Speak': A team approach to augmentative communication*. London: Hospitals for Sick Children and the Institute of Child Health.

Perry, A., Anderson, K., Lean, R., Cotton, S. (2002). Elevation of the soft palate in speech and swallowing in normal female participants and females with motor neuron disease: an innovative procedure for measuring palatal elevation. *International Journal of Language and Communication Disorders* **37;2**: 197–214.

Peter, M., Barnes, R. (1982). *Signs, Symbols and Schools: An introduction to the use of non-vocal communication systems and sign language in schools*. Chester: NCSE.

Peterson, S.L., Bondy, A.S., Vincent, Y., Finnegan, C.S. (1995). Effects of altering communicative input for students with autism and no speech. *Augmentative and Alternative Communication* **11;2**: 93–100.

Pit Corder, S. (1973). *Introducing Applied Linguistics*. London: Penguin.

Plant, G. (1993). The speech of adults with acquired profound hearing losses. I: A perceptual evaluation. *European Journal of Communication Disorders* **8**: 273–288.

Plaza, M. (1997). Phonological impairment in dyslexic children with and without early speech-language disorder. *European Journal of Disorders of Communication* **32**: 277–290.

Porkess, R. (1988). *Dictionary of Statistics*. Glasgow: Collins.

Pracy, R., Siegler, J., Stell, P.M. (1974) *A Short Textbook of Ear, Nose and Throat*. London: Hodder and Stoughton.

Pulvermüller, F., Roth, V.M. (1991). Communicative aphasia treatment as a further development of PACE therapy. *Aphasiology* **5;1**: 39–50.

Purser, H. (1982). *Psychology for Speech Therapists.* London: MacMillan Press.

Quirk, R., Greenbaum, S. (1979). *A University Grammar of English.* London: Longman.

Rachman, S.J., Wilson, G.T. (1980). *The Effects of Psychological Therapy.* Oxford: Pergamon Press.

Raghavendra, P., Allen, G.D. (1993). Comprehension of synthetic speech with three text-to-speech systems using a sentence verification paradigm. *Augmentative and Alternative Communication* 9;2: 119–225.

Ramsden, R., Axon, P. (2001). Objective audiometry. In J. Graham, M. Martin (eds) *Ballantyne's Deafness* (6th edn). London: Whurr.

Rapin, I., Allen, D.A. (1983). Developmental language disorders: nosological considerations. In U. Kirk (ed.) *Neuropsychology of Language, Reading and Spelling.* New York: Academic Press.

Rapin, I., Allen, D.A. (1987). Developmental dysphasia and autism in preschool children: characteristics and shape. In J. Martin, P. Fletcher, P. Grunwell, D. Hall (eds) *Proceedings of the First International Symposium on Specific Speech and Language Disorders in Children* (pp. 20–35). London: AFASIC.

Rapin, I., Allen, D.A. (1992). Developmental language disorders. In S.J. Segalowitz, I. Rapin (eds) *Child Neuropsychology,* (pp. 111–137). Amsterdam: Elsevier Science.

Rapin, I., Allen, D.A. (1998). The semantic-pragmatic deficit disorder: classification issues. *International Journal of Disorders of Communication* 33;1: 82–87.

Ratcliff, A., Coughlin, S., Lehman, M. (2002). Factors influencing ratings of speech naturalness in Augmentative and Alternative Communication. *Augmentative and Alternative Communication* 18;1: 11–19.

Razzell, R.E., Harding, A., Harland, K. (1996). Cleft palate speech audit: Turner project 95/96. *Paper presented at the Carniofacial Society of Great Britain Annual Conference, Egham, Surrey.*

Reber, A.S. (1995). *The Penguin Dictionary of Psychology.* London: Penguin.

Reed, C., Delhorne, L., Durlach, N., Fischer, S. (1990). A study of tactual and visual reception of fingerspelling. *Journal of Speech and Hearing Research* 33: 786–797.

Reeves, J., Harris, S. (2001). AAC and aphasia. *Communication Matters* 15;3: 23–27.

Reichard, S., Livson, F., Peterson, P.G. (1962). *Aging and Personality: A study of eighty-seven older men.* New York: John Wiley.

Renfrew, C. (1966). Persistence of the open syllable in defective articulation. *Journal of Speech and Hearing Disorders* 31: 370–373.

Repo, M. (1991). The holistic approach to rehabilitation: a commentary. *Aphasiology* 5;6: 571–572.

Reynolds, I. (2001). Can AAC promote communication and language in children with autism? *Communication Matters* 15;2: 25–28.

Reynolds, M.E., Isaacs-Duvall, C., Sheward, B., Rotter, M. (2000). Examination of the effects of listening practice on synthesized speech comprehension. *Augmentative and Alternative Communication* 16;4: 250–259.

Reynolds, M.E., Jefferson, L. (1999). Natural and synthetic speech comprehension: comparison of children from two age groups. *Augmentative and Alternative Communication* 15;3: 174–182.

Reynolds, M.E., Jones, H.A. (1996). Synthetic speech intelligibility: comparison of native and non-native speakers of English. *Augmentative and Alternative Communication* 12;1: 32–36.

Riedel, K. (1981). Auditory comprehension in aphasia. In M.T. Sarno (ed.) *Acquired Aphasia.* London: Academic Press.

Robertson, J. (1995). *Stepping Stones.* Swinstead: Liberator Ltd.

Robertson, J. (2000). *Getting Started with a Core Low Technology Augmentative and Alternative Communication (AAC) Vocabulary.* Knebworth: Independent Expressions.

Robertson, J. (2002). Dynamic Minspeak. *Proceedings of Communication Matters Conference 2002.*

Robertson, S.J., Thomson, F. (1986). *Working with Dysarthrics.* London: Winslow Press.

Robins, R.H. (1971). *General Linguistics: An introductory survey.* London: Longman.

Robins, R.H. (1979). *A Short History of Linguistics.* London: Longman.

Robinshaw, H.M. (1996). Acquisition of speech, pre- and post-cochlear implantation: longitudinal studies of a congenitally deaf infant. *European Journal of Communication Disorders* **31**;2: 121–139.

Robinson, J. (2001). Causes of conductive hearing loss and their non-surgical management. In J. Graham, M. Martin (eds) *Ballantyne's Deafness* (6th edn). London: Whurr.

Robson, J., Marshall, J., Chiat, S., Pring, T. (2001). Enhancing communication in jargon aphasia: a small group study of writing therapy. *International Journal of Disorders of Communication* **36**;4: 471–488.

Robson, J., Pring, T., Marshall, J., Morrison, S., Chiat, S. (1998). Written communication in undifferentiated jargon aphasia: a therapy study. *International Journal of Disorders of Communication* **33**;3: 305–328.

Romski, M.A., Sevcik, R.A., Adamson, L.B. (1997). Framework for studying how children with developmental disabilities develop language through augmented means. *Augmentative and Alternative Communication* **13**;3: 172–178.

Rondal, J.A., Perera, J., Nadel, L. (1999). *Down Syndrome: A review of current knowledge.* London: Whurr.

Rosenbek, J.C., LaPointe, L.L., Wertz, R.T. (1989). *Aphasia: A clinical approach.* Texas: Pro-ed.

Rosenbloom, L. (1997). A neurological commentary. *European Journal of Communication Disorders* **32**: 81–82.

Rotholz, D., Berkowitz, S., Burberry, J. (1989). Functionality of two modes of communication in the community by students with developmental disabilities: a comparison of signing and communication books. *Journal of the Association for Persons with Severe Handicaps* **14**: 227–233.

Rowland, C., Schweigert, P. (1989). Tangible symbols: symbolic communication for individuals with multisensory impairments. *Augmentative and Alternative Communication* **6**: 226–234.

Rowland, C., Stremell-Campbell, K. (1987). Share and share alike: conventional gestures to emergent language for learners with sensory impairments. In L. Goetz, D. Guess, K. Stremell-Campbell (eds) *Innovative Program Design for Individuals with Dual Sensory Impairments.* Baltimore: Paul Brookes.

Ruiter, I. (2000). *Allow Me: A guide For counsellors of adults with developmental delays.* Toronto: Hanen Centre.

Rumble, G.D., Larcher, J. (1998). *AAC Device Review.* Marlow, Bucks: Vocation

Rumble, G.D., Robertson, J. (1995). *Lesson Plans for Minspeak Application Programmes.* Swinstead: Liberator Ltd.

Rupprecht, S.L., Beukelman, D.R., Vrtiska, H. (1995). Comparative intelligibility of five synthesized voices. *Augmentative and Alternative Communication* **11**;4: 244–248.

Rustin, L., Purser, H., Rowley, D. (1987). *Progress in the Treatment of Fluency Disorders.* London: Whurr.

Rustin, L., Spence, R., Cooke, F. (1995). *Management of Stuttering in Adolescence.* London: Whurr.

Rutter, M. (1975). *Helping Troubled Children.* London: Penguin.

Ryan, B.P., Van Kirk, B. (1978). *Monterey Fluency Program.* Palo Alto, California: Monterey Learning Systems.

Salkie, R. (1990). *The Chomsky Update: Linguistics and politics.* London: Routledge.

Salmon, M.A. (1978). *Developmental Defects and Syndromes.* Chichester: HM+M Publishers.

Sanders, D.A. (1977). *Auditory Perception of Speech.* London and New York: Prentice-Hall.

Sarno, M.T. (1969). The Functional Communication Profile: manual of directions. *Rehabilitation Monograph* **42**. New York: Institute of Rehabilitation Medicine.

Sarno, M.T. (ed.) (1991). *Acquired Aphasia* (2nd edn). London: Academic Press.

Satz, P., Bullard-Bates, C. (1981). Acquired aphasia in children. In M.T. Sarno (ed.) *Acquired Aphasia.* London: Academic Press.

Sauber, G.R., L'Abate, L., Weeks, G.R., Buchanan, W.L. (1993). *The Dictionary of Family Psychology and Family* (2nd edn). California: Sage Publications.

Saussure, F. de (1916). *Cours de Linguistique Générale.* Paris: Payot.

Scherz, J.W., Beer, M.M. (1995). Factors affecting the intelligibility of synthesized speech. *Augmentative and Alternative Communication* **11;2**: 79–88.

Schlosser, R.W., Lloyd, L.L. (1991). Augmentative and Alternative Communication: an evolving field. *Augmentative and Alternative Communication* **7;3**: 154–160.

Schlosser, R.W., Lloyd, L.L. (1997). Effects of paired-associate learning versus symbol explanations on Blissymbol comprehension and production. *Augmentative and Alternative Communication* **13;4**: 226–238.

Scott, S., Caird, F.I. (1981). Speech therapy for patients with Parkinson's disease. *British Medical Journal* **283**: 1088.

Scott, S., Caird, F.I., Williams, B.O. (1985). *Communication in Parkinson's Disease.* London: Croom Helm.

Searle, J.R. (1969). *Speech Acts: An essay in the philosophy of language.* Cambridge: Cambridge University Press.

Sell, D., Grunwell, P. (1994). Speech studies and the unoperated cleft palate subject. *European Journal of Communication Disorders* **29;2**: 151–164.

Sell, D., Harding, A., Grunwell, P. (1994). A screening assessment of cleft palate speech (Great Ormond Street Speech Assessment). *European Journal of Communication Disorders* **29;1**: 1–16.

Sell, D., Harding, A., Grunwell, P. (1999). GOS.SP.ASS.'98: an assessment for speech disorders associated with cleft palate and/or velopharyngeal dysfunction (revised). *International Journal of Language and Communication Disorders* **34;1**: 17–33.

Shakespeare, R. (1975). *The Psychology of Handicap.* London: Methuen.

Shearer, D.E., Shearer, M.S. (1974). The Portage Project. A paper presented at the *Conference on Early Intervention for High Risk Infants and Young Children*, N. Carolina.

Shepherd, T.A., Haaf, R.G. (1995). Comparison of two training methods in the learning and generalization of Blissymbolics. *Augmentative and Alternative Communication* **11;3**: 154–164.

Shipster, C., Hearst, D., Dockrell, J.E., Kilby, E., Hayward, R. (2002). Speech and language skills and cognitive functioning in children with Apert syndrome: a pilot study. *International Journal of Language and Communication Disorders* **37;3**: 325–343.

Shore, C., O'Connel, B., Bates, E. (1984). First sentences in language and symbolic play. *Developmental Psychology* **20**: 872–880.

Sigafoos, J. (1999). Creating opportunities for augmentative and alternative communication: strategies for involving people with developmental disabilities. *Augmentative and Alternative Communication* **15;3**: 183–190.

Silver, L.B. (1992). *The Misunderstood Child: A guide for parents of children with learning disabilities.* Florida: McGraw Hill.

Silverman, E.H., Elfant, I.L. (1979). An evaluation and treatment program for the adult. *American Journal of Occupational Therapy* **33;6**: 382–392.

Silverman, F. (1995). *Communication for the Speechless* (3rd edn). Needham Heights, MA: Allyn & Bacon.

Simmons, N.N., Buckingham Jr., H.W. (1992) Recovery in Jargon aphasia. *Aphasiology* **6;4:** 403–414.

Skelly, M. (1979). *Amer-Ind Gestural Code Based on Universal American Hand Talk.* New York: Elsevier.

Skelly, M., Schinsky, L., Smith, R., Donaldson, R., Griffin, P. (1975). American Indian sign: agestural communication for the speechless. *Archives of Physical and Rehabilitation Medicine* **56:** 156–160.

Skelly, M., Schinsky, L., Smith, R., Fust, R. (1974). American Indian sign (Amer-Ind) as a facilitator of verbalisation in the oral apraxic. *Journal of Speech and Hearing Disorders* **39:** 445–456.

Smith, D.W. (1985). *Recognizable Patterns of Human Malformation.* Volume VII In the series *Major Problems of Clinical Pediatrics.*

Smith, E.E., Nolen-Hoeksema, S., Fredrickson, B., Loftus, G.R. (2003). *Atkinson & Hilgard's Introduction to Psychology* (14th edn). Belmont, CA: Wadsworth/Thomson Learning.

Soto, G., Toro-Zambrana, W. (1995). Investigation of Blissymbol use from a language research paradigm. *Augmentative and Alternative Communication* **11;2:** 118–130.

Sparks, R.W. (1981). Melodic intonation therapy for aphasia. In R. Chapey (ed.) *Language Intervention Strategies in Adult Aphasia.* Baltimore: Williams & Wilkins.

Sparks, R., Helm, N., Albert, M. (1974). Aphasia rehabilitation resulting from melodic intonation therapy. *Cortex* **10:** 303.

Sparks, R.W., Holland, A.L. (1976). Method, melodic intonation therapy for aphasia. *Journal of Speech and Hearing Disorders* **41:** 287–297.

Springer, L. (1991). Facilitating group rehabilitation. *Aphasiology* **5;6:** 563–565.

Stackhouse, J. (1992). Developmental verbal dyspraxia. I: A review and critique. *European Journal of Disorders of Communication* **27;1:** 19–34.

Stackhouse, J., Snowling, M. (1992). Developmental verbal dyspraxia. II: A developmental perspective on two case studies. *European Journal of Disorders of Communication* **27;1:** 35–54.

Stackhouse, J., Wells, B. (1993). Psycholinguistic assessment of developmental speech disorders. *European Journal of Disorders of Communication* **28;4:** 331–348.

Stafford-Clark, D., Bridges, P. (1990). *Psychiatry for Students* (7th edn). London: George Allen Unwin.

Stampfl, T.C. and Lewis, D.J. (1967) Essentials of implosive therapy: a learning therapy based psychodynamic behaviour therapy. *Journal of Abnormal Behaviour* **73:** 496–503.

Steinberg, D.D. (1982). *Psycholinguistics: Language, mind and world.* London: Longman.

Steinberg, D.D. (1993). *An Introduction to Psycholinguistics.* London: Longman.

Stevens, S.J. (1992). Differentiating the language disorder in dementia from dysphasia – the potential of a screening test. *European Journal of Disorders of Communication* **27;4:** 275–288.

Stockwell, R.P. (1977). *Foundations of Syntactic Theory.* New Jersey: Prentice-Hall.

Stoel-Gammon, C., Dunn, C. (1985). *Normal and Abnormal Phonology in Children.* Austin, Texas: Peo-Ed.

Stott, C.M., Merricks, M.J., Bolton, P.F., Goodyer, I.M. (2002). Screening for speech and language disorders: the reliability, validity and accuracy of the General Language Screen. *International Journal of Language and Communication Disorders* **37;2:** 133–151.

Strang, M.H. (1968). *Modern English Structure.* London: Edward Arnold.

Stuart-Smith, V.G., Wilks, V. (1979). Gesture program: a supplement to verbal communication for severely aphasic individuals. *Australian Journal of Human Communication Disorders* **7:** 2.

Sturn, A., Johnston, J. (1999). Thinking out loud: an explanation of problem-solving language in preschoolers with and without language impairment. *International Journal of Language and Communication Disorders* 34;1: 1–15.

Sussman, F. (1999). *More than Words: Helping parents promote communication and social skills in children with autism spectrum disorder.* Toronto: Hanen Centre.

Sutton, B., King, J., Hux, K., Beukelman, D.R. (1995). Younger and older adults' rate performance when listening to synthetic speech. *Augmentative and Alternative Communication* 11;3: 147–153.

Swiffin, A.L., Arnott, J.L., Pickering, A., Newell, A.F. (1987). Adaptive and predictive techniques in a communication prosthesis. *Augmentative and Alternative Communication* 3;4: 181–191.

Tallal, P., Dukette, D., Curtiss, S. (1989). Behavioural/emotional profiles of preschool language-impaired children. *Development and Psychopathology* 1: 51–67.

Tallal, P., Miller, S., Fitch R.H. (1993). Neurobiological basis of speech: a case study for the preeminence of temporal processing. In P. Tallal, A.M. Galaburda, R.R. Llinás, C. von Euler (eds). *Temporal Information Processing in the Nervous System: Special reference to dyslexia and dysphasia* (pp. 27–47). New York: New York Academy of Sciences.

Taverner, D. (1983). *Taverner's Physiology.* London: Hodder & Stoughton.

Taylor, A., Sluckin, W., Davies, D.R., Reason, J.T., Thomson, R., Colman, A.M. (1982). *Introducing Psychology.* London: Penguin.

Thoonen, G., Maassen, B., Gabraëls, F., Schreuder, R., de Swart, B. (1997). Towards a standardised assessment procedure for developmental apraxia of speech. *European Journal of Disorders of Communication* 32: 37–60.

Thordardottir, E.T., Weismer, S.E. (2001). High-frequency verbs and verb diversity in the spontaneous speech of school-age children with specific language impairment. *International Journal of Language and Communication Disorders* 36;2: 221–244.

Tjellström, A. (2001) Implantable hearing aids. In J. Graham, M. Martin (eds) *Ballantyne's Deafness* (6th edn). London: Whurr.

Tortora, G.J., Grabowski, S.R. (2000). *Principles of Anatomy and Physiology* (9th edn). New York: Harper & Row.

Travis, L.E. (ed.) (1971). *Handbook of Speech Pathology and Audiology.* New York: Appleton-Century-Crofts.

Trower, P., Bryant, B., Argyle, M. (1978). *Social Skills and Mental Health.* London: Methuen.

Trudgill, P. (1995). *Sociolinguistics: An introduction to language and society.* London: Penguin.

Tudor, C., Selley, W.G. (1974). A palatal training appliance and visual aid for use in the treatment of hypernasal speech. *British Journal of Disorders of Communication* 9: 117–122.

Valot, L. (1995). *BUILLD: Bringing Unity Into Language and Learning Development.* Wooster, OH: Prentke Romich.

Van Borsel, J., Van Snick, K., Leroy, J. (1999). Macroglossia and speech in Beckwith-Wiedemann syndrome: a sample survey study. *International Journal of Language and Communication Disorders* 34;2: 209–221.

Van der Gaag, A., Dormandy, K. (1993). *Communication and Adults with Learning Disabilities.* London: Whurr.

Van der Lely, H.K.J. (1993). Specific language impairment in children: research findings and their therapeutic implications. *European Journal of Disorders of Communication* 28: 247–261.

Van Dijk, T.A. (1980). *Text and Context: Exploration in the semantics and pragmatics of discourse.* London: Longman.

Van Mourik, M., Verschaeve, M., Boon, P., Paquier, P., van Harskamp, F. (1992). Cognition in global aphasia: indicators for therapy. *Aphasiology* **6;5**: 491–500.

Van Oosterum, J., Devereux, K. (1985). *Learning with Rebuses*. Black Hill, Ely, Cambs: EARO, The Resource Centre.

Van Tattenhove, G. (1989). Power in play. *Proceedings of 1st UK Minspeak Conference*. Sept.

Vance, M. (1991). Education and therapeutic approaches used with a child presenting with acquired aphasia with convulsive disorder (Landau-Kleffner syndrome). *Child Language Teaching and Therapy* **7**: 1.

Vanderheiden, G.C., Lloyd, L. (1986). Communication systems and their components. In S. Blackstone (ed.) *Augmentative Communication: An introduction* (pp. 49–162). Rockville, MD: American Speech-Language Hearing Association.

Venkatagari, H.S. (1991). Effects of rate and pitch variations on the intelligibility of synthesized speech. *Augmentative and Alternative Communication* **7;4**: 284–289.

Venkatagari, H.S. (1994). Effect of sentence length and exposure on the intelligibility of synthesized speech. *Augmentative and Alternative Communication* **10;2**: 96–104.

Venkatagari, H.S., Ramabadran, T.V. (1995). Digital speech synthesis: a tutorial. *Augmentative and Alternative Communication* **11;1**: 14–25.

von Tetzchner, S., Martinsen, H. (2000). *Introduction to Augmentative and Alternative Communication in Primary Education* (2nd edn). London: Whurr.

Walker, M., Armfield, A. (1982). What is the Makaton vocabulary? In M. Peter, R. Barnes (eds) *Signs, Symbols and Schools: An introduction to the use of non-vocal communicative systems and sign language in schools*. Stratford-upon-Avon: NCSE.

Waller, A., Dennis, F., Brodie, J., Cairns, Y.A. (1998). Evaluating the use of TalksBac, a predictive communication device for nonfluent adults with aphasia. *International Journal of Disorders of Communication* **33;1**: 45–70.

Wardhaugh, L.R. (2002). *An Introduction to Sociolinguistics* (4th edn). Mass: Oxford Blackwell.

Ware, J. (1996). *Creating a Responsive Environment for People with PMLD*. London: David Fulton.

Warner, J. (1981). *Helping the Handicapped Child with Early Feeding: A checklist and manual for parents and professionals*. Oxon: PTM Winslow.

Watkin, P. (2001). The causes of childhood deafness and its identification and confirmation. In J. Graham, M. Martin (eds) *Ballantyne's Deafness* (6th edn). London: Whurr.

Watkin, P., Dufy, A. (2001). The management of deafness in childhood. In J. Graham, M. Martin (eds) *Ballantyne's Deafness* (6th edn). London: Whurr.

Watson, A., Sell, D., Grunwell, P. (2001). *Management of Cleft Lip and Palate*. London: Whurr.

Wells, G, (1985). *Language Development in the Pre-school Years*. Cambridge: Cambridge University Press.

Wells, J.C. (1982). *Accents of English 1: An introduction*. Cambridge: Cambridge University Press.

Wertz, R.T. (1981). Neuropathologies of speech and language: an introduction to patient management. In D.F. Johns (ed.) *Clinical Management of Neurogenic Communicative Disorders*. Boston: Little Brown and Company.

Wetherby, A.M., Cain, D.H., Yonclas, D., Walker V.G. (1988). Analysis of intentional communication of normal children from the prelinguistic to the multiword stage. *Journal of Speech and Hearing Research* **31**: 240–252.

Wheldall, K. (1987). Assessing young children's receptive language development: a revised edition of the sentence comprehension test. *Child Language Teaching and Therapy* **3;1**: 72–85.

White, M. (1985). *Good Basic Programming with the BBC Microcomputer*. London: MacMillan Publishers.

Whittle, H., Detheridge, T. (2001). The Rebus Symbols Development Project. *Communication Matters* 15;3: 14–15.

Whitton, M., Zloch, R. (1995). *Talking Lifestyles*. Lancaster: Mardis.

Wiedemann, H.R. (1964). Complex malformatif familial avec hernie ombilicale et macroglossie – un syndrome nouveau? *Journal Génétique Humaine* 13: 223–232.

Wietzman, E. (1992). *Learning Language and Loving It: A guide promoting children's social and language development in early childhood settings*. Toronto: Hanen Centre.

Williamson, I. Sheridan, C. (1994). The development of a test of speech reception disability for use in 5- to 8-year-old children with otitis media with effusion. *European Journal of Communication Disorders* 29;1: 27–37.

Wilson, D.K. (1979). *Voice Problems in Children*. Baltimore: Williams & Wilkins

Wilson, R., Teague, G., Teague, M. (1984). The use of fingerspelling to improve spelling performance with hearing children. *Reading Psychology* 5: 267–273.

Wing, L. (1980). *Autistic Children, a Guide for Parents. 3rd. ed*. London: Constable.

Wing, L. (1996). *The Autistic Spectrum: A guide for parents and professionals*. London: Constable.

Wing, L., Gould, J. (1979). Severe impairments of social interaction and associated abnormalities in children: epidemiology and classification. *Journal of Autism and Childhood Schizophrenia* 9: 11–29.

Wolff, S. (1981). *Children under Stress*. London: Penguin.

Woll, B., Barnett, S. (1998). Toward a sociolinguistic perspective on augmentative and alternative communication. *Augmentative and Alternative Communication* 14;4: 200–211.

Wood, M.E. (1981). *The Development of Personality and Behaviour in Children*. London: Harrap.

Woodcock, R., Clark, C., Davies, C. (1968). *Peabody Rebus Reading Program*. Circle Pines, MN: American Guidance Service.

Woolf, G. (1967). The assessment of stuttering as struggle, avoidance, and expectancy. *British Journal of Disorders of Communication* 2: 158–171.

World Health Organisation (1967). *Manual of the International Statistical Classification of Diseases, Injuries and Causes of Death*. Geneva: WHO.

Wright, T. (2001). Structure and function of the ear: its anatomy and how we hear. In J. Graham, M. Martin (eds) *Ballantyne's Deafness* (6th edn). London: Whurr.

Wyke, M. (ed.) (1978). *Developmental Dysphasia*. London: Academic Press.

Yorkston, K.M. (1989). Early intervention in amyotrophic lateral sclerosis. *Augmentative and Alternative Communication* 5;1: 67–70.

Yorkston, K.M., Miller, R.M., Strand, E.A. (1995). *Management of Speech and Swallowing Disorders in Degenerative Disease*. San Antonio, TX: The Psychological Corporation.

Yovetich, W.S., Young, T.A. (1988). The effects of representativeness and concreteness in the 'guessability' of Blissymbols. *Augmentative and Alternative Communication* 4;1: 35–39.

Zangari, C., Kangas K.A., Lloyd, L.L. (1988). Augmentative and Alternative Communication – a field in transition. *Augmentative and Alternative Communication* 4;2: 60–65.

Zangari, C., Lloyd, L., Vicker, B. (1994). Augmentative and Alternative Communication: an historic perspective. *Augmentative and Alternative Communication* 10;1: 27–59.